Pocket Guide to
Nutrition and Diet Therapy

Pocket Guide to
Nutrition and Diet
Therapy

Mary Courtney Moore, RN, RD, PhD, CNSN
Clarksville, Tennessee

Second Edition

With 27 illustrations

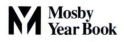

**Mosby
Year Book**

St. Louis Baltimore Boston Chicago London Philadelphia Sydney Toronto

Mosby
Year Book
Dedicated to Publishing Excellence

Executive Editor: Don Ladig
Managing Editor: Robin Carter
Assistant Editor: Fran Wulfers
Project Manager: Karen Edwards
Production Editor: Amy Adams Squire Strongheart
Designer: Jeanne Wolfgeher

Second Edition
Copyright © 1993 by Mosby–Year Book, Inc.
A Mosby imprint of Mosby–Year Book, Inc.

Previous edition copyrighted 1988

Printed in the United States of America

Mosby–Year Book, Inc.
11830 Westline Industrial Drive, St. Louis, Missouri 63146

Library of Congress Cataloging in Publication Data

Moore, Mary Courtney.
    Pocket guide to nutrition and diet therapy / Mary Courtney Moore.
    —2nd ed.
        p.   cm.
    Includes bibliographical references and index.
    ISBN 0-8016-6690-2
    1. Diet in disease—Handbooks, manuals, etc.   2. Diet therapy-
-Handbooks, manuals, etc.   3. Nutrition—Handbooks, manuals, etc.
I. Title.
    [DNLM: 1. Diet Therapy—handbooks.   2. Nutrition—handbooks.   WB
39 M823p]
RM217.2.M66   1992
615.8′54—dc20
DNLM/DLC   92-8484
for Library of Congress   CIP

95 96 97 CL/DC/DC 9 8 7 6 5 4 3

Consultant Board

Dedicated to *Bill*
whose gifts
of time and support
made this book possible

Preface

A growing awareness of the importance of nutrition to the health of well individuals and the care of ill ones has created a need for a brief, yet comprehensive, resource that can easily be carried to the clinical setting and consulted as needed. The *Pocket Guide to Nutrition and Diet Therapy* is designed to be such a resource. Many of the features of the first edition have been retained, particularly the emphasis on performing a thorough nutritional assessment as a basis for planning nutrition teaching and interventions. Each chapter includes practical, concrete suggestions for intervention and client teaching and an example demonstrating application of concepts presented in the chapter. The first part of the book describes nutritional care of well individuals of all ages; the second part serves as a guide to the care of clients with a variety of disease states. A chapter is devoted to nutrition support, and wherever a disease state warrants the use of specialized nutrition support, parenteral feeding and tube feeding are discussed in relation to that disease. Throughout the *Pocket Guide,* efforts have been made to demonstrate that nutritional care is generally multidisciplinary with physicians, nurses, dietitians, pharmacists, and other health care professionals contributing to the process. These features make the book especially well suited to serve as a resource for dietetic and nursing students, nurses and dietitians in inpatient and outpatient settings.

This edition of the book has been extensively revised and updated. Some of the most significant changes relate to nutritional teaching and care in pregnancy, heart disease, and diabetes. The latest available authoritative recommendations regarding weight gain and nutritional supplementation during pregnancy; dietary modifications for individuals with elevated serum cholesterol and/or triglycerides; and diet, hypoglycemic agents, and exercise in diabetes have been incorporated.

This edition also contains several new features. Among the most prominent is Chapter 10, devoted to acquired immunodeficiency syndrome (AIDS), a growing problem with a substantial impact on nutrition. In addition, the number of illustrations has been increased to make the text easier to understand, and, in response to reader requests, a key to the major abbreviations used throughout the book has been included on the inside front cover for easy reference. Moreover, content relating to nutritional care and teaching of healthy individuals in the early and middle adult years has been added, reflecting the importance of health promotion and health maintenance during these pivotal years. This content is congruent with and builds upon the *Dietary Guidelines for Americans,* ed 3, published by the U.S. Department of Agriculture and the U.S. Department of Health and Human Services in 1990.

It is my hope that the *Pocket Guide* will serve as a portable, up-to-date reference for health professionals, simplifying their tasks and improving the nutritional care of their clients.

Mary Courtney Moore

Contents

Appendixes

NUTRITION THROUGHOUT THE LIFE CYCLE

Nutrition Assessment

An individual's nutritional status affects performance, well-being, growth and development, and resistance to illness. Nutrition assessment is the process used to evaluate nutritional status, identify malnutrition, and determine which individuals need aggressive nutritional support.

Terms Describing Nutritional Status

Malnutrition refers to impaired nutrition, which can result from inadequate intake, disorders of digestion or absorption, or overeating. Undernutrition and overnutrition are types of malnutrition.

Undernutrition

Protein calorie malnutrition (PCM)

PCM is a type of undernutrition resulting from inadequate intake, digestion, or absorption of protein or calories. There are two types of PCM, kwashiorkor and marasmus. Table 1-1 provides guidelines for distinguishing between the two.

Vitamin and mineral deficiencies

Vitamin and mineral deficiencies rarely occur in isolation. Most commonly, these deficiencies occur in groups or in conjunction with PCM. For example, the individual who consumes no animal products is at risk of deficiency of vitamin B_{12}, protein, calcium, iron, and zinc.

Overnutrition

Excess of kilocalories

Obesity and overweight result from intake of more kilocalories, or kcal (a unit of measure used to express the energy value of

Table 1-1   Protein calorie malnutrition (PCM)

Distinguishing Characteristics	Marasmus	Kwashiorkor
Primary causative factors	↓ kcal (primarily)	↓ Protein and stress (e.g., injury, surgery, infection)
Time course for development	Months or years	Weeks
Physical findings		
General appearance	Wasted	Well-nourished
Weight Loss*	Present	Absent or minimal (edema may mask a loss of body mass)
Edema	Absent	Present
Hair	Normal	Easily plucked, loss of pigmentation
Serum albumin, transferrin, or prealbumin	Normal	Decreased
Mortality	Low (unless caused by underlying disease)	High (↓ wound healing, immunocompetence, ↑ infections)

*Severe loss may be defined as loss of more than 2% of body weight in 1 week, more than 5% in 1 month, more than 7.5% in 3 months, and more than 10% in 6 months.

foods), than are needed. These terms refer to excess body fat, but for simplicity, they are often defined in terms of body weight. Overweight is defined as a weight of at least 10% greater than ideal or desirable. Obesity is defined as a weight of at least 20% greater than ideal. Appendix E includes a table of desirable body weights for height. Another way of determining ideal body weight (IBW) is to use the following formulas:

Women: IBW = 100 lb for the first 5′ of height + 5 lb for every inch over 5′

Men: IBW = 106 lb for the first 5′ of height + 6 lb for every inch over 5′

Another commonly used method for expressing appropriateness of weight for height is the body mass index (BMI), or Quetelet score. Following is the equation most commonly used for calculating BMI*:

BMI = weight in kg/(height in m)^2

The National Health and Nutrition Examination Survey defined women with a BMI of 27.3 or greater as overweight and those with a BMI of 32.3 or more as severely overweight. Men with a BMI of 27.8 or greater were considered overweight, and those with a BMI of 31.1 or greater were considered severely overweight.

Obesity and overweight are discussed further in Chapter 19.

Excess of vitamins and minerals

Fat-soluble vitamins and some minerals can be toxic when consumed in excess. For example, excessive intake of vitamin A can cause increased intracranial pressure. Excessive amounts of water-soluble vitamins, however, are usually excreted in the urine without ill effects.

Assessment Procedures

Assessment of nutritional status has four components: anthropometric measurements, physical assessment, nutritional history, and laboratory analyses.

Anthropometric Measurements

Anthropometric measurements are measurements of the human body. Essential measurements include height (or length for children less than 24 to 36 months) and weight.

Skinfold measurements provide an estimate of body fat, which is used in the identification of obesity or marasmus. Triceps skinfold (TSF) is the most commonly used (Fig. 1-1).

---

*1 kg = 2.2 lb; 1 m = 39.37 in; 1 cm = 0.39 in.

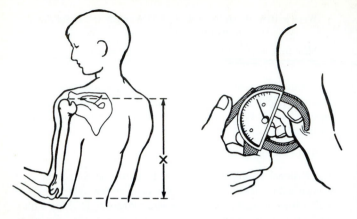

Fig. 1-1
TSF and AMC measurements.

Arm muscle circumference (AMC) reflects muscle mass. It is determined by measuring arm circumference (AC) and TSF at the midpoint of the upper arm (Fig. 1-1) and using this equation:

AMC (cm) = AC (cm) − [0.314 × TSF (mm)]

Both TSF and AMC may be altered by edema of the arm.

Interpretation in adults

The best use of anthropometric measurements is to compare changes in one individual over time. Anthropometric measurements are sometimes compared with standard measurements. Standard (desirable) weights have already been discussed. Standards for TSF and AMC are found in Appendix G. Generally, these measurements are considered low if less than the 5th percentile and excessive if greater than the 95th. However, there are exceptions, such as the manual laborer with an AMC greater than the 95th percentile because of increased muscle bulk.

BMI is usually considered low (underweight) if it is less than 19.1 for women or 20.7 for men.

Interpretation in children

Height and weight are compared with standard growth charts (see Appendix F). According to the Waterlow Criteria (see the Bibliography at the end of this chapter), two types of undernutrition exist:

1. Growth retardation: Height is low in relation to expected height for age, which reflects chronic undernutrition. To evaluate, determine the percentage of standard height, using the following equation:

$$\left(\text{actual height} \div \dfrac{\text{50th percentile value of}}{\text{height for the child's age}}\right) \times 100$$

Degree of Retardation	Expected Height for Age (%)
0 (not growth retarded)	>95*
1	87.5-95
2	80-87.5
3	<80

2. Malnutrition: Weight is low in relation to height, which reflects acute undernutrition. To evaluate, determine percentage of expected weight for height, using the following equation:

$$\left(\text{actual weight} \div \dfrac{\text{50th percentile value of}}{\text{weight for the child's height}}\right) \times 100$$

Degree of Malnutrition	Expected Weight for Height (%)
0 (not undernourished)	>90
1	80-90
2	70-80
3	<70

Both growth retardation and malnutrition can be present in the same child.

Physical Assessment

Many nutrient deficiencies and excesses become apparent during careful physical assessment of the individual. Table 1-2 describes findings that may indicate malnutrition.

Nutritional History

Several methods can be used to obtain information about nutritional history. With all methods, the interviewer should determine whether there have been changes in food intake over the past few months.

---

*This value corresponds to approximately the 3rd percentile on the growth charts.

Table 1-2   Signs that suggest nutrient imbalance

Area of Concern	Possible Deficiency	Possible Excess
Hair		
Dull, dry, brittle	Pro	
Easily plucked (with no pain)	Pro	
Hair loss	Pro, Zn, biotin	Vit A
Flag sign (loss of hair pigment in strips around the head)	Pro, Cu	
Head and Neck		
Bulging fontanel (infants)		Vit A
Headache		Vit A, D
Epistaxis (nosebleed)	Vit K	
Thyroid enlargement	Iodine	
Eyes		
Conjunctival and corneal xerosis (dryness)	Vit A	
Pale conjunctiva	Fe	
Blue sclerae	Fe	
Corneal vascularization	Vit B_2	
Mouth		
Cheilosis or angular stomatitis (lesions at corners of mouth)	Vit B_2	
Glossitis (red, sore tongue)	Niacin, folate, vit B_{12}, other B vit	
Gingivitis (inflamed gums)	Vit C	
Hypogeusia, dysgeusia (poor sense of taste, bad taste)	Zn	
Dental caries	Fluoride	
Mottling of teeth		Fluoride
Atrophy of papillae on tongue	Fe, B vit	

Pro, Protein; *Vit,* vitamin(s); *EFA,* essential fatty acids; *Ca,* calcium; *Cu,* copper; *Fe,* iron; *K,* potassium; *Mg,* magnesium; *Na,* sodium; *P,* phosphorus; *Se,* selenium; *Zn,* zinc.

Table 1-2   Signs that suggest nutrient imbalance—cont'd

Area of Concern	Possible Deficiency	Possible Excess
Skin		
Dry, scaly	Vit A, Zn, EFA	Vit A
Follicular hyperkeratosis (resembles gooseflesh)	Vit A, EFA, B vit	
Eczematous lesions	Zn	
Petechiae, ecchymoses	Vit C, K	
Nasolabial seborrhea (greasy, scaly areas between nose and upper lip)	Niacin, vit B_2, B_6	
Darkening and peeling of skin in areas exposed to sun	Niacin	
Poor wound healing	Pro, Zn, vit C	
Nails		
Koilonychia (spoon-shaped nails)	Fe	
Brittle, fragile	Pro	
Heart		
Enlargement, tachycardia, failure	Vit B_1	
Small heart	kcal	
Sudden failure, death	Se	
Arrhythmia	Mg, K, Se	
Hypertension	Ca, K	Na
Abdomen		
Hepatomegaly	Pro	Vit A
Ascites	Pro	
Musculoskeletal, Extremities		
Muscle wasting (especially temporal area)	kcal	
Edema	Pro, vit B_1	
Calf tenderness	Vit B_1 or C, biotin, Se	

Continued.

Table 1-2   Signs that suggest nutrient imbalance—cont'd

Area of Concern	Possible Deficiency	Possible Excess
Musculoskeletal, Extremities—cont'd		
Beading of ribs, or "rachitic rosary" (child)	Vit C, D	
Bone and joint tenderness	Vit C, D, Ca, P	Vit A
Knock knees, bowed legs, fragile bones	Vit D, Ca, P, Cu	
Neurologic		
Paresthesias (pain and tingling or altered sensation in the extremities)	Vit B_1, B_6, B_{12}, biotin	
Weakness	Vit C, B_1, B_6, B_{12}, kcal	
Ataxia, decreased position and vibratory senses	Vit B_1, B_{12}	
Tremor	Mg	
Decreased tendon reflexes	Vit B_1	
Confabulation, disorientation	Vit B_1	
Drowsiness, lethargy	Vit B_1	Vit A, D
Depression	Vit B_1, biotin	

Methods

24-hour recall

The individual is asked to recall everything he or she consumed the previous day. A sample tool for collection of a 24-hour recall is shown in the box on p. 11.

Advantages. The 24-hour recall is easily and quickly done.

Disadvantages. The person may not be able to recall his or her intake accurately.

The interviewer must be trained in prompting and questioning the individual to obtain complete and accurate information.

The previous day's intake may be atypical for the person.

Sauces, gravies, and snack items tend to be omitted or reported inaccurately.

24-Hour Recall

The following questions may be used to elicit a 24-hour recall.

1. What time did you get up yesterday? _____
   Was this the usual time? _____

2. When was the first time you had anything to eat or drink? _____
   (Avoid mentioning specific meals, e.g., "What did you have for breakfast?")
   What did you have? How much? (For each food, ask for details if type or preparation method is unclear, e.g., was chicken fried or baked; was milk whole, low-fat, or skim?)

3. When did you eat or drink something again?
   What did you have and how much?
   (Repeat question 3 until the individual has described the entire day.)

4. Did you eat or drink anything else? (Review the day with the individual to see if any snacks have been omitted.)

5. Was this day's intake different from usual?
   If so, in what way? _____

6. Do you eat differently on weekends than on weekdays?
   _____ If so, in what way?

Food frequency questionnaire

The health professional collects information regarding the number of times per day, week, or month the individual eats particular foods. A sample tool is shown in the box on p. 12.

Advantages. When used with the 24-hour recall, the food frequency questionnaire can help validate the accuracy of the recall and provide a more complete picture of the individual's intake.

This method can be tailored to particular nutrients of interest (e.g., cholesterol and saturated fat).

Disadvantages. The food frequency questionnaire provides no quantitative information.

This method provides no information except for foods consumed. Other methods can reveal time and circumstances of food

Food Frequency List for Cholesterol and Fat Intake

How often do you consume each of the following?

	Times/ wk	Times/ mo	<Once/ mo	Never
Eggs	_____	_____	_____	_____
Liver	_____	_____	_____	_____
Shellfish	_____	_____	_____	_____
Other fish	_____	_____	_____	_____
Beef or pork	_____	_____	_____	_____
Poultry	_____	_____	_____	_____
Cheese	_____	_____	_____	_____
Butter	_____	_____	_____	_____
Whole milk	_____	_____	_____	_____
Cream	_____	_____	_____	_____
Pastries	_____	_____	_____	_____
Gravies	_____	_____	_____	_____
Ice cream	_____	_____	_____	_____
Stick margarine	_____	_____	_____	_____
Soft margarine	_____	_____	_____	_____
Corn, sunflower, or safflower oils	_____	_____	_____	_____

intake, which may be of help in identifying and changing poor eating habits (e.g., nighttime snacking during television viewing).

Food record

The individual records all the foods he or she consumed, with portions weighed, measured, or estimated. Usually this is done for three days—a weekend day and two weekdays.

Advantages

The food record provides more information than the 24-hour recall, particularly about amounts eaten.

Disadvantages. The food record relies heavily on client cooperation.

Intake may be atypical during the recording period.

In some cases, the act of recording one's intake results in a change in eating patterns.

Diet history
The individual is extensively interviewed to elicit detailed information about nutritional status, as well as general health, socioeconomic status, and cultural impact on nutrition. The diet history usually includes information similar to that collected by the 24-hour recall and food frequency questionnaire, as well as other information listed in the box on p. 14.

Advantages. The diet history gives an indication of food habits over several months or years.

This method provides more information than either the 24-hour recall or the 3-day food record.

Disadvantages. The diet history requires an experienced interviewer.

This method is time consuming.

Interpretation of dietary information
Dietary intake can be evaluated by the food group plan and nutrient composition.

Food group plan
The number of servings from each of the four food groups is determined and compared with the Daily Food Guide (see Appendix A).

Advantages. Poor intake of protein, iron, vitamin C, vitamin A, and calcium is easily detected.

This method is easily and quickly done.

Disadvantages. Combination foods are difficult to categorize.

Nutrient composition
Tables of food composition or computer data bases can be used to calculate the amount of each nutrient in the diet. Nutrient intake is then compared with some standard, usually the Recommended Dietary Allowances (RDAs) (see Appendix I).

Advantages. The nutrient composition process provides specific information about a wider group of nutrients (e.g., sodium, potassium).

Computer data bases make the process very rapid and easy.

Diet History

I. Socioeconomic data
  A. Income
    1. Adequacy for food purchasing
    2. Eligibility for food stamps or other public assistance
  B. Ethnic or cultural background
    1. Influence of culture or religion on eating habits
    2. Educational level
II. Food preparation
  A. Problems in shopping for or preparing food
    1. Skill of person who shops and cooks
    2. Availability of market(s)
    3. Adequacy of facilities for cooking, food storage, and refrigeration
  B. Use of convenience foods
III. Physical activity
  A. Occupation—type, number of hours per week, activity level
  B. Exercise—type and frequency
  C. Handicaps
IV. Appetite and perception of taste and smell—quality, any changes over the last 12 months
V. Allergies, intolerances, food avoidances, and special diets
  A. Foods avoided and reason
  B. Special diet—what kind, why followed, and who recommended it
VI. Oral health/swallowing
  A. Dentures; completeness of dentition
  B. Problems with chewing, swallowing, and salivation
VII. Gastrointestinal problems
  A. Heartburn, bloating, gas, diarrhea, vomiting, constipation—frequency of problems; any association with food intake or other occurrences
  B. Remedies used—laxatives, antacids
VIII. Medical or psychiatric illnesses
  A. Type of disease
  B. Type and duration of treatment

Diet History — cont'd

  IX. Medications
      A. Vitamins, minerals, or other nutritional supplements—frequency, type, amount, and recommended or prescribed by whom
      B. Other medications—frequency, type, amount, and duration of use
   X. Recent weight change
      A. Amount of loss or gain and over what period of time (most significant if during past year)
      B. Intentional or unintentional; if intentional, what method was used
  XI. Usual food intake—description of a "typical" day's intake, or 24-hour recall with use of food frequency questionnaire

Disadvantages. Use of food composition tables for manual calculations can be a laborious process.

Foods consumed may not have the same nutrient composition as those in the table or data base because of variations in growing and storage conditions, food processing, and cooking procedures.

The RDAs are intended for planning and evaluating the diets of *groups* of people. They are not always appropriate for evaluation of intake of an individual.

Gaps exist in the information available in tables and data bases of nutrient composition. Many foods have not been analyzed for all trace elements, for example.

The output is only as good as the input. The accuracy of the analysis is limited by the accuracy of the 24-hour recall or food record.

The computer hardware and software can be expensive.

Table 1-3 illustrates nutritional history findings that may indicate nutritional deficits.

Laboratory Analyses

Analysis of blood, urine, and other body tissues provides useful information about nutritional status. Table 1-4 lists some tests
Text continued on p. 20.

Table 1-3 Evaluation of nutritional history

Areas of Concern	History	Possible Deficiency
Inadequate intake	Alcohol abuse	kcal, pro, vit B_1, niacin, folate
	Avoidance of food groups:	
	Fruits and vegetables	Vit A, C
	Breads and cereals	Vit B_1 and B_2, fiber
	Meat, eggs, dairy products	Vit B_{12}, protein, Fe, Zn
	Dairy products	Ca, vit B_2
	Constipation, hemorrhoids, diverticulosis	Fiber
	Poverty, disadvantaged environment	Various nutrients, especially pro and Fe
	Multiple food allergies	Depends on specific allergies
	Weight loss	kcal, other nutrients
Inadequate absorption	Drugs (especially antacids, cimetidine, anticonvulsants, cholestyramine, neomycin, antineoplastics, laxatives)	Various nutrients (see Chapter 18)
	Malabsorption (diarrhea, weight loss, steatorrhea)	kcal; vit A, D, E, K; pro; Ca; Mg; Zn
	Parasites	Fe
	Surgery	
	Gastrectomy	Vit B_{12}, Fe, folate
	Intestinal resection	kcal; vit A, D, E, K; Ca; Mg; Zn; vit B_{12} if distal ileum

Modified from Weinsier RL, Butterworth CE Jr: *Handbook of clinical nutrition*, St Louis, 1981, Mosby–Year Book.
Pro, Protein; *Vit,* vitamin(s); *Fe,* iron; *Ca,* calcium; *Mg,* magnesium; *Zn,* zinc; *Cr,* chromium.

Table 1-3   Evaluation of nutritional history—cont'd

Areas of Concern	History	Possible Deficiency
Impaired utilization	Drugs (especially anti-neoplastics, oral contraceptives, isoniazid, colchicine, corticosteroids)	Various nutrients (see Chapter 18)
	Inborn errors of metabolism (by family history)	Depends on disorder
Increased losses	Diabetes	Zn, Cr
	Alcohol abuse, cirrhosis of the liver	Mg, Zn
	Blood loss	Fe
	Diarrhea, fistula	Pro, Zn, fluid, electrolytes
	Draining abscesses or wounds	Pro, Zn
	Nephrotic syndrome	Pro, Zn
	Peritoneal dialysis or hemodialysis	Pro, water-soluble vit, Zn
	Vomiting (persistent)	Fluid, electrolytes, kcal, other nutrients
Increased requirements	Fever	kcal, vit B_1
	Hyperthyroidism	kcal
	Physiologic demands (infancy, adolescence, pregnancy, lactation)	Fe, Ca, other nutrients
	Surgery, trauma, burns, infection	kcal, pro, vit C, Zn
	Neoplasms (some types)	kcal, pro, other nutrients

Table 1-4 Laboratory analyses used in routine nutritional assessment

Area of Concern	Possible Deficiency	Comments
Serum Proteins (1 or more are usually evaluated in nutritional assessment)		
↓ Albumin	Protein	Long half-life (14-20 days), slow to change during malnutrition and repletion; ↓ in liver disease and nephrosis
↓ Transferrin (iron transport protein)	Protein	Shorter half-life than albumin (7-8 days); prevalence of iron deficiency limits usefulness in diagnosing PCM (↑ in iron deficiency)
↓ Prealbumin	Protein	Half-life 2-3 days; ↓ in trauma, inflammation
Hematologic Values		
Anemia (↓ Hct, Hgb)		
Normocytic (normal MCV,* MCHC)*	Protein	
Microcytic (↓ MCV, MCH*, MCHC)	Fe, Cu	
Macrocytic (↑ MCV)	Folate, vitamin B_{12}	

*MCV, mean cell volume; *MCH,* mean cell hemoglobin; *MCHC,* mean cell hemoglobin concentration.

†The equation for the calculation of nitrogen balance is:

[24-hour protein intake (g) ÷ 6.25] − [24-hour urine urea nitrogen (g) + 4g]

‡Skin testing involves intradermal injection of 3 to 5 antigens, often including *Candida,* trichophytin (a fungus), PPD (tuberculosis), and mumps. Response ("reactivity") is evaluated at 24, 48, and 72 hours after injection. Induration (and sometimes erythema) of greater than or equal to 10 mm diameter is considered a positive reaction.

NOTE: Reference values for biochemical parameters are given in Appendix H.

Table 1-4 Laboratory analyses used in routine nutritional assessment—cont'd

Area of Concern	Possible Deficiency	Comments
Total lymphocyte count (TLC) (WBC × % lymphocytes)		
↓ TLC	Protein	↓ In severe debilitating disease (e.g., cancer, renal disease)
Urinary Values		
↓ Creatinine-height index (CHI)	Protein (reflects lean body mass)	Expected creatinine excretion is 20 mg/kg body weight for children, 17 mg/kg for women, and 23 mg/kg for men; CHI is expressed as percent of the expected value; *Problems:* difficult to collect accurate 24-hr urine; wide variation in day-to-day creatinine excretion
Negative nitrogen balance†	Protein	Used in evaluation of nutrition therapy; negative values occur when more nitrogen is lost than is consumed (inadequate intake or physiologic stress); positive values occur when more is consumed than lost (e.g., during nutritional repletion); *Problems:* difficult to collect accurate 24-hr urine; retention of nitrogen does not necessarily mean that it is being used for anabolism

Continued.

Table 1-4 Laboratory analyses used in routine nutritional assessment—cont'd

Area of Concern	Possible Deficiency	Comments
Skin Testing‡		
Nonreactivity	Protein	Indicator of immune function; response may be impaired in diabetes, elderly; use of corticosteroids or general anesthetics; trauma; elevated BUN

used in routine nutritional assessment. Specific tests used for evaluation of vitamin and mineral nutrition are listed in Appendix H along with reference values for nutrition-related laboratory tests.

Laboratory tests are not infallible, and good clinical judgment must be used in selecting tests to be performed and interpreting test results. Some studies have shown that a thorough physical assessment and nutritional history are as effective in identifying malnutrition as a battery of laboratory analyses.

Estimating Nutrient Needs

Determining the individual's degree of malnutrition and physiologic stress through nutritional assessment makes it possible to estimate nutrient needs.

Caloric Needs

There are several methods of estimating kcal needs, three of which follow:
1. Use of the RDA. This has at least two shortcomings. First, as previously mentioned, the RDAs are designed to be applied to *groups* of people; they may not be appropriate for an individual. Second, they are designed for healthy people, not sick ones.

2. Use of formulas to estimate kcal needs based on basal energy expenditure (BEE).
   a. BEE includes the energy required for basic life processes such as respiration, cardiac function, and maintenance of body temperature.

   Women: BEE = 655 + (9.6 × W) + (1.7 × H) − (4.7 × A)

   Men: BEE = 66 + (13.7 × W) + (5 × H) − (6.8 × A)

   W = Weight in kg; H = Height in cm; A = Age in years

   b. Once the BEE is determined, the daily energy needs for the healthy individual can be determined from it by multiplying by an activity factor.

Type of Activity	Amount of Increase in kcal Needs (%)	Multiply BEE by
Bed rest	20	1.2
Light activity	30	1.3
Moderate activity	40	1.4
Strenuous activity	50 or more	1.5 or more

   c. If the individual is malnourished or under physiologic stress, energy needs are further increased. They can be calculated by multiplying by an appropriate factor.

Condition	Amount of Increase in kcal Needs (%)	Multiply Energy Needs in Health (Step b) by
Pneumonia	20	1.2
Major injury	30	1.3
Severe sepsis	50-60	1.5-1.6
Major burns	80-100	1.8-2

3. Measurement of resting energy expenditure (REE) by indirect calorimetry. Although this is the most accurate method, it is not available in all institutions.

Protein Needs

Protein needs vary with degree of malnutrition and stress. To calculate an adult's daily protein need, use the following guidelines:

Condition	Multiply *Ideal* Body Weight (kg) by
Healthy individual or elective surgery patient (well-nourished)	0.8 to 1 g protein
Malnourished or catabolic state (sepsis, major injury, burns)	1.2 to 2+ g protein

---

CASE STUDY

Ms. L., a 65-year-old woman, was admitted to the hospital with pneumonia. She was noted to have moderate sacral and lower extremity edema, and her hair was dull and easily pluckable. On questioning, she admitted that her appetite had been poor since the death of her husband 5 months earlier. Her usual diet consisted largely of canned soups, toast, and tea. Laboratory testing revealed decreased serum albumin, hematocrit (Hct), MCV, MCH, and MCHC. Anthropometric measurements were notable for:

Height: 160 cm (5'3")   Current weight: 54.5 kg (120 lb)

Weight 6 mo ago: 58.2 kg (128 lb)

TSF 15 mm (normal)   AMC 22.3 cm (<5th percentile)

Nutritional Diagnoses

1. Combined kwashiorkor ($\downarrow$ albumin, hair changes, edema) and marasmus (weight loss, some of which is masked by edema; $\downarrow$ AMC)
2. Microcytic anemia

Calculation of Nutrient Needs

1. Daily kcal needs:
   BEE = 655 + (9.6 × 54.5 kg) + (1.7 × 160 cm) − (4.7 × 65 yr) = 1145
   Energy needs for light activity = 1152 × 1.3 = 1498
   Energy needs during illness = 1498 × 1.2 = 1798
2. Daily protein needs
   IBW (use formula on p. 5): 52 kg (115 lb)
   Protein needs = 52 kg × 1.2 g = 63 g

Bibliography

Grant, JP: Nutritional assessment in clinical practice, *Nutr Clin Prac* 1:3, 1986.

Himes JH, ed: *Anthropometric assessment of nutritional status,* New York, 1991, Wiley-Liss.

Jeejeebhoy KN, Detsky AS, and Baker JP: Assessment of nutritional status, *J Parenter Enteral Nutr* 14:193S, 1990.

McMahon MM, Bistrian BR: The physiology of nutritional assessment and therapy in protein-calorie malnutrition, *Dis Mon* 36:373, 1990.

National Center for Health Statistics, Najjar MF, Rowland M: *Anthropometric reference data and prevalence of overweight,* United States, 1976-80. Vital and Health Statistics. Series 11, No 238. DHHS Pub No (PHS) 87-1688. Public Health Service, Washington, DC, 1987, US Government Printing Office.

Waterlow JC: Classification and definition of protein-calorie malnutrition, *Br Med J* 3:566, 1972.

Pregnancy and Lactation

2

Pregnancy

The idea that the pregnant woman is "eating for two" has been largely discredited, at least in terms of quantity. However, the quality of food intake during pregnancy deserves special attention to promote optimal health for both the mother and the child.

Special Concerns

Nutritional needs

Nutritional deficiencies during pregnancy can have adverse effects on both the mother and her infant. Maternal diets are most likely to be low in iron, zinc, folate, and vitamin D. Some of the more serious effects of deficiencies are provided in Table 2-1. Requirements for some important nutrients are described later in this chapter. Food sources of these nutrients are listed in Appendix B.

Preconceptual weight, weight gain, and energy needs

Both the preconceptual weight of the mother and the amount of weight she gains during pregnancy influence the outcome of pregnancy. Risks are increased in the following cases: (1) *Underweight:* Women who are underweight before pregnancy are more likely to experience preterm labor and to deliver low birth weight (LBW; less than 2500 g or 5.5 lb) infants. LBW is the single greatest risk factor for the survival of the newborn. (2) *Overweight:* Women who are overweight before pregnancy are more likely to have hypertension and diabetes. Fetal death rates are highest in pregnancies where the mother weighs more than 77.3 kg (170 lb). (3) *Inadequate gain:* For normal-weight and underweight women, maternal weight gain is directly related to infant

Table 2-1   Nutritional deficiencies during pregnancy

| Nutrient | Potential Effects of Deficiency | |
	Maternal	Fetal
Kcal*	Anemia Endometritis	Prematurity Low birth weight (LBW)
Protein	Hypoproteinemia with edema ? Increased incidence of preeclampsia	? LBW (difficult to separate from effects of kcal deprivation)
Iron	Microcytic, hypochromic anemia	Fetal death; LBW; premature birth
Zinc	Amnionitis	Fetal malformations, including neural tube defects
Calcium	Acceleration of osteoporosis	Decreased bone density (unlikely)
Folic acid	Megaloblastic or macrocytic anemia	Neural tube defects

*Especially if underweight before pregnancy.

birth weight, and the risk of delivering a LBW infant is increased by inadequate gain. Gain of 1 kg (2.2 lb) or less per month in the second or third trimester by normal-weight women and 0.5 kg or less (1 lb) by obese women should be investigated. (4) *Excessive gain:* Gain of 3 kg (6.6 lb) or more per month can result from excessive food intake, accumulation of fluid and possibly onset of pregnancy-induced hypertension, and multiple gestation. Very high total weight gain, especially in short women (less than 157 cm or 62 in) is associated with increased risk of fetopelvic disproportion, operative delivery, birth trauma, and infant mortality. Moreover, excessive fat stores tend to be retained after pregnancy, increasing the woman's likelihood of being overweight or obese.

The optimum amount of weight gain in a singleton pregnancy is determined largely by the mother's preconceptual weight. Recommendations have been developed for desirable ranges for total weight gain and rate of weight gain based on body mass index (BMI), an indicator of the appropriateness of weight for height

Table 2-2   Recommended weight gain during pregnancy based on prepregnancy body mass index (BMI)*

Weight-for-Height Category	Recommended Total Gain in kg (lb)	Recommended Weekly Gain During Second and Third Trimesters in kg (lb)
Low (BMI <19.8)	12.5-18 (28-40)	0.5 (1.1)
Normal (BMI 19.8 to 26.0)	11.5-16 (25-35)	0.4 (1.0)
High (BMI 26.0 to 29.0)	7-11.5 (15-25)	0.3 (0.66)
Obese (BMI >29.0)	>6.8 (15)	Determine on individual basis

From Institute of Medicine: *Nutrition during pregnancy,* Washington, DC, 1990, National Academy Press.

*BMI = weight in kg/(height in m)^2. For example, a woman weighing 51 kg (112 lb), 1.57 m (5′2″) in height, would have a BMI = $51/(1.57)^2$ = 20.7.

(Table 2-2). The composition of this weight gain is shown in Fig. 2-1. Progressive gain is important, but there should not be undue concern if weight gain is slightly more or less than the desirable amount because there is much individual variability. Young adolescents (less than 2 years past menarche) and black women should be encouraged to make their weight gain goal the upper end of the recommended range, since their infants are smaller than those of white adult mothers for any given amount of maternal gain. If gestational age is uncertain, the focus should be on ensuring an appropriate rate of weight gain. Outcome of a twin pregnancy appears to be best if weight gain is approximately 16 to 20.5 kg (35 to 45 lb), a total that can be achieved with a gain of 0.75 kg (1.65 lb) per week during the second and third trimesters.

The 1989 Recommended Dietary Allowances (RDAs) suggest that during the second and third trimesters the woman should consume 300 kcal/day more than her nonpregnant intake to promote an adequate gain. (See Appendix I for RDA.)

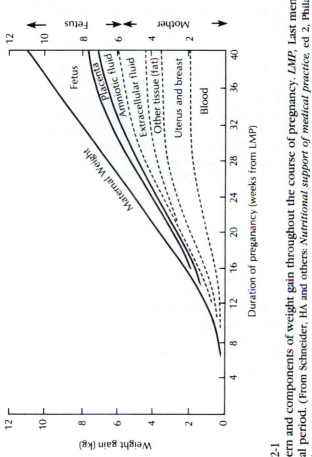

Fig. 2-1
Pattern and components of weight gain throughout the course of pregnancy. *LMP,* Last menstrual period. (From Schneider, HA and others: *Nutritional support of medical practice,* ed 2, Philadelphia, 1983, Harper & Row.)

Protein

A total of 60 g of protein per day is recommended. This amount, which is easily provided by the average diet in the United States, is necessary for normal growth of the fetus, enlargement of the uterus and breasts, formation of blood cells and proteins as the blood volume expands, and production of amniotic fluid.

Iron

The red blood cell mass expands by about 15% during pregnancy, and this requires a substantial increase in the maternal content of iron. Iron is also needed for deposition of fetal stores.

Pica, the consumption of substances usually considered nonfoods, is especially common in women with iron deficiency. Soil, clay, chalk, glue, cornstarch, laundry starch, and ice are some of the substances often eaten. Pica substances may replace nutritious foods in the diet and may interfere with absorption of nutrients from foods and nutritional supplements.

Zinc

Absorption of zinc is inhibited by large intakes of iron and folic acid. Women taking iron and folic acid supplements need to consume rich sources of zinc daily. Vegetarians are especially apt to have marginal zinc status, both because animal products are generally richer sources of zinc than plant foods and because phytates and oxalates found in grains and some vegetables inhibit zinc absorption.

Calcium

Demands imposed by fetal calcification increase daily calcium needs; the RDA for pregnant women is 1200 mg.

Folic acid (folate or folacin)

The recommended intake of folic acid increases from 180 μg in the nonpregnant state to 400 μg in pregnancy. It is needed for both maternal red blood cell production and the DNA synthesis entailed in fetal and placental growth. Some data indicate that women with folate deficiency are more likely to give birth to infants with neural tube defects.

Potential toxins

Caffeine

The effect of caffeine intake on the fetus is not fully known. Some investigators have reported that heavy caffeine use is associated with increased stillbirths, spontaneous abortions, and premature deliveries. Other studies have failed to find an association between coffee consumption and adverse pregnancy outcome.

Alcohol

Heavy drinking during pregnancy can result in fetal alcohol syndrome, which may include some or all of the following features: microcephaly; prenatal and postnatal growth failure; mental retardation; ocular abnormalities, such as narrow palpebral fissures and presence of epicanthic folds; micrognathia; cleft palate; skeletal-joint abnormalities; abnormal palmar creases; and cardiac defects. Moderate drinkers may give birth to infants with some features of fetal alcohol syndrome. There is no known safe level of alcohol intake during pregnancy, and thus alcohol is best avoided altogether by pregnant women.

Cigarette smoking

Infants of women who smoke during pregnancy have lower birth weights than infants of nonsmoking mothers. In addition, women who smoke have an increased risk of preterm delivery, perinatal mortality, and possibly spontaneous abortion. The mechanism by which smoking affects the fetus is not completely understood, but it is likely that it causes intrauterine hypoxia, perhaps through reduced placental blood flow. Also, smoking increases the metabolic rate and thus caloric needs. Weight gain and prepregnant weight tend to be lower in smokers than in nonsmokers. Women who smoke have been reported to have decreased levels and/or increased needs for several nutrients, including vitamin C, folic acid, zinc, and iron. Assisting women to quit smoking is of far more benefit than merely providing vitamin and mineral supplementation, and women who cease smoking during pregnancy have been successful in increasing the birth weights of their infants.

Illicit drugs

Increased risk of intrauterine growth retardation (IUGR) and preterm labor is associated with both marijuana and cocaine abuse. The risk of abruptio placentae is also increased by co-caine. Moreover, infants of mothers who abuse crack cocaine often display persistent learning and behavioral abnormalities. It is difficult to determine exactly what impact illicit drugs have on the nutritional status of the pregnant woman, since drug abuse is often accompanied by abuse of other substances, such as alcohol or cigarettes; poverty; and poor education, all of which have detrimental influences on nutritional status. Vitamin and mineral supplements are recommended for women who abuse drugs, but supplements cannot be expected to correct the problems associated with drug use during pregnancy. Every effort should be made to convince the pregnant woman to stop using drugs.

Pregnancy Complications with Nutritional Implications

Nausea and vomiting

Nausea and vomiting, or "morning sickness," are common during the first trimester of pregnancy. Although annoying, nausea and vomiting are rarely severe and prolonged enough to impair nutritional status. Severe vomiting, known as *hyperemesis gravidarum,* occurs occasionally. This results in loss of fluids and electrolytes and limits intake of all other nutrients.

Constipation

Constipation is most common during the last half of pregnancy. It results from decreased gastrointestinal (GI) motility, resulting from increased progesterone levels, increased pressure on the GI tract by the bulky uterus, and decreased physical activity.

Pregnancy-induced hypertension (preeclampsia or toxemia)

Pregnancy-induced hypertension (PIH) is characterized by hypertension, albuminuria, and excessive edema. It generally occurs in the third trimester. The cause is unknown, but diets adequate in protein, kcal, calcium, and sodium are associated with the lowest incidence of PIH. Bed rest and antihypertensive medications are used in the treatment of PIH.

Diabetes

For the diabetic woman who becomes pregnant or the woman who develops glucose intolerance or "gestational diabetes" during pregnancy, the goal is to maintain normoglycemia during pregnancy. Insulin requirements usually decline during early pregnancy but increase during the second trimester and remain high until delivery. Gestational diabetes often can be managed by dietary modification alone, but some women with type II (non-insulin-dependent) diabetes who become pregnant may require insulin during pregnancy.

Poor control of blood glucose levels during pregnancy is associated with an increased number of congenital malformations and fetal deaths. In fact, it is important for diabetic women to achieve good control before conception, because those who do not will have an increased risk of preeclampsia as well as an increased risk of producing infants with malformations.

Nutritional Care

Assessment

Assessment is summarized in Table 2-3.

Intervention and client teaching

Objectives of intervention and teaching during pregnancy are for the client to:

1. Recognize and alter any practices or findings that could interfere with optimal nutritional status and pregnancy outcome
2. Establish with the health care provider a goal for weight gain within the recommended range and achieve this goal with an appropriate rate of gain
3. Cope with physiologic changes during pregnancy that interfere with optimal nutritional intake or comfort

Selecting a balanced diet

For most healthy women, nutritional needs during pregnancy, except perhaps those for iron, can be met through a varied diet of normal foods. The food group plan (see Appendix A) can be used as a guideline for teaching the pregnant woman to plan an adequate diet. Where income is inadequate, the client can be referred to the Special Supplemental Food Program for Women, Infants, and Children (WIC), which provides vouchers for selected food items. Low-income clients may also be eligible for the Food Stamp program.

When the woman's diet is found to be poor, and there is little

Text continued on p. 36.

Table 2-3 Assessment of nutrition in pregnancy and lactation

Areas of Concern	Significant Findings
Inadequate Kcal Intake and Weight Gain	*History* Limited income; body image concerns; nausea and vomiting; lack of knowledge about optimum gain during pregnancy, nutritional needs during pregnancy and lactation; stress or fatigue; prepregnant weight <90% of ideal or BMI < 19.8; poor obstetric history during previous pregnancies (e.g., spontaneous abortion, delivery of an LBW infant); heavy smoking; illicit drug use; unmarried; adolescent pregnancy *Physical examination* Pregnancy: failure to demonstrate adequate weight gain (Table 2-2); lactation: poor milk production, inadequate gain by infant
Excessive Kcal Intake	*History* Emotional stress, indulgence, and boredom from interruption of job routine; decrease in activity because of awkwardness during pregnancy or interruption of job routine; prepregnant weight > 120% of ideal or BMI > 26 *Physical examination* Pregnancy: weight gain > recommended range (Table 2-2); lactation: weight gain or maintenance of weight > 120% of ideal body weight or BMI > 26
Inadequate Protein Intake	*History* Limited income, strict vegetarianism,* nausea and vomiting during pregnancy, lack of knowledge about needs, or fatigue (es-

*Strict vegetarians consume no milk products, eggs, meat, poultry, or fish. Lactovegetarians use milk products, and ovolactovegetarians use both milk products and eggs.

Table 2-3   Assessment of nutrition in pregnancy and lactation—cont'd

Areas of Concern	Significant Findings
Inadequate Protein Intake—cont'd	pecially during lactation); frequent pregnancies (>3 within 2 years) or high parity; poor obstetric history during previous pregnancies (e.g., spontaneous abortion, delivery of an LBW infant); alcohol or illicit drug use; multiple gestation *Physical examination* Edema (some lower extremity edema is normal during pregnancy; look for edema in hands and periorbital area); changes in hair color and texture; hair loss *Laboratory analysis* Serum albumin < 3.2 g/dl; ↓ lymphocyte count
Inadequate Vitamin Intake	
Vitamin C	*History* Failure to consume vitamin C-containing foods daily because of poverty, alcohol or drug abuse, or dislike of these foods; increased needs because of smoking, long-term oral contraceptive or salicylate use, multiple gestation *Physical examination* Bruising, petechiae, bleeding gums *Laboratory analysis* ↓ serum vitamin C
Folic acid	*History* Failure to use a daily supplement or foods rich in folic acid; delivery of a previous infant with a neural tube defect; increased needs because of alcohol or drug abuse, smoking, or multiple gestation *Physical examination* Pallor; glossitis

Continued.

Table 2-3 Assessment of nutrition in pregnancy and lactation—cont'd

Areas of Concern	Significant Findings
Folic acid—cont'd	*Laboratory analysis*
	Hct < 33%; ↑ MCV; ↓ serum folate
Vitamin B_{12}	*History*
	Strict vegetarian with failure to use a supplement or foods fortified with vitamin B_{12}
	Physical examination
	Maternal findings: glossitis, pallor, ataxia; infant breastfed by strict vegetarian: delayed growth, pallor, glossitis, developmental delay
	Laboratory analysis
	↓ Hct; ↑ MCV (in mother or infant); ↓ serum vitamin B_{12} (in mother or infant)
Vitamin D	*History*
	Failure to consume vitamin D-fortified milk because of strict vegetarianism, lactose intolerance, dislike of milk, or cultural practices; little exposure of skin to sunlight because of residence in northern latitudes in winter or cultural prohibitions against exposing the body
Inadequate Mineral Intake	
Iron (Fe)	*History*
	Failure to consume a daily supplement and foods rich in Fe because of vegetarianism, limited income, or dislike of these foods; frequent pregnancies or high parity with depletion of stores; adolescent client with increased needs for her growth as well as that of the fetus; anemia during a previous pregnancy; pica; menorrhagia; multiple gestation
	Physical examination
	Pallor, especially of conjunctiva; blue sclerae; koilonychia (spoon-shaped nails)
	Laboratory analysis
	Hct < 33%; Hgb < 11 g/dl; ↓ MCV, MCH, MCHC, serum ferritin, serum Fe; ↑ free erythrocyte protoporphyrin (FEP)

Table 2-3 Assessment of nutrition in pregnancy and lactation—cont'd

Areas of Concern	Significant Findings
Zinc (Zn)	*History* Use of supplement containing >30 mg Fe (competition between Zn and Fe for absorption); use of supplement containing 400 μg or more of folate; avoidance of animal protein foods because of vegetarianism or limited income; frequent pregnancies or high parity with depletion of stores; adolescent client with increased needs for her growth as well as that of the fetus; pica; alcoholism with increased excretion *Physical examination* Seborrheic dermatitis; alopecia; diarrhea *Laboratory analysis* ↓ Serum Zn
Calcium (Ca)	*History* Lactose intolerance; dislike of milk products; strict vegetarianism; or cultural food patterns that avoid milk (e.g., Japanese, Mexican); frequent pregnancies or high parity with depletion of stores; adolescent client with increased needs for her growth as well as fetus

Potentially Harmful Substances (During Pregnancy)

Caffeine	*History* Daily consumption of coffee, tea, and soft drinks (other than caffeine-free); use of over-the-counter cold or analgesic medications (not usually recommended during pregnancy; client should consult her physician before using)
Alcohol	*History* Use of alcoholic beverages, especially if > 1 oz/day or more than 3 or 4 times/wk
Cocaine/other illicit drugs	*History* Use of drugs, especially on a regular basis, during pregnancy *Laboratory analysis* Positive urinary drug screen

likelihood of its improving, or when other risk factors (adolescent pregnancy; maternal smoking, use of illicit drugs, or heavy use of alcohol; multiple gestation) exist, vitamin-mineral supplementation may be required (see the discussion that follows).

Kilocalories

Women may be surprised to learn how large the desirable weight gain in pregnancy is. Explanation of the components of that weight gain (Fig. 2-1) may help them to understand the importance of weight gain. The extra 300 kcal needed are easily obtained by increasing intake of milk products by two servings per day and making small increases in intake of protein foods, fruits, or vegetables. There is little room in the diet for high kcal foods that are low in nutrients. Excessive weight gain is undesirable because it is associated with the development of diabetes and hypertension and can be difficult to correct after delivery.

If activity levels decrease, kcal needs may actually decline during pregnancy. Pregnant women need to plan time for exercise at least 3 or 4 days a week. Non-weight-bearing activities such as bicycling and swimming may be the most comfortable.

Pregnant women should avoid increasing their heart rates to more than 140 beats/min, limit exercise periods to no more than 35 minutes, and avoid becoming overheated. Other advice for pregnant women planning aerobic exercise programs is: discuss exercise plans with the obstetrician before beginning to exercise; avoid risky activities or those that rely heavily on coordination and balance such as diving, surfing, and skydiving; break activities into 10- to 15-minute periods with 2- to 3-minute rest periods in between; wear a supportive bra and shoes; drink adequate fluids during and after exercise to replace losses in perspiration; and stop exercising immediately and notify the physician if any untoward symptoms (dizziness, abdominal pain, shortness of breath, or vaginal bleeding) develop.

Protein

The extra protein needed in addition to the prepregnant intake can be provided by 1 cup of milk and 1 oz of meat or an equivalent meat substitute per day. Protein intake in excess of the recommendations has not been shown to be beneficial.

Minerals and vitamins

A supplement of 30 mg of ferrous iron is recommended for the general population of pregnant women during the second and third trimesters. Ferrous sulfate, 150 mg, provides 30 mg of elemental iron and is often prescribed because it is inexpensive and relatively well absorbed. To maximize absorption of iron from the supplement, women should be taught to take it between meals or at bedtime and to take it with liquids other than milk, coffee, and tea, which inhibit iron absorption. (The 30-mg supplement is less likely to cause gastrointestinal [GI] distress than the 60 mg supplement often used in the past, but taking the supplement at bedtime will help to minimize any GI discomfort.) Even with supplementation, the pregnant woman needs to include in her daily diet good sources of iron, such as meats, and vitamin C sources, which enhance iron absorption. In teaching about the supplement, remind your client to keep it out of the reach of children.

Good sources of other minerals, especially zinc, should be consumed daily in the diet. Sources of zinc include oysters and other shellfish, red meats, poultry, fish, dairy products, legumes, and whole grains (see Appendix B).

Dairy products, particularly milk, buttermilk, yogurt, and cheese, are the best calcium sources available. Three to four daily servings meet most of the needs of pregnant adults. Ice cream and cottage cheese provide lesser amounts of calcium, as do most deep green, leafy vegetables, baked beans, and tofu. Women who do not use dairy products are unlikely to get enough dietary calcium. The following suggestions can help these women meet their calcium needs:

1. Women with lactose intolerance (cramping, bloating, and diarrhea following milk consumption, resulting from lack of lactase, the enzyme that digests lactose) can use milk that has been treated with a commercial enzyme preparation (Lact-Aid or Lactrase). Also they usually tolerate yogurt and hard cheeses.
2. Women who do not drink enough milk can add ⅓ cup of powdered milk to each glass to double the calcium and protein consumed. They can also add it to cream soups, meat loaf, whipped potatoes, and cooked cereals.

Vitamins of greatest concern for the pregnant woman are folic acid, ascorbic acid, and vitamin D. Women who ingest fruit, juices, green vegetables, and whole grains are likely to receive enough dietary folate. One to two servings of citrus fruits, broccoli, green peppers, or other good source of ascorbic acid (see Appendix B) daily is sufficient to meet needs during pregnancy. Regular exposure of the skin to sunlight or consumption of vitamin D-fortified milk provides a reliable source of vitamin D.

Where there are unusual nutritional risks, additional vitamin and mineral supplementation is recommended by the National Academy of Sciences (1990).

Multivitamin-multimineral supplements: A daily multivitamin and multimineral supplement is recommended for women who consume poor diets and those who are at high nutritional risk (such as women carrying more than one fetus, using cigarettes or alcohol heavily, or using illicit drugs). Specifically, this supplement should provide:

Iron	30 mg	Vitamin B$_6$	2 mg
Zinc	15 mg	Folate	300 μg
Copper	2 mg	Vitamin C	50 mg
Calcium	250 mg	Vitamin D	5 μg

In teaching the client about the supplement, emphasize that it should be taken between meals or at bedtime to avoid inhibition of absorption by foods in the GI tract. A supplement will not avert potential complications associated with drinking or drug abuse or smoking, and all possible efforts should be made to assist the woman to abstain from these practices.

Single-nutrient supplementation in special circumstances: In a few instances, women may be deficient in or at risk for deficiency of one specific nutrient.

Vitamin D (10 μg or 400 IU a day) is recommended daily for strict vegetarians or other women with little intake of vitamin D-fortified milk, especially for women with little exposure of the skin to sunlight.

Calcium (600 mg daily) is recommended for women under age 25 who consume less than 600 mg of calcium (two 8-oz glasses of milk) daily, since the bones of these women may still be increasing in density. Calcium carbonate, which is 40% calcium, is a commonly used supplement. To maximize absorption, it should not be taken with the iron supplement.

Vitamin B$_{12}$ (2 μg daily) is suggested for strict vegetarians.

Zinc and copper (15 mg and 2 mg daily, respectively) is advised for women who require therapeutic doses of iron (more than 30 mg daily) to treat anemia, since iron may inhibit absorption and utilization of these minerals.

Avoiding or limiting agents that may harm the fetus

There are insufficient data available to make a recommendation regarding caffeine use during pregnancy. However, until such data are available, it would be wise to abstain from caffeine use if possible. If the mother does choose to continue caffeine use, it would be advisable to limit intake to no more than 300 mg (approximately two 6-oz cups of coffee) daily. Sources of caffeine other than coffee may be found in Appendix D. Decaffeinated coffee, tea, or soft drinks may be used during pregnancy.

Abstinence from alcohol should be strongly advised. If the mother does not find this possible, she should be urged to limit her intake to small amounts consumed infrequently and never to exceed one drink a day. Smoking and drug abuse have extremely adverse effects on the fetus, and the woman should be assisted to stop these practices if at all possible.

Aspartame (NutraSweet), an artificial sweetener, has not been found to have adverse effects on the normal mother or fetus, but its use should be avoided by pregnant women homozygous for phenylketonuria (PKU). Another artificial sweetener, saccharin, has not been shown to be safe for use during pregnancy.

Using nutritional measures to cope with common discomforts

Nausea and vomiting. Suggestions for coping include:

1. Eat small, frequent meals; hunger can worsen nausea.
2. Avoid fluids for 1 to 2 hours before and after meals.
3. Consume plain, starchy foods (crackers, dry toast, Melba toast, rice or noodles, potatoes, cooked cereal) before rising in the morning and during times of nausea because they are easily digested and unlikely to cause nausea. Spicy foods tend to worsen nausea.
4. Decrease intake of fats and fried foods. Fat delays gastric emptying and may increase nausea.
5. Minimize exposure to strong food odors. Avoid cooking foods with strong odors during times of nausea, maintain adequate ventilation in the kitchen, and use lids on pots during cooking.

The woman suffering from hyperemesis gravidarum may require hospitalization to receive intravenous fluids for rehydration. Peripheral parenteral nutrition (containing glucose, amino acids, vitamins, and electrolytes) may be used initially. When vomiting has diminished, small amounts of low-fat, easily digested starches, skinless poultry, and lean meats are reintroduced orally, and the diet is gradually advanced as tolerated. Occasionally, nausea and vomiting will be so severe and unrelenting that total parenteral nutrition will be required (see Chapter 6).

Constipation. Increased intake of fiber (found in whole grains, legumes, and fresh fruits and vegetables [see Appendix C]) and at least 50 ml/kg/day of fluid helps relieve constipation. Regular physical activity also helps improve GI function.

Using nutritional measures to help control PIH and diabetes

PIH. A moderate restriction of sodium to 2 to 3 g/day may be prescribed to help control PIH. This level of intake can be achieved by omitting the following foods and seasonings from the diet: salt and obviously salty foods, such as potato chips and pretzels; smoked or canned meats, fish, and poultry; condiments and seasonings, such as prepared mustard, catsup, Worcestershire or soy sauce; canned soups and vegetables (unless they are low sodium); bouillon; prepared mixes for cakes, casseroles, breads and muffins, gravies or sauces; frozen entrees; salted butter, margarine, peanut butter, and cheese; garlic, onion, and celery salt; and celery seeds. Fresh, canned, or frozen fruits; fresh vegetables and those canned or frozen without salt (check label); and unprocessed meats, poultry, and fish are good choices for a low-sodium diet.

Diabetes. The diet for diabetes in pregnancy is discussed in Chapter 12. Strict control of blood glucose is currently advocated in many centers, with insulin-dependent women receiving several daily injections or continuous insulin infusions.

Lactation

Human milk is an ideal food for the infant, and any mother who is interested in breastfeeding should be encouraged to do so. The advantages of breastfeeding are summarized in the box on p. 41.

Advantages of Breastfeeding

Benefits for the Infant

Antiinfective factors: Human milk contains a variety of antiinfective factors and immune cells such as IgA, IgM, IgG, B- and T-lymphocytes, neutrophils, macrophages, and complement. These properties are more important in countries where sanitation and immunization are suboptimal than in industrialized nations.

Fewer food allergies.

Avoidance of obesity: Breastfed infants are less likely to be overfed than bottlefed infants.

Nutritional advantages: Protein and fat are in an optimal form for digestion, absorption, and utilization. Zinc and iron are more readily absorbed from human milk than from formula.

Benefits for the Mother

Convenience (once lactation is established).

Economy: Breastfeeding is generally less expensive than commercial infant formulas.

Acceleration of the return to prepregnant weight.

Mutual benefit

Promotion of maternal-child bonding.

Special Concerns

Nutritional requirements

Kilocalories

The RDAs suggest that the lactating woman consume about 500 kcal per day more than her nonpregnant intake. Because this is inadequate to meet the energy cost of producing milk, maternal stores deposited during pregnancy are used to provide the extra kcal required. Thus return to prepregnant weight is often more rapid in women who breastfeed.

Protein

Recommendations for protein are 65 g during the first 6 months of lactation and 62 g during the second 6 months.

Calcium

The RDA for calcium during lactation remains the same as during pregnancy—1200 mg/day.

Fluid

Lactating women should drink 50 ml/kg of body weight of fluid per day plus an additional 800 to 1000 ml in order to produce adequate milk.

Vitamin B_{12}

Women who have followed strict vegetarian diets for several years may produce milk with very low vitamin B_{12} levels. Megaloblastic anemia, poor growth, and neurologic abnormalities have occurred in infants breastfed by such mothers.

Foods to avoid

Lactating women are sometimes told to avoid "gas-forming" foods such as onions, cabbage, legumes, chocolate, and spicy foods. There is little basis for these prohibitions. Very rarely a mother will note that some foods she consumes cause a rash, diarrhea, or irritability in her infant on a *consistent* basis. Elimination of this food from her diet readily corrects this problem.

Maternal alcohol intake during lactation appears to have a detrimental effect on infant motor development.

Diabetes

Breastfeeding may have a positive effect on blood glucose control in insulin-dependent diabetes. Successful breastfeeding is associated with a kcal prescription of at least 31 kcal/kg maternal weight. Women with diabetes should be carefully monitored for mastitis, since it is more common in diabetic than in nondiabetic women.

Nutritional Care

Assessment

Assessment is summarized in Table 2-3.

Intervention and client teaching

The objectives of intervention and teaching are for the client to:
1. Maintain an adequate diet to replenish her stores that were diminished during pregnancy and produce sufficient milk for growth of the infant

2. Lose the weight gained during pregnancy
3. Avoid nutritional practices that could harm the infant

Eating a balanced diet and achieving prepregnant weight

The food pattern followed during pregnancy (see Appendix A) is appropriate during lactation. Once again, emphasis should be placed on a variety of foods from all food groups.

Kilocalories. The increased kcal needs should be met by use of additional milk products and small increases in meat and meat substitutes, fruits and vegetables, and whole grain or enriched breads and cereals. Fatigue and the demands of the infant on the client's time may interfere with food preparation. Judicious use of commercially prepared foods such as new low-salt and low-fat frozen meals may be helpful during the early postpartum period.

It is important to maintain an exercise program after the birth of the baby to promote weight control, reshape the figure, and foster a feeling of health and well-being. The lactating woman can participate in any activity she enjoys. The information in Chapter 5 can be used to help the client plan an exercise program.

Protein. As with pregnancy, most of the extra protein needed is provided by the consumption of 4 cups of milk or equivalent products per day, rather than the 2 cups suggested for nonpregnant, nonlactating women.

Calcium. Those individuals who do not consume dairy products should follow the suggestions given for pregnant women.

Fluid. Water, milk, tea, decaffeinated coffee, soft drinks, fruit juices, and ices can be used to meet fluid needs. If kcal intake is likely to be excessive, emphasis should be placed on skim milk and unsweetened beverages.

Vitamin B_{12}. Strict vegetarian mothers need a supplement or soy milk fortified with vitamin B_{12}.

Avoiding practices that could harm the infant

In a few circumstances, mothers should not be encouraged to breastfeed. These include:

1. Galactosemia (congenital inability to metabolize galactose, a component of lactose) in the newborn.
2. Serious maternal infections that pose a threat to the infant, such as sputum-positive tuberculosis. In the United States and other industrialized nations women positive for the hu-

Drugs and Breastfeeding

Drugs that Are Contraindicated During Breastfeeding

Most antineoplastics and antimetabolites*
Bromocriptine
Chloramphenicol (especially in younger infants)
Cimetidine
Clemastine
Ergotamine
Ethyl biscoumacetate

Gold salts
Isotretinoin
Methimazole

Phenindione
Primidone
Thiouracil
Tolbutamide

Drugs that Require Temporary Cessation of Breastfeeding

Gallium-67 (24 hr to 2 wk)†
Iodine-123 (24 to 36 hr)
Iodine-125 (3 to 4 wk)
Iodine-131 (36 hr for test dose, 2 wk for therapeutic dose)
Metronidazole (24 hr, if mother receives a single dose)
Radioactive sodium (1 to 4 days)
Technetium-99m (1 to 3 feedings)

Drugs with Potential Adverse Effects that May Be Used with Close Observation

May suppress lactation:
  Thiazide diuretics
  Oral contraceptives
May exacerbate hyperbilirubinemia:
  Sulfa drugs‡
May produce sedation:
  Barbiturates (e.g., chlorpromazine)
  Benzodiazepines (e.g., meprobamate, chlordiazepoxide, diazepam, desmethyldiazepam, and oxazepam)

Modified from American Academy of Pediatrics Committee on Drugs: The transfer of drugs and other chemicals into human breast milk, Pediatrics 72:375, 1983, and Lawrence RA: Breastfeeding: a guide for the medical profession, ed 3, St Louis, Mosby–Year Book, 1989. Consult these sources for further information about maternal drug usage and breastfeeding.
*Includes azathioprine, busulfan, chlorambucil, cisplatin, cyclophosphamide, cytarabine, doxorubicin, mercaptopurine, and methotrexate, although for most of these drugs very limited information is available regarding safety during lactation.
†Until gallium is cleared from the milk.
‡Avoid during neonatal period.

man immunodeficiency virus (HIV) are advised not to breastfeed because the virus is present in milk. In developing countries, however, the issue is more complicated. Contacts other than breastfeeding (e.g., the process of birth) are more likely than breastfeeding to transmit the virus, and the antiinfective properties of human milk, which protect the infant from many diarrheal and respiratory infections associated with high mortality, may outweigh the additive risk of transmission of HIV posed by breastfeeding.

3. Maternal need for certain drugs that are secreted in milk (see box on p. 44).
4. Unusually severe maternal exposure to pollutants such as polychlorinated biphenyls (PCBs) and polybrominated biphenyls (PBBs).
5. Maternal disinclination to breastfeed.

Certain medical conditions are compatible with breastfeeding as long as there is careful medical supervision:

1. Phenylketonuria (PKU). Human milk is relatively low in phenylalanine. Many PKU infants can be totally or partially breastfed if their phenylalanine levels are closely monitored. A resource designed for physicians by AE Ernest and others (1980) provides detailed information regarding managing the care of these infants.
2. Severe "breast milk jaundice" (serum bilirubin concentration approaching 20 mg/dl). Human milk contains an inhibitor of bilirubin conjugation and excretion, and severe hyperbilirubinemia may require temporary interruption of breastfeeding. After 12 to 24 hours of formula feeding, bilirubin usually declines, and breastfeeding can continue. The mother should be reassured that her milk is not bad for the infant and assisted in pumping her breasts if necessary during the interruption of breastfeeding.
3. Carriers of hepatitis B may breastfeed as long as their infants have received hepatitis B immune globulin at birth and hepatitis B vaccine before hospital discharge.

Certain personal practices could potentially be harmful during breastfeeding. There are insufficient data available regarding the effects of alcohol intake during lactation, but women should be encouraged to avoid regular and heavy drinking. The breastfeeding mother should also be advised to quit smoking, if applicable.

Nicotine does appear in milk, but the major risk to the infant is from "passive smoking"—exposure to tobacco pollutants within the home environment.

CASE STUDY

Ms. M., a typist, was pregnant for the first time. At her 28-week checkup, the nurse noted that she had gained only 2.3 kg (5 lb). Ms. M. admitted that she had been eating only two small meals a day to save money. Her husband was a law student, and her paycheck was the couple's only income. The nurse determined that she was eligible for WIC benefits and helped her enroll in the program. The nurse also helped Ms. M., who had little experience in food purchasing and meal planning, plan low-cost, nutritious meals. Two weeks later, she had gained 1.4 kg; her 24-hour recall revealed an adequate diet.

Bibliography

Aaronson LS, Macnee CL: The relationship between weight gain and nutrition in pregnancy, *Nurs Res* 38:223, 1989.

Abrams B and others: Maternal weight gain and preterm delivery, *Obstet Gynecol* 74:577, 1989.

Berger A: Effects of caffeine consumption on pregnancy outcome: a review, *J Reprod Med* 33:945, 1988.

Centers for Disease Control: Recommendations for assisting in the prevention of perinatal transmission of human T-lymphotrophic virus type III/lymphadenopathy: associated virus and acquired immune deficiency syndrome, *MMWR* 34:681, 1985.

Ernest AE and others: Guide to breast feeding the infant with PKU, Washington DC, 1980, US Government Printing Office.

Ferris AM and others: Lactation outcome in insulin-dependent diabetic women, *J Am Diet Assoc* 88:317, 1988.

Goldman JA and others: Pregnancy outcome in patients with insulin-dependent diabetes mellitus with preconceptual diabetic control: a comparative study, *Am J Obstet Gynecol* 155:293, 1986.

Gorski J: Exercise during pregnancy: maternal and fetal responses. A brief review, *Med Sci Sports Exerc* 17:407, 1985.

Hediger ML and others: Patterns of weight gain in adolescent pregnancy: effects on birth weight and preterm delivery, *Obstet Gynecol* 74:6, 1989.

Horner RD and others: Pica practices of pregnant women, *J Am Diet Assoc* 91:34, 1991.

Institute of Medicine, National Academy of Sciences: *Nutrition during pregnancy,* Washington, DC, 1990, National Academy Press.

Leventhal JM and others: Does breastfeeding protect against infections in infants less than 3 months of age? *Pediatrics* 78:896, 1986.

Lindenberg CS and others: A review of the literature on cocaine abuse in pregnancy, *Nurs Res* 40:69, 1991.

Little RE and others: Maternal alcohol use during breast-feeding and infant mental and motor development at one year, *N Engl J Med* 321:425, 1989.

London RS: Saccharin and aspartame: Are they safe to consume during pregnancy? *J Reprod Med* 33:17, 1988.

National Center for Health Statistics: *Maternal weight gain and the outcome of pregnancy,* United States, 1980. Vital and Health Statistics, Series 21, No 44 DHHS Publ No (PHS) 86-1922, 1986.

Oxtoby MJ: Perinatally acquired human immunodeficiency virus infection, *Pediatr Infect Dis J* 9:609, 1990.

Parham ES, Astrom MF, and King SH: The association of pregnancy weight gain with the mother's postpartum weight, *J Am Diet Assoc* 90:550, 1990.

Pederson AI, Worthington-Roberts B, and Hickok DE: Weight gain patterns during twin gestation, *J Am Diet Assoc* 89:642, 1989.

Simmer K and others: Are iron-folate supplements harmful? *Am J Clin Nutr* 45:122, 1987.

Infancy, Childhood, and Adolescence

3

During infancy, childhood, and adolescence, adequate nutrition is essential for the promotion of growth and the establishment of a framework for lasting health. Growth is the simplest and most basic parameter for evaluation of nutritional status in children.

Evaluation of Growth

Adequate nutrition is reflected in a child's progress on standardized growth charts depicting height for age, weight for age, height for weight, and head circumference. Sex- and age-specific charts are available for children from birth through 18 years (see Appendix F).

Each child establishes an individual growth pattern and should follow this pattern consistently. Children should be evaluated for nutritional or medical disorders when:

1. They are consistently below the 5th or above the 95th percentile for any growth parameter. Some normal children fall outside the boundaries of the 5th and 95th percentile markings, but all children outside these boundaries should be evaluated to be sure that their growth patterns are reasonable for them (e.g., consistent with the size of their parents and other family members).
2. They fail to stay within one percentile marking of their previous growth parameter (e.g., weight has been at 75th percentile marking, and it then declines below the 50th percentile).

Infancy

Special Concerns

Human milk and infant formula

Either human milk or iron-fortified infant formula meets the nutritional needs of term infants for the first 4 to 6 months of life. Commercial formulas closely resemble human milk, but there are some nutritional differences (Table 3-1). Both products provide about 20 kcal/oz. Commercial formulas are available in three forms: ready-to-feed, concentrate (to be diluted with an equal volume of water), and powder.

Frequency and amount of feedings

Infants vary considerably in their feeding patterns, but most breastfed infants feed at approximately 3-hour intervals and formula-fed infants feed at 4-hour intervals. Although overfeeding is more likely than underfeeding, parents frequently worry about whether they are feeding their infants enough, especially if the infants are breastfed. Infants who are gaining steadily and are wetting at least 6 to 8 diapers a day are usually taking enough. Table 3-2 shows the approximate amount of formula needed for infants less than 6 months old who are not receiving solid foods.

Nutritional Problems in Infancy

Acute gastroenteritis

Acute episodes of diarrhea and vomiting, usually associated with viral illness, are common during infancy and early childhood. These illnesses damage the intestinal mucosa, and diminish the activity of the lactase enzyme needed for lactose (milk sugar) digestion, because lactase is located in the mucosal cells. Foods containing lactose are poorly digested and absorbed, and water is drawn into the gastrointestinal tract as a consequence of the osmolality of the unabsorbed lactose, worsening diarrhea. In addition, the rapid transit of nutrients through the GI tract does not allow sufficient time for fat absorption. Fatty foods often worsen diarrhea and delay gastric emptying, which may increase vomiting.

Maltase, an enzyme which is involved in digestion of maltose, glucose oligosaccharides (corn syrup solids), and starch, retains much of its activity during gastroenteritis. Salivary and pancreatic amylases (enzymes active in starch digestion) are also ad-

Table 3-1 Comparison of human milk and cow's milk formulas

Nutrient	Infant Formula	Human Milk
Protein	Higher content	Primarily α-lactalbumin, an extremely high quality protein*
Calcium	Content is about 1.5 times that of human milk; infant retains about one fourth to one third	Infant retains about two thirds
Iron (Fe)	Fe-fortified formula contains about 24 times as much as human milk; only about 4% is absorbed	Infant absorbs about 49%; Fe deficiency is rare before 6 mo in infants given only human milk
Zinc	Content is about 3-4 times that of human milk; about 30% is absorbed	About 60% is absorbed
Vitamin D	Contains 400 IU/qt, sufficient to prevent rickets	Contains little or none
Bifidus factor†	Not present	Present‡
Immune factors	Not present	Present‡ (immunoglobins, lysozyme)

*Previously the predominant protein in most formulas was casein, a protein less easily digested and assimilated. All major manufacturers now market a formula in which whey, or lactalbumin, predominates.

†Promotes growth of lactobacilli, which inhibit growth of pathogenic microorganisms.

‡Potentially decrease the incidence of respiratory and gastrointestinal infections.

Table 3-2   Approximate daily amount of 20 kcal/oz formula
needed by infants younger than 6 months

Infant Weight			
kg	lb	Caloric Need	Ounces of Formula Needed
3	6.6	324	16.2
4	8.8	432	21.6
5	11	540	27
6	13.2	648	32.4
7	15.4	756	37.8
8	17.6	864	43.2

equate. Therefore it is best to choose foods low in lactose and fat
and high in glucose oligosaccharides or starch during and immediately after a bout of gastroenteritis.

Allergy

As a preventive measure, infants with a strong family history of
allergies who are to be formula fed are often fed soy formulas,
which are less allergenic than cow's milk formulas. However, infants known to be allergic to cow's milk formulas should receive
protein hydrolysate formulas such as Nutramigen, which are even
less allergenic than soy.

Nutritional Care

Assessment

Assessment is summarized in Table 3-3.

Intervention and parent teaching

Goals of intervention and teaching are to assist the infant to:
1. Consume an adequate diet for optimum growth and development
2. Avoid practices that may contribute to obesity, poor dentition, or other health problems
3. Eat a wide variety of foods

Table 3-3   Assessment in growth and development

Areas of Concern	Significant Findings
Inadequate Kcal or Protein Intake	*History* Poverty; chronic illness or frequent acute illnesses; altered parent-infant relationship manifested by failure to feed infant adequately; fear of becoming obese; obsession with thinness (older children and adolescents); poorly planned vegetarian diet *Physical examination* Length, height, or weight <5th percentile, or decrease in these parameters by > one percentile marking; edema, ascites; hair changes: alopecia, loss of pigmentation (flag sign), altered texture; muscle wasting; TSF <5th percentile for age; tooth erosion, gastric bleeding, weak and flabby muscles, poor skin turgor (signs of self-induced vomiting) *Laboratory analysis* Serum albumin, transferrin, and prealbumin, lymphocyte count, serum K^+ (self-induced vomiting)
Excessive kcal Intake	*History* Overfeeding; sedentary life-style: frequent and prolonged television viewing, lack of regular physical activity *Physical examination* Weight >95th percentile for length/height; TSF >95th percentile for age
Adequate Mineral Intake	
Iron (Fe)	*History* Poverty; dislike of iron-containing foods; vegetarianism; increased needs (especially adolescent females); excessive milk consumption by toddlers; infant receiving cow's milk before 12 months of age

Table 3-3 Assessment in growth and development—cont'd

Areas of Concern	Significant Findings
Iron (Fe) —cont'd	*Physical examination* Pallor; blue sclerae; koilonychia (spoon-shaped nails); short attention span; diminished learning ability *Laboratory analysis* ↓ Hgb, Hct, MCV, MCH, MCHC, serum Fe, serum ferritin; ↑ free erythrocyte protoporphyrin (FEP), serum transferrin
Zinc (Zn)	*History* Poverty; dislike of zinc-containing foods; vegetarianism (large intake of grains and vegetables containing phytates and oxalates that impede absorption); abnormal losses (severe or prolonged diarrhea) *Physical examination* Seborrheic dermatitis; anorexia; weight or length <5th percentile for age, or decline in these parameters by > one percentile marking; diarrhea *Laboratory analysis* ↓ Serum Zn
Calcium (Ca)	*History* Failure to consume milk products, calcium-fortified soy milk or formula, or a calcium supplement daily because of food preferences, vegetarianism, dieting, or frequent reliance on fast foods *Laboratory analysis* Radiographic evidence of bone thinning; ↓ serum Ca } Only in very severe cases

Inadequate Vitamin Intake

A	*History* Failure to consume vitamin A (liver, deep green, leafy, or deep yellow vegetables) at least every other day; frequent reliance on fast foods

Continued.

Table 3-3 Assessment in growth and development—cont'd

Areas of Concern	Significant Findings
A—cont'd	*Physical examination*
	Dry skin, mucous membranes, or cornea; follicular hyperkeratosis (resembles gooseflesh); poor growth, susceptibility to infection
	Laboratory analysis
	↓ Serum retinol
B_{12}	*History*
	Child or adolescent following strict vegetarian diet without a supplement or use of fortified soy milk*; infant breastfed by strict vegetarian mother
	Physical examination
	Pallor; glossitis; neurologic abnormalities (altered sensation, altered sense of balance)
	Laboratory analysis
	↓ Serum vitamin B_{12}, Hct; ↑ MCV

*Children should not follow strict vegetarian regimens because of the difficulty of ensuring that the diet contains adequate kcal and protein for growth. Lactovegetarian diets and ovolactovegetarian diets can be adequate for children.

Introduction of solid foods

There is no need to introduce solid foods before 4 to 6 months of age. Reasons for delaying solid food intake include:

1. The tongue extrusion reflex, which tends to push solid foods out of the mouth, doesn't fade until the infant is about 4 months of age.
2. Production of pancreatic amylase, an important enzyme for digestion of starches in infant foods, is low before 4 months.
3. Infants can maintain good head control at 4 months of age and can sit fairly well by 6 months of age. Thus they are better prepared to participate in the feeding process.
4. Eczema and other atopic diseases are more common in infants who have undergone early introduction of solid foods; the greater the diversity of foods introduced, the greater the risk.

5. Early introduction of solid food has no effect on sleep patterns. Many lay people introduce solid foods early, believing that this will cause the infant to sleep through the night.
6. Solid foods can inhibit absorption of iron and other nutrients from human milk.
7. Introduction of solid foods before 4 to 6 months of age is associated with a shorter duration of lactation.

Method of introducing solid foods

When introducing solid foods, the parents should:

1. Begin with foods that provide a good source of iron and that are least likely to result in allergy. Iron-fortified infant cereals, especially rice, fulfill both of these criteria. Foods that are more likely to cause allergy, such as egg white and fish, should be introduced late in infancy. A suggested sequence for adding foods to the infant's diet is shown in Table 3-4.
2. Introduce only one new food every 3 to 5 days, and observe for allergic reactions after each food. If a reaction is thought to have occurred, stop that food for several weeks and then try again. If the same thing occurs after second or third trial, the infant is probably sensitive to this food.
3. Begin with about 1 tsp at a time, and advance the amount as the infant seems ready.
4. Offer solid foods at the beginning of feedings while the infant is hungry.

Table 3-4   Suggested sequence for adding solid foods to infant's diet

Age (Months)	Foods Introduced
4-6	Iron-fortified infant cereal (dry type); strained vegetables and fruits
6-8	Strained beef, lamb, and poultry; cheese, yogurt; toast, crackers, zwieback; mashed or chopped fruits and vegetables
9-11	Chopped table foods (meat, vegetables, and fruits); juice (given by cup)
≥12	Egg white, shellfish

5. Thin foods slightly with formula initially to help the infant make the transition from human milk or formula to foods with thicker consistencies.
6. Never add foods to formula in a bottle. Feed the infant with a spoon.
7. Never feed the infant from the jar. If any food is left over, enzymes in the saliva will digest starches in the food, making it watery, and bacteria from the mouth can multiply in the food.
8. Avoid serving desserts regularly; these are usually low in nutrients and establish a desire for sweets.

Home preparation of infant foods (if parent desires)

When preparing infant foods at home, the parents should:
1. Use fresh or frozen fruits, vegetables, and meats. Canned foods may contain lead, and canned vegetables and meats contain salt, unless they are "no salt added" products.
2. Cook foods in as little water as possible, and do not overcook; this preserves the vitamin content.
3. Do not add sugar or salt. Infants have a well-developed sense of taste and require no flavor enhancers. Routine use of sugar and salt also establishes poor habits.
4. Puree foods in a blender or food grinder initially; chop or mash foods once the infant has more teeth and can chew lumpier foods.
5. Freeze prepared foods in ice trays for later use; 1 to 2 cubes can be used each time for an infant-sized serving.

Minimizing risk of obesity

Parents should reduce formula and milk intake as infants consume more solids and should recognize cues that the infant has reached satiety. Satiety cues from a younger infant include withdrawing from the nipple, falling asleep, closing the lips tightly, and turning the head away. Cues from an older infant include closing the lips tightly, shaking the head "no," playing with or throwing utensils or food, and handing the cup or bottle back to the parent.

Transition from formula to cow's milk

Whole cow's milk can cause gastrointestinal blood loss in infants, for reasons that are not completely understood. Also, cow's milk has excessive amounts of protein, calcium, phosphorus, and sodium as well as inadequate iron for young infants. Infants given cow's milk before 12 months of age are likely to develop iron deficiency anemia.

Children less than 1 year of age should not drink skim milk. It contains excess protein and minerals in proportion to its caloric content and lacks essential fatty acids, which are needed for optimal growth, as well as maintenance of skin integrity.

Appropriate supplements

Vitamins. Breastfed infants not exposed to sun need approximately 400 IU of vitamin D daily. Milk from strict vegetarian mothers is likely to be low in vitamin B_{12}, and their infants need supplements of this vitamin.

Minerals. Breastfed infants need iron-fortified infant cereals or a supplement of 10 mg of iron daily by the time they are 6 months old. Infants should receive 0.25 mg fluoride daily if they are fed human milk, ready-to-feed formula, or formula reconstituted with water containing less than 0.3 ppm fluoride.

Promote dental health

Nursing bottle caries results from prolonged contact of sugar-containing fluids (milk, juice, fruit drinks) with developing teeth. When infants are put to bed with a bottle, they suck on it periodically and keep the mouth full of fluid. If infants are put to bed with a bottle, it should contain water only so that exposure of the teeth to sweet fluids is minimized.

Promote feeding safety

Infants less than 1 year of age should not consume honey. *Clostridium botulinum* spores in honey can cause infant botulism. Symptoms range from constipation through progressive weakness and hyporeflexia to sudden death. Older persons are unlikely to develop botulism from spores.

Coping with gastroenteritis

A regimen frequently used for managing mild gastroenteritis would be to offer clear liquids, usually glucose-electrolyte solutions such as Pedialyte or Lytren, in small amounts (0.5 to 1 oz) every 30 to 60 minutes. Vomiting and stool frequency should decrease during this time. When vomiting stops, begin plain starchy foods (cereals, potatoes, toast, rice) without any added fat, avoiding lactose-containing foods, except breast milk. Soy formula, which is lactose-free, can be used. Gradually add vegetables, fruits, and finally meats until the infant is receiving his usual diet. The usual formula can then be reintroduced. Infants with more severe gastroenteritis that does not respond to this therapeutic program or that causes dehydration may need to be hospitalized for oral rehydration with closer monitoring or for intravenous fluids.

Toddlers and Preschoolers

Special Concerns

Caloric intake

As the growth rate slows during the toddler and preschool years, caloric needs (per kg) are not as high as they are during infancy, and the appetite also declines. The rule of thumb is that caloric needs in early childhood equal 1000 kcal + 100 kcal per year of life. That is, a 3-year-old needs about 1300 kcal/day. Needs for protein, vitamins, and minerals remain high, however. Thus there is little room for "empty calories" from high-fat or high-sugar foods.

Mineral intake

The highest incidence of iron deficiency in the United States is found in children under age 5. Children at special risk include Mexican-Americans, Native Americans, the poor, and those who consume a quart or more of milk per day. Milk, which is low in iron, may take the place of iron-rich foods in the diet. Iron deficiency is associated with decreased attentiveness, narrow attention span, and impaired problem-solving ability.

Calcium needs of children are high (800 mg/day). Development of bones and teeth depend on adequate calcium intake. Furthermore, the habit of consuming a diet rich in calcium is important for the prevention of osteoporosis in later life.

Nutritional Care

Assessment

Assessment is summarized in Table 3-3.

Table 3-5   Food preferences of young children

Likes	Dislikes
Crisp, raw vegetables	Strong-flavored vegetables such as cabbage and brussels sprouts; overcooked vegetables
Foods that can be served and eaten without help, such as finger foods (sandwiches cut into strips or shapes, raw fruit or vegetables cut into small pieces, cheese cubes) and milk and other beverages that can be poured from a child-sized pitcher	Highly spiced foods
	Large servings of beverages or foods
	Foods served at temperature extremes
Foods served lukewarm	Combination foods (e.g., mixed vegetables) where flavors mingle and textures become similar; exceptions: pizza, spaghetti, macaroni and cheese
Single foods that have a characteristic color and texture; preferably, different foods should not even touch each other on the plate	

Parent teaching

The goals of teaching are to foster development of good eating habits that will ensure adequate nutrient intake and minimize the risk of obesity and other health problems. Specific topics follow.

Develop good eating habits

Children need to consume a diet with a variety of foods from all food groups to ensure a balanced diet (see Appendix A). Parental food habits strongly influence those of children, so parents may need to make an effort to eat a balanced and varied diet and avoid voicing distaste for any foods. Young children begin to develop food likes and dislikes (Table 3-5). Parents should continue to encourage their children to eat a variety of foods, while respecting children's preferences as much as possible. Children sometimes refuse foods simply because they are unfamiliar with them. Children's opinions of particular foods improve after repeated exposure to those foods.

Food jags

Food jags, during which children consume only one or two foods for several days, are common. This is not usually harmful; intake over a period of several weeks balances out.

Feeding skills

Young children want to feed themselves and need to learn the necessary skills. Although the process is messy, it should be encouraged. Overemphasis on neatness creates stress at mealtimes and could interfere with the development of good eating habits.

Mineral intake

To ensure an adequate intake of iron, the child needs to consume at least two servings of meat, poultry, fish, or legumes and four servings of enriched or whole-grain breads and cereals daily. Deep green, leafy vegetables can also supply some iron.

Calcium

To ensure adequate intake of calcium, children should:

Drink milk regularly. Chocolate milk can be used if the child will not drink unflavored milk, although chocolate inhibits calcium absorption slightly.

Eat cheese often. Offer cheese for snacks, use cheese in main dishes such as macaroni and cheese or Welsh rarebit, or use cheese sauce over vegetables. Low-fat or "part skim" versions of some cheeses are available and should be used when possible.

Use instant milk powder. This can be added to foods such as meatloaf, mashed potatoes, and cream soups.

Eat yogurt. Yogurt can be eaten for breakfast, snacks, or a light main dish.

Minimize the risk of obesity

Parents may be concerned about what they perceive as poor food intake. They need to be reminded that the growth rate is slowing, and appetite will reflect this. A general rule is that serving sizes should be about 1 tbsp per year of life. More can be served if the child is still hungry. An appropriate food guide for children is provided in Appendix A. Most foods should be chosen from the five food groups, since caloric needs are too low to allow for consumption of many sweets or high-fat foods. Routine use of sweet desserts should be discouraged, and fresh fruits should be served instead. Fried foods should be strictly limited.

Parents should limit the amount of time that young children watch television and encourage daily activities that use large muscle groups. Excessive television watching promotes inactivity and exposes children to multiple cues to eat. Food advertisements make up more than half of all advertising during children's programming, and advertisements often promote foods with low nutrient density.

Promote dental health

The following factors promote the development of good dentition:

1. Adequate calcium, phosphorus, and fluoride for development of caries-resistant teeth. Four servings of milk daily provide the calcium and phosphorus needed. If the local water supply is not fluoridated, the child needs a daily supplement of 0.25 mg fluoride before age 2, 0.5 mg between ages 2 and 3, and 1 mg after age 3.
2. Avoidance of sticky carbohydrates such as chewy candies, cookies, and pastries, which cling to the teeth.
3. Developing the habit of regular brushing and flossing as soon as the child has teeth.

Promote feeding safety

Most deaths resulting from asphyxiation by food occur in children under age 3. The following guidelines will help to prevent asphyxiation:

1. For children under age 3, avoid foods such as hot dogs, hard candy, caramels, jelly beans, gum drops, nuts or peanuts, grapes, and raw carrots, which are difficult to chew or swallow and are an appropriate size to block the airway.
2. When possible, modify foods to make them less likely to obstruct the airway. Grapes can be quartered, carrots cooked, and meat cut into very small pieces. Hot dogs can be cut lengthwise into four strips.
3. Provide adult supervision for very young children while they eat.
4. Insist that children sit down while they eat.
5. Keep eating times as calm as possible. A child who is laughing or extremely excited could inhale food.

School-Age Children

Special Concerns

Influences on food consumption

Peers, teachers, and other significant adults begin to influence food choices during the school years, and home influences decline. As children grow older and have more money to spend, they consume more snacks and meals outside the home. Vending machines and fast food restaurants offer foods that are likely to be high in fat, salt, and sugar and low in vitamins and minerals.

Furthermore, there are a growing number of latchkey children, who may spend several hours of each day without adult supervision. Among the many issues regarding the welfare of these children is a concern about the quality of their food intake.

Attention deficit disorders (hyperkinesis, or hyperactivity)

Attention deficit disorders (ADDs) are characterized by focusing on irrelevant stimuli, impulsive behavior, overactivity (not in all children with hyperkinesis), inconsistency, and lack of persistence. The Feingold diet has been recommended as a treatment for ADDs. It excludes foods containing salicylates, compounds that cross-react with salicylates, artificial flavors, colors, and preservatives. Controlled studies have not provided clear-cut evidence that this diet is effective. Positive effects from the diet may be a result of the placebo effect or of the fact that it takes pressure off the child (placing the blame for his behavior on the diet, rather than on the child). Unfortunately, some of the supposed salicylate-containing foods such as oranges, peaches, grapes, raisins, apples, berries, and cherries are nutritious and are commonly enjoyed by children.

A modified Feingold diet, restricting only food additives, allows a more varied diet, even though it, too, increases the difficulty of food purchasing and preparation. There should be no objection if the family wants to follow such a diet, unless they substitute the diet for medication or mental health care needed by the child, or unless emphasis on the diet promotes behavioral problems by forcing the child to be "different" from his peers.

Sugar has also been proposed as a cause of ADDs, but studies done thus far do not support this hypothesis.

Preventive diet

Eating habits with long-lasting impacts are set during childhood. Dietary intake can influence the incidence of chronic health problems such as obesity, heart disease, cancer, and osteoporosis. The ideal diet is low in fat, high in calcium and complex carbohydrate (starch and fiber), and adequate but not excessive in kcal.

Nutritional Care

Assessment

Assessment is summarized in Table 3-3.

Client/family teaching

The goals of teaching are to develop sound eating habits that will minimize the risk of obesity and other health problems while providing adequate amounts of all nutrients and fiber. Specifically, teaching should include choosing a balanced diet and encouraging physical activity.

Choose a balanced diet

Children need to eat foods from all food groups (see Appendix A) daily. Their diet should be low in fat, high in calcium, and adequate but not excessive in kcal. Do the following to encourage children to eat a nutritious diet:

1. Establish a rule that all family members eat at least one meal together daily. The example of parents, as well as exposure to new foods, encourages children to eat a variety of foods. Also, it is easier to control the amount of sodium, sugar, and fat in home-prepared foods than in items obtained outside the home.
2. Involve children in food preparation. This helps children to be aware of what is in the food they eat and is a good way to introduce elementary nutrition.
3. At fast food restaurants, encourage children to choose fresh salads and baked or broiled fish or chicken, rather than fried foods.
4. Make nutritious snacks available at all times, especially for latchkey children, to discourage the consumption of high-kcal, low-nutrient foods. Good choices for snacks include fresh or dried fruits; yogurt; popcorn; cheese, especially low-fat varieties; cottage cheese with raisins or other fruits; unsalted, dry roasted seeds or nuts; bran or oat muf-

fins; fruit juice frozen into pops; and peanut butter in moderation, because of the high fat content.

Encourage physical activity

The degree of overweight in children is correlated with lack of activity, particularly with the amount of time spent watching television. Children need daily physical activity that involves use of large muscle groups—either team sports or individual aerobic exercises.

Adolescence

Special Concerns

Calories

Caloric needs for growth during adolescence are high—approximately 2200 kcal for girls and 2500 to 3000 kcal for boys. Because caloric intake in boys is so high, they are likely to consume adequate amounts of most nutrients, even though their food choices may not be the wisest. Girls have more difficulty obtaining adequate vitamins and minerals within their kcal allowance, and this problem is aggravated by the widespread interest of girls in weight control.

Dieting

About three fourths of girls in high school have dieted at least once, and 40% are on diets at any one time. Fad diets are popular but are more likely to promote transient water loss than lasting changes in eating habits.

Minerals

Lack of calcium and iron is particularly common among teenage girls. Bone growth requires an increase in calcium intake to 1200 mg/day. Growth and menstruation necessitate an iron intake of 15 mg/day. Fast foods and traditional snack foods tend to be low in calcium and iron. Also, girls concerned about their weight often consider dairy products, the best source of calcium, too fattening to include in their diets.

Food habits of adolescents

Snacks furnish about 40% of kcal in adolescent diets. While snacking is not bad in itself, traditional snack foods such as chips, cookies, and soft drinks are low in nutrients. Ice cream, shakes, hamburgers, and pizza provide important nutrients, but they are also high in fat, sodium, and kcal. Adolescents rely heavily on fast food restaurants, which have very limited menus and often emphasize foods high in kcal, fat, and sodium.

Vegetarianism

The teen years are a time of experimentation, and this may take the form of adopting vegetarianism. There are many types of vegetarians, with some of the most common being strict vegetarians (vegans), those who consume no animal products; lactovegetarians, those who use milk products but no other animal products; and ovolactovegetarians, those who use milk products and eggs. Unless they are carefully planned, vegetarian diets may be nutritionally inadequate.

Protein

Most plant proteins are lacking in one or more amino acids. Combining two proteins with differing amino acid patterns produces "complementary" (complete) protein. For example, grains are low in lysine but high in methionine. Legumes are rich in lysine but lack methionine. Thus grains and legumes are complementary proteins. Fig. 3-1 shows the types of protein foods and gives examples of foods providing complementary proteins.

Minerals

Vegetarians who avoid dairy products will have difficulty consuming enough calcium. Furthermore, plant foods are usually lower in zinc and iron than animal products, and phytate (in whole grains) and oxalate (in chocolate; green, leafy vegetables; and rhubarb) form complexes with minerals and inhibit their absorption.

Vitamin B_{12}

Vitamin B_{12} is found naturally only in animal products. Vegetarians who consume no eggs or dairy products are unlikely to receive enough vitamin B_{12}.

Nutritional Care

Assessment

Assessment is summarized in Table 3-3.

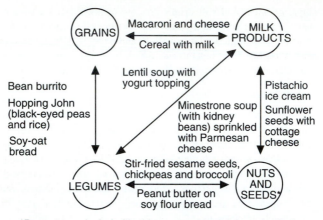

*Peanuts are included in this group, although botanically they are legumes.

Fig. 3-1

Complementary proteins for vegetarian diets. The major types of proteins included in a lactovegetarian diet are circled. Where two types of protein are connected by arrows, those proteins are complementary. Examples of dishes providing complementary proteins are shown beside each arrow. (It probably is not necessary for complementary proteins to be consumed at the same meal, but they should be consumed sometime during the day.)

Client/family teaching

The goal is to help adolescents learn to make wise food choices that will provide the necessary nutrients while maintaining a desirable body weight. Following are some specific teaching topics.

Eat a balanced, nutritious diet to maintain desirable body weight

A food guide for adolescents is provided in Appendix A. It is especially important for them to learn to select diets with a wide variety of foods that are low in fat and cholesterol; high in vitamins, minerals, and fiber; and moderate in kcal. Following are some guidelines that will help them to achieve these diets.

Fat and cholesterol. Limit use of fried foods to one serving per day or less. Eat only two to three servings of red meat a week; choose poultry, fish, or grain and legume main dishes on the other days. Limit meat intake to about 5 oz/day. This is sufficient even for most athletes in training. Use dairy products made with skim milk whenever possible. Chapter 13 provides additional information.

Vitamins and minerals. To promote optimum growth and prevent later osteoporosis, it is very important that teenage girls consume four servings of milk or milk products daily. Skim milk and yogurt, cheese, or cottage cheese made of skim milk are low in kcal and may be acceptable to dieting teens. Plain yogurt with unsweetened fresh fruit or fruit canned in water or juice is lower in kcal than commercial fruit yogurt. Those who do not use milk products need a daily supplement, for example, calcium carbonate, which is 40% calcium. Supplements are best taken at bedtime, when they are least likely to have to compete for absorption with other minerals or vitamins.

Meat, poultry, fish, enriched or whole grains, and deep green, leafy vegetables provide dietary iron (see Appendix B). Even if they use a variety of these foods daily, adolescent girls may still have an inadequate or marginal iron intake. A daily supplement (15 mg) may be warranted. Ferrous sulfate, 20% iron, is available without prescription, inexpensive, and well absorbed.

Kilocalories. Limiting fat and cholesterol intake also helps control kcal intake. High-fiber foods (see Appendix C) may help to reduce kcal intake, since they are bulky and require more chewing than low-fiber, refined foods. The person feels full after eating fewer kcal. Whole grains, legumes, and crisp salads without excessive additions such as dressing, eggs, meat, and bacon are nutritious, low kcal foods.

Eat nutritious snacks

Since snacks are such an important part of the adolescent's diet, they need to provide their share of nutrients. Some tasty and nutritious snacks include fresh or dried fruits; fresh vegetables with a dip made of yogurt and curry, oregano, garlic, or other spices; popcorn; bran or oat muffins; fruit ices; and yogurt, cottage cheese, or cheese (made with skim milk if kcal intake is a concern).

Encourage regular physical activity

Establishing a pattern of physical activity at least 3 or 4 days per week is a valuable habit for later life. Some teens wish to participate in team sports, and this can be encouraged. Others need to choose individual activities that they will continue on a long-term basis. Chapter 5 shows how to calculate the target heart rate for cardiovascular fitness and includes recommendations for becoming and remaining physically fit.

Discourage unhealthy weight loss practices

Since teens are so interested in weight reduction diets, they need to be taught to recognize a safe and effective diet. Fad diets promise and often deliver quick results, but the weight loss is usually fluid and muscle. A good diet meets the criteria given on p. 345.

Eating disorders often appear during adolescence. Weight should be plotted on the growth charts at regular intervals, and any teen whose weight declines by at least one percentile marking should be evaluated for a possible eating disorder. For further information about recognition and treatment of eating disorders, see Chapter 20.

Encourage nutritious choices by clients who choose vegetarianism

Protein. Fig. 3-1 gives guidance for using complementary proteins to ensure that protein intake is adequate.

Minerals. Whole grains, legumes, and deep green, leafy vegetables contain iron and zinc. Additional iron can be obtained from dried fruits, molasses, soy sauce, and use of iron cookware. Calcium sources include dark green, leafy vegetables, except spinach and chard; grains; legumes; soy milk fortified with calcium; tofu; and baked beans.

Improving absorption of minerals. Nonheme iron from plant sources is better absorbed if it is consumed with a vitamin C-containing food such as citrus fruit. Coffee and tea inhibit iron absorption, thus it is best not to consume these products with meals.

Lactose in dairy products stimulates calcium absorption. Vegetarians should be encouraged to use dairy products daily or to take a calcium supplement.

Vitamin B_{12}. Vegetarians need to consume vitamin B_{12}-con-

Table 3-6   Lactovegetarian meal plan

Foods and Amounts	Milk	Meat Substitutes	Vegetables	Fruits	Grains
Breakfast					
⅔ cup orange juice	—	—	—	1	—
⅔ cup bran cereal	—	—	—	—	1
1 cup skim milk	1	—	—	—	—
Sliced banana	—	—	—	1	—
Lunch					
1 cup bean soup	—	1	—	—	—
Toasted cheese sandwich (1 oz cheese, 2 slices whole-grain bread)	⅔	—	—	—	2
1 cup carrot and celery sticks	—	—	2	—	—
Apple	—	—	—	1	—
Snack					
1 cup blueberry yogurt	1	—	—	—	—
½ cup granola	—	—	—	—	1
Dinner					
2 bean burritos	—	1	—	—	2
1 cup spinach salad	—	—	1	—	—
1 cup skim milk	1	—	—	—	—
½ cup peach ice cream	⅓	—	—	—	—
TOTALS	4	2	3	3	6

taining products several times a week. Some soy milk and nutritional yeast is fortified with vitamin B_{12}. Consult the label to determine whether the product is fortified. Where fortified soy milk or nutritional yeast are not used, the individual will need a vitamin B_{12} supplement.

Encourage safe use of nutritional supplements

High doses of vitamin A, including synthetic vitamin A products used in treatment of acne (isotretinoin), are teratogenic. Sexually active girls taking vitamin A supplements need instruction in effective methods of contraception (as do all other sexually active teens).

CASE STUDY

Jenny K., who is 15 years old, and her mother disagreed because Jenny had decided to become a lactovegetarian, and her mother was concerned about her diet. With help, they were able to plan menus that satisfied Jenny and were nutritionally adequate. Table 3-6 gives an example of a lactovegetarian meal plan.

Bibliography

Barness LA: Infant feeding: formula, solids, *Pediatr Clin North Am* 32:355, 1985.

Birch LL and others: The variability of young children's energy intake, *N Engl J Med* 324:232, 1991.

Brown KH: Dietary management of acute childhood diarrhea: optimal timing of feeding and appropriate use of milks and mixed diets, *J Pediatr* 118:S92, 1991.

Casteel HB, Fiedorek SC: Oral rehydration therapy, *Pediatr Clin North Am* 37:295, 1990.

Committee on Nutrition: Soy-protein formulas: recommendations for use in infant feeding, *Pediatrics* 72:359, 1983.

Committee on Nutrition, AAP: Prudent life-style for children: dietary fat and cholesterol, *Pediatrics* 78:521, 1986.

Committee on Nutrition, AAP: Fluoride supplementation, *Pediatrics* 77:758, 1986.

Dietz WH Jr, Gortmaker SL: Do we fatten our children at the television set? *Pediatrics* 75:807, 1985.

Farthing MC: Current eating patterns of adolescents in the United States, *Nutrition Today* 26(2):35, 1991.

Fergusson DM, Horwood LJ, and Shannon FT: Early solid feeding and recurrent childhood eczema: a 10-year longitudinal study, *Pediatrics* 86:541, 1990.

Harris CS and others: Childhood asphyxiation by food: a national analysis and overlook, JAMA 251:2231, 1984.

Hill PD, Aldag J: Potential indicators of insufficient milk supply syndrome, *Res Nurs Health* 14:11, 1991.

Klesges RC and others: Parental influence on food selection in young children and its relationships to childhood obesity, *Am J Clin Nutr* 53:859, 1991.

Kruesi MJP: Carbohydrate intake and children's behavior, *Food Technol* 40:150, 1986.

Lammer EJ and others: Retinoic acid embryopathy, *N Engl J Med* 313:837, 1985.

Manipulation of children's eating preferences, *Nutr Rev* 44:327, 1986.

Moses NS and others: Fear of obesity among adolescent females, *Am J Clin Nutr* 43:664, 1986.

Pridham KF: Feeding behavior of 6- to 12-month-old infants: assessment and source of parental information, *J Pediatr* 117:S174, 1990.

Stekel A and others: Absorption of fortification iron from milk formulas in infants, *Am J Clin Nutr* 43:917, 1986.

Vyhmeister IB, Register UD, and Sonnenberg LM: Safe vegetarian diets for children, *Pediatr Clin North Am* 24(1):203, 1977.

Zeigler EE and others: Cow milk feeding in infancy: further observations on blood loss from the gastrointestinal tract, *J Pediatr* 116:11, 1990.

Adulthood and Aging

4

Many people recognize the central role of optimal nutrition in growth and development of children but are less aware of the importance of good nutrition throughout adulthood.

Special Concerns

Diet and Disease Relationships

Cardiovascular disease, hypertension, cancer, and diabetes, as well as other chronic illnesses, are related to dietary factors. The following is a summary of some of the most common diet-disease relationships among adults in the United States.

Coronary heart disease

Excessive intake of saturated fat and cholesterol increases the risk of coronary heart disease. Overweight and obesity are also factors. Conversely, some types of dietary fiber bind bile salts (formed from cholesterol in the body), prevent their absorption in the intestine, and contribute to reduction of the total body cholesterol pool.

Hypertension

Both overweight/obesity and sodium intake contribute to the development of high blood pressure. In addition, there is evidence that low calcium, magnesium, and potassium intakes may play a role. Alcohol abuse increases the risk of hypertension and cerebrovascular accident (stroke).

Carcinogenesis

Intake of vitamin A or carotenoids (including β-carotene, a precursor of vitamin A), vitamin C, and vitamin E appears to be inversely related to the development of certain neoplasms (e.g., lung cancer). Moreover, epidemiologic studies indicate that cruciferous vegetables, such as broccoli, cauliflower, brussels sprouts, and cabbage, have a protective effect against colon and other types of gastrointestinal (GI) cancers. Whether this is due to their carotene and vitamin C content or to nonnutritive components is unknown.

Evidence points to obesity and excessive dietary fat as factors in the causation of cancer of the breast, colon, rectum, prostate, endometrium, kidney, cervix, ovary, thyroid, and gallbladder. In addition, heavy alcohol consumption contributes to the development of oral, esophageal, rectal, and breast neoplasms.

Preservation of foods with nitrates (used in most salt or smoke curing processes) and charring of foods, as in grilling or broiling, increases the risk of stomach and esophageal tumors.

On the other hand, some types of dietary fiber apparently reduce the risk of cancer, probably by stimulating colonic motility and reducing exposure of the mucosa to carcinogenic agents within the feces.

Diabetes

Non-insulin-dependent diabetes is more common among the overweight and obese. In addition, epidemiologic evidence links diabetes with diets low in fiber.

Prevalence of Osteoporosis

Throughout life, bone is constantly being formed and resorbed. At about 35 years of age in women and 45 years in men, maximum bone mass is reached. After that point, more bone is lost than is formed. Because women generally have smaller, less dense bones than men, they are more likely to develop osteoporosis. Bone loss is accelerated by the decline in estrogen levels at the time of menopause. The most vulnerable individuals are white women or those who have had oophorectomies or who are immobile for prolonged periods. Inadequate calcium intake over a long period of time predisposes people to osteoporosis. About one third of women and one sixth of men who reach age 90 will have a hip fracture related to osteoporosis.

Physiologic and Psychosocial Impacts of Aging on Nutrition

Many physiologic changes that affect nutritional status occur with aging. Some of these are summarized in Table 4-1. Nutritional status is also influenced by the psychosocial impacts of aging and retirement (Table 4-2).

Nutritional Care

The goals of care are to alter nutritional factors that may increase the risk of chronic illness and to help the individual maintain health, well-being, and functional capacity.

Assessment

Assessment of nutrition in adulthood and in the aging are summarized in Tables 4-3 and 4-4, respectively.

The institutionalized elderly have been reported to be especially vulnerable to weight loss and other nutritional problems. This is probably related to the prevalence of chronic diseases and medication usage in the institutionalized elderly. Thus thorough assessment and appropriate nutritional intervention is especially important for elderly individuals in long-term care facilities.

Obtaining accurate values for height in the elderly can be problematic, since loss of vertebral mineralization and volume in intervertebral disks results in loss of height. Long bones, however, retain their mature adult length. Chumlea, Roche, and Steinbaugh (1985) developed equations for estimating height based on knee height (length from sole of foot to anterior thigh with both ankle and knee bent at 90-degree angle).

> For women:
> Estimated height in cm = 84.88 + (1.83 × knee height in cm) +
> (−0.24 × age in years)
>
> For men:
> Estimated height in cm = 60.65 + (2.04 × knee height in cm).

For men, the inclusion of age in the equation adds nothing to the predictive value; for women, age does increase accuracy.

It may be impossible to measure knee height accurately if the individual has severe contractures or other handicaps. For those

Table 4-1   Physiologic changes during aging

Physiologic Change	Nutritional Implications
Decline in basal metabolic rate (BMR) by about 2%/decade after age 30; decrease in physical activity is also documented in aging	Daily caloric need declines; potential for obesity
Loss of taste buds, decrease in taste acuity; impaired sense of smell	Disinterest in food, anorexia; some individuals salt or sugar their food heavily to compensate for loss of taste
Periodontal disease (occurs in about 80% of older adults); loss of teeth	Difficulty eating; restricted food choices (avoidance of raw or crisp fruits and vegetables and high-fiber grains with selection of softer, low-fiber, and often high-calorie alternatives)
Decreased secretion of hydrochloric acid, pepsin, and bile	Potential for impaired absorption of calcium, iron, zinc, protein, fat, and fat-soluble vitamins
Decreased gastrointestinal motility	Constipation, hemorrhoids; diverticulosis
Frequent use of medications	Potential for impaired appetite, decreased absorption or utilization of nutrients, or increased requirements for nutrients; see Chapter 18 for nutritional implications of specific drugs
Impaired motor abilities (not a problem for all elderly people)	Difficulty shopping for or preparing foods; difficulty feeding oneself; decreased energy expenditure, which contributes to weight gain

Table 4-2   Psychosocial changes during aging and retirement

Psychosocial Change	Nutritional Implications
Fixed income	Decreased food consumption, particularly milk, meats, fruits, and vegetables, which are important sources of calcium, riboflavin, protein, iron, and vitamins C and A
Lack of socialization; loneliness	Apathy about meals; poor intake
Vulnerability to advertising and food fads, which can be appealing when touted as methods of alleviating the effects of aging	27%-72% of older Americans use vitamin supplements, although studies indicate that their diets are usually not low in the vitamins they are supplementing; wasting of limited income on diet or health aids with dubious value; potential for toxic intakes of vitamins, particularly A and D

Table 4-3   Assessment of nutrition in adulthood

Areas of Concern	Significant Findings
Obesity	*History* Sedentary life-style; in the elderly, decrease in activity with retirement or chronic illness; decrease in metabolic rate; increase in intake of kcal-dense refined foods because of difficulty in chewing higher fiber foods with periodontal disease; high-fat diet (e.g., heavy use of meats, fried foods, fast foods, many snack foods) *Physical examination* Weight > 120% of ideal for height or BMI >27.3 (women) or >27.8 (men); TSF > 95th percentile

Table 4-3 Assessment of nutrition in adulthood—cont'd

Areas of Concern	Significant Findings
Inadequate Vitamin C Intake	*History* Failure to consume citrus or other vitamin C source daily because of inadequate income, lack of knowledge of nutrient needs, or failure to plan diet wisely *Physical examination* Ecchymoses, petechiae, bleeding gums *Laboratory analysis* ↓ Serum vitamin C
Inadequate Vitamin A Intake	*History* Failure to consume at least one serving of a vitamin A- or β-carotene-rich food daily (see Appendix B), (same reasons as for inadequate vitamin C intake) *Physical examination* Dry, scaly skin; hyperkeratosis (resembles gooseflesh); poor night vision *Laboratory analysis* ↓ Serum vitamin A (retinol)
Inadequate Fiber Intake	*History* Low-fiber diet because of reliance on processed and refined foods (e.g., most fast foods, many convenience foods), difficulty chewing high-fiber foods because of periodontal disease or poorly fitting dentures *Physical examination* Constipation, hemorrhoids *Laboratory analysis* Radiographic evidence of colonic diverticuli
Inadequate Mineral Intake	
Calcium (Ca)	*History* Lactose intolerance: bloating, cramping, flatus, or diarrhea following milk consumption; lack of knowledge of continuing need for milk intake in adulthood *Laboratory analysis* ↓ Bone density on radiographs

Table 4-4   Assessment of nutrition in aging

Areas of Concern	Significant Findings
Protein Calorie Malnutrition (PCM)	*History* Fixed income; lack of socialization: living alone, loss of spouse or friends; difficulty chewing; poorly fitting dentures; difficulty getting to market or transporting purchases home; lack of food preparation skills; lack of facilities for food storage or preparation; frequent use of medications that impair appetite (e.g., digoxin); anorexia and wasting because of chronic disease (e.g., chronic obstructive pulmonary disease or cancer); unpalatable therapeutic diets; food offered unfamiliar or unappealing *Physical examination* Weight < 90% of standard for height or BMI < 19.1 (women) or 20.7 (men), lack of body fat; TSF < 5th percentile; muscle wasting; edema; thinning of hair; changes in hair texture *Laboratory analysis* ↓ Serum albumin, transferrin, prealbumin, lymphocyte count; nonreactive skin tests
Inadequate Fluid Balance (Potential for Fluid Deficit)	*History* Altered mental status (confusion or coma) with inability to feel or express thirst; febrile illness or extremely hot weather with increased fluid needs *Physical examination* Poor skin turgor; dry, sticky mucous membranes; rapid weight loss over 1-2 wk; oliguria; lethargy, hypotension *Laboratory analysis* ↑ Hct, BUN

Table 4-4   Assessment of nutrition in aging—cont'd

Areas of Concern	Significant Findings
Inadequate Vitamin D Intake	*History* Institutionalization or chronic illness with little sun exposure; inadequate intake of vitamin D-fortified milk products *Laboratory analysis* ↓ Bone density on radiographs
Inadequate Zinc (Zn) Intake	*History* Decreased animal protein intake because of fixed income or difficulty chewing *Physical examination* Hypogeusia, dysgeusia; alopecia; dermatitis *Laboratory analysis* ↓ Serum Zn

individuals, Haboubi, Hudson, and Pathy (1990) have developed a nomogram for estimating height based on arm length.

Intervention and Client Teaching

Health care professionals can help the adult to:
1. Obtain adequate nutrients through a diet of regular foods, recognize the impact of dietary choices on health, and decide whether dietary supplements are needed
2. Achieve and maintain a desirable weight
3. Cope with altered GI function accompanying aging
4. Prevent or delay the progression of osteoporosis

Guidelines for choosing a healthful diet

The following suggestions can be used for all adults:
1. Choose a varied diet with at least three servings of vegetables, two servings of fruits, and six servings of grain products daily (see Appendix A). No single food supplies all the nutrients needed, so selection of many different foods from each food group is the best method of ensuring adequate intake of nutrients. Fruits and vegetables are good sources of vitamin C, carotenoids, and fiber and thus may

reduce cancer risk. In addition, fruits and vegetables are generally low in sodium (unless salt or other sodium-containing ingredients are added in their preparation) and are fair to excellent sources of potassium, qualities that may reduce the risk of hypertension. Fruits, vegetables, and grains also tend to be low in fat and moderate to high in fiber and thus may reduce the risk of obesity, heart disease, and cancer and improve bowel function.

On a typical day, 45% of U.S. adults are estimated to consume no fruit or juice and 22% consume no vegetables. Thus a change in adult food habits is badly needed.

2. Maintain weight at a healthy level. Desirable weight ranges for adults are given in Appendix E. These "desirable" weights increase with age, because moderate increases in weight appear to pose less risk as adults age than similar degrees of overweight would pose for young adults. As many as one out of every four U.S. adults is estimated to be overweight. Abdominal fat is associated with more health risk than fat in the thighs and hips. The waist/hip ratio is one method of determining whether abdominal fat is excessive and identifying those individuals most in need of weight reduction.

$$\text{Waist/hip ratio} = \frac{\begin{array}{c}\text{Waist circumference} \\ \text{(near the umbilicus)}\end{array}}{\begin{array}{c}\text{Hip circumference (at the largest} \\ \text{point, over the buttocks)}\end{array}}$$

Table 4-5   Fat content of selected foods

Food and Serving Size	Fat (g)	Kcal from Fat (%)
Bacon, broiled, 2 slices	6.0	78
Cheddar cheese, 1 oz	9.5	74
Cottage cheese, creamed, ½ cup	5.0	39
Cottage cheese, 1% fat, ½ cup	1.2	13
Cream cheese, 2 tbsp	10.0	90
Ground beef, extra lean, broiled, 1 oz	4.7	57
Milk, low-fat (2% fat), 1 cup	4.7	35
Milk, whole (3.5% fat), 1 cup	8.0	48

Ratios greater than or equal to 1 seem to be most closely associated with heart disease. Chapter 19 contains information regarding weight reduction.

Underweight is much less common than overweight in the United States, but it is associated with osteoporosis in women and increased risk of early death in both sexes.

3. Choose a diet with no more than 30% of the kcal from fat. Fat provides 9 kcal/g; carbohydrate and protein each provide 4 kcal/g. Therefore if total intake is 2100 kcal/day, fat intake should be no more than 630 kcal, or 70 g. Butter, margarine, oil, mayonnaise, and salad dressings are the most concentrated sources of fat, with approximately 10 to 14 g/tbsp. However, other foods, particularly meats and milk products, can be surprisingly high (Table 4-5). Nutrition labeling is an aid to individuals wanting to restrict their fat intake, as demonstrated in the accompanying box.

Sample Food Label

Frozen Pepperoni Pizza

Serving size	5 oz (150 g)
Servings per pizza	4
Nutrition information per serving	
Calories, total	380
Calories from fat	189
Fat, total (g)	21
Saturated fat (g)	16
Cholesterol (mg)	350
Total carbohydrates (g)	30
Complex carbohydrates (g)	26
Sugars (g)	3
Dietary fiber (g)	1
Protein (g)	15
Sodium (mg)	650
	Percent of daily value
Vitamin A	20
Vitamin C	5
Calcium	25
Iron	15

Note that in this example 50% of the kcal (189 of 380) come from fat.

Saturated fat should be limited to less than or equal to 10% of the kcal, and cholesterol intake should also be limited. To reduce intake of these, choose lean cuts of meat and poultry without skin; use cold cuts, hot dogs, bacon, and sausage only occasionally; limit use of egg yolks (although egg whites, which contain no fat or cholesterol, can be used frequently; two egg whites are the equivalent of one whole egg in cooking); limit use of cream, sour cream, cream cheese, and creamed cottage cheese; and choose margarine rather than butter. Cheeses made with skim milk and hard cheeses, such as Parmesan, are lower in saturated fat and cholesterol than cheeses such as regular American, cheddar, or Swiss.

4. Use only moderate amounts of salt or sodium. Sodium intake can be reduced by avoiding salt at the table and using it sparingly, if at all, in cooking. In addition, use of processed foods containing sodium should be limited. These foods are listed in the box on p. 261 in Chapter 13. Smoked, cured, and grilled foods should be used infrequently, since they are associated with increased risk of GI cancers.

5. If alcoholic beverages are used at all, use them in moderation. "Moderate" alcohol intake is no more than one drink per day for women and two drinks per day for men, with a "drink" referring to 12 oz (360 ml) of beer, 5 oz (150 ml) of wine, or 1½ oz (45 ml) distilled spirits. In addition to increasing the risk of hypertension and some types of neoplasia, heavy drinking can result in cirrhosis of the liver, malnutrition, and pancreatitis.

Some individuals should not drink at all: pregnant women and those trying to conceive; individuals planning to drive, operate heavy equipment, or perform other activities requiring coordination and rapid responses; individuals taking medications; those who cannot control their drinking; and adolescents and children.

6. Maintain an adequate calcium intake. An intake of at least 800 to 1000 mg/day (equivalent to about 3 cups of milk or yogurt or 4 oz cheese), especially for women, may help to reduce the risk of osteoporosis. Milk products are the richest source of calcium. Individuals with lactose intolerance may be able to tolerate yogurt, buttermilk, cheese, choco-

late milk or cocoa, or milk treated with commercial lactase enzyme (Lact-Aid or Lactrase) to hydrolyze the lactose. Additional calcium is provided by dark green, leafy vegetables, such as kale or mustard greens; sardines and other small fish in which bones are eaten; baked beans; and tofu. Where dietary calcium intake is inadequate, the physician may prescribe a supplement providing 1000 to 1500 mg/day. This is best absorbed if taken with a small amount of milk, since lactose improves absorption, or with no food at bedtime to avoid competition with other nutrients for absorption. Supplementation is used with caution in individuals with a history of renal lithiasis (kidney stones); calcium citrate seems to be the form of supplement that is least likely to cause a recurrence of stone formation.

7. Obtain aerobic exercise at least three to five times a week (20 to 60 minutes per session, depending on intensity of exercise). Exercise is a valuable adjunct to a weight-control regimen, and it improves cardiovascular function and encourages a feeling of well-being. In addition, weight-bearing exercise, such as brisk walking, helps to delay the progression of osteoporosis.

Nutritional Interventions Especially Relevant to the Elderly

Maintaining or increasing weight in underweight individuals

Clients with health or dentition problems are especially likely to be underweight. To help correct this:

1. Offer small, frequent feedings rather than three large meals a day.
2. Be aware of drugs taken regularly by the elderly client and their potential side effects. If medication usage appears to be decreasing the appetite, the physician may be able to substitute another drug or reduce the dosage.
3. If food intake is inadequate because of poverty, help the client obtain funds or food through community services. Arrange for Food Stamps; encourage participation in the National Nutrition Program for the Elderly, which provides meals at congregate feeding sites, or arrange for Meals on Wheels if the individual is homebound.
4. If the client lives alone or has limited social outlets, en-

courage opportunities for group meals. Congregate feeding sites, church functions, or other social activities offer opportunities for socialization.

5. If periodontal disease is responsible for poor intake, help the client obtain proper dental care, including well-fitted dentures, if needed.

6. Involve elderly clients in the planning of menus for extended care facilities or congregate feeding sites. Attempt to accommodate the clients' culture(s) and preferences as much as possible.

7. Light the dining area well so that food can be clearly seen.

8. Provide assistance in eating, if necessary. This may range from opening packages of condiments to feeding the person. Plates with high outer rims make it easier for the elderly with physical handicaps to scoop up food.

9. Instruct the client in simple food preparation techniques, if appropriate. Elderly men who have never cooked until late in life are especially vulnerable to nutritional deficits. The county home demonstration agent and the Expanded Nutrition Program are good resources for food purchasing and preparation materials or classes.

Coping with altered GI function

To reduce the risk of constipation, hemorrhoids, and diverticulosis:

1. Suggest daily use of high-fiber foods, such as fresh fruit and vegetables, whole-grain breads and cereals, and legumes, to produce bulky, easy to evacuate stools. Cooked whole grains, such as oatmeal, bulgur, brown rice, and Wheatena, are good sources of fiber for the elderly who have difficulty chewing.

2. Encourage the client to drink at least 8 cups of fluid (water, juice, tea, coffee) daily to soften stools.

3. Discourage routine use of laxatives, since the client may develop dependence on them.

Impairment of digestion and absorption with aging is rarely severe enough to produce deficiency states. However, the individual who develops achlorhydria often needs supplements of calcium, iron, and vitamin B_{12}.

Preventing or delaying the progression of osteoporosis

Encourage an elderly woman to follow the diet and exercise recommendations just described. In addition, her physician may prescribe medications if osteoporosis is evident or the risk is very high. The nurse and dietitian should encourage the client to take these as prescribed. A vitamin D supplement (usually 400 to 800 IU daily) is sometimes prescribed to ensure calcium absorption, particularly for women who receive little sun exposure. (Exposure of the skin to sunlight is an essential step in the activation of vitamin D.) Estrogen, which delays bone loss, is commonly used, especially for women who are less than 10 years postmenopause, since they seem to derive the most benefit. It is associated with increased risk of breast cancer; thus women taking it should be urged to examine their breasts and have mammograms regularly. Other medications sometimes used include calcitonin, fluoride, bisphosphonates, and thiazide diuretics. Thiazide diuretics decrease calcium excretion in the urine and are sometimes prescribed when calcium loss is increased, in long-term steroid use, for example. Individuals taking thiazide diuretics need to be reminded to maintain a fluid intake of 35 to 50 ml/kg daily to avoid dehydration, and to consume rich sources of potassium daily to avoid potassium depletion. Meats and most fruits and vegetables, particularly citrus fruits, bananas, and tomatoes, are rich in potassium.

Supplementation

No supplements, except calcium as described above, are needed routinely by the elderly or other adults. However, if assessment reveals specific deficiencies, supplements may be needed to correct them.

CASE STUDY

Mr. H., a 72-year-old retired carpenter, was admitted to the hospital for treatment of pneumonia. At the time of his admission, he was noted to be thin and frail, with large ecchymoses almost covering his lower extremities and arms. He had marked gingivitis. His weight was 84% of ideal, serum albumin was low normal, and serum ascorbic acid was 0.2 mg/dl (low).

The health care team learned that Mr. H. had lived alone since his wife's death 15 months ago. He had never cooked before her death and knew little about food preparation or meal planning. His usual meal plan follows.

Breakfast

Black coffee and cereal with whole milk (one or two times per week)

Lunch

Peanut butter or cheese on crackers and soft drink or tea

Dinner

Fried hamburger patty and instant mashed potatoes or canned green beans

Nutrition Diagnoses

1. Protein calorie malnutrition (marasmus)
2. Scurvy (vitamin C deficiency)

Intervention

During hospitalization, Mr. H. consumed a regular diet with good appetite, along with a daily vitamin C supplement. At the time of discharge, he was referred to a congregate feeding site two blocks from his home. The site offered a noon meal that provided approximately one third of the RDA for the major nutrients. The dietitian worked with him to plan nutritious breakfast and dinner meals that would require little skill to prepare. Mr. H.'s revised meal plan follows.

Breakfast

Oatmeal, whole wheat toast with jam, coffee, and orange juice

Dinner

Toasted cheese sandwich, cream of tomato soup (canned), milk, fresh fruit cup (pear and banana)

Bibliography

Butrum RR, Clifford CK, and Lanza E: NCI dietary guidelines: rationale, *Am J Clin Nutr* 48(suppl 3):888, 1988.

Chumlea WC, Roche AF, and Steinbaugh ML: Estimated stature from knee height for persons 60-90 years of age, *J Am Geriatr Soc* 33:116, 1985.

Collinsworth R, Boyle K: Nutritional assessment of the elderly, *J Gerontol Nurs* 15:17, 1989.

Dietary guidelines for healthy American adults: a statement for physicians and health professionals by the Nutrition Committee, American Heart Association, *Circulation* 77:721A, 1988.

Haboubi NY, Hudson PR, and Pathy MS: Measurement of height in the elderly, *J Am Geriatr Soc* 38:1008, 1990.

Mobarhan S, Trumbore LS: Nutrition problems of the elderly, *Clin Geriatr Med* 7:191, 1991.

Nutrition and your health: dietary guidelines for Americans, ed 3, Washington, DC, 1990, USDA and DHHS.

Patterson BH and others: Fruit and vegetables in the American diet: data from the NHANES II survey, *Am J Public Health* 80:1443, 1990.

Sahyoun NR and others: Dietary intakes and biochemical indicators of nutritional status in an elderly, institutionalized population, *Am J Clin Nutr* 47:524, 1988.

Vaughan L, Zurlo F, and Ravussin E: Aging and energy expenditure, *Am J Clin Nutr* 53:821, 1991.

Weinerman SA, Bockman RS: Medical therapy of osteoporosis, *Orthop Clin North Am* 21:109, 1990.

Physical Fitness and Athletic Competition

5

A nutritious diet and exercise are among the major factors contributing to physical fitness and health. Habits that promote physical fitness should be developed during childhood and maintained throughout life.

Special Concerns

Physical Fitness

Exercise

Aerobic exercise is required for developing and maintaining cardiorespiratory fitness and desirable body composition. To promote fitness, exercise must be intense enough to raise the heart rate to 60% to 90% of the maximum (HR_{max}), or 50% to 85% of the maximum heart rate reserve (HR_{max} reserve). The Case Study on pp. 96 and 97 demonstrates calculation of HR_{max} and HR_{max} reserve. In addition, the exercise must be carried out continuously for 20 to 60 minutes, and it must be performed 3 to 5 days a week. Any activity that uses large muscle groups, can be maintained continuously, and is rhythmic and aerobic can be used to develop and sustain cardiovascular fitness. To develop and maintain muscular fitness, strength training should also be performed at least 2 days a week. It should consist of at least 8 to 12 repetitions of 8 to 10 different exercises that condition the major muscle groups (e.g., weight training).

Protein needs

It is commonly believed that markedly increased amounts of certain nutrients, particularly protein, are needed to build muscle mass. However, this is not the case. The protein RDA for adults is 0.8 g/kg/day. Most exercising individuals do well with 1 to 1.5 g/kg/day as long as kcal intake is adequate to meet energy needs. This amount is contained in the average American diet, which provides 80 to 110 g/day.

Kilocalories

Caloric needs vary because of differences in physical activities and the intensity of exercise. Table 5-1 gives an indication of the caloric expenditure during various types of activities.

Increased caloric needs resulting from exercise can be met through a diet of regular foods. Fat should provide no more than 30% of the kcal, and carbohydrate should provide approximately 55%, with emphasis being placed on complex carbohydrates (fibers and starches, found primarily in grains, legumes, vegetables, and fruits).

Exercise facilitates weight reduction in at least two ways. First, it tends to cause fat loss, even with little or no reduction in kcal intake. Second, regular aerobic exercise averts the decline in resting energy expenditure, which often occurs as weight is lost. This decline in resting energy expenditure can undermine weight loss efforts, even for individuals who adhere to low kcal diets.

Vitamins

Supplemental vitamins do not improve performance. A balanced diet provides all necessary vitamins. B vitamin needs increase

Table 5-1   Approximate energy expenditure during exercise

Activity	Kcal/kg/min	Kcal Used During 30 Min of Exercise	
		54.5 kg (120 lb) Person	87.3 kg (192 lb) Person
Bicycling 12 mph	0.17	276	442
Running 5 mph	0.14	228	364
Swimming (fast freestyle)	0.13	212	340
Jumping rope	0.11	180	288
Skating (ice or roller)	0.08	130	208
Walking 3 mph	0.06	102	164

during vigorous activity, but they will be met by the increased caloric intake needed during heavy exercise.

Minerals

Vigorous exercise increases iron needs. Iron deficiency, which is prevalent among female athletes, impairs physical performance by interfering with energy production and allowing lactate accumulation in muscle. If iron intake appears inadequate, athletes should have a complete blood count done and possibly have their serum iron, total iron-binding capacity, free erythrocyte protoporphyrin, or serum ferritin measured to rule out iron deficiency.

Nutrition for Competition

Carbohydrate loading

Carbohydrate loading can double muscle glycogen stores, increasing endurance during competition. It is of benefit only to athletes in endurance events (marathons, long-distance cycling, cross-country skiing).

Traditionally, the technique of carbohydrate loading involved the following: (1) exercising to exhaustion 7 days before the competition to deplete muscle glycogen stores, (2) consuming a high-fat, high-protein, low-carbohydrate diet for the next 3 days, and (3) discontinuing athletic training for the 3 days just before the event, while consuming a high-carbohydrate diet. However,

Table 5-2   Food guide for carbohydrate loading*

Type of Food	Amount
Meat, fish, poultry, eggs, cheese	6-8 oz
Bread, pasta, cereals (1 slice or ½ -¾ cup)	18-24 servings
Vegetables (½ cup)	8 servings
Fruits and juices (½ cup)	6 servings
Fats and oils (tbsp)	1-2
Milk (cup)	3 (skim)
Beverages	Sweetened, unlimited to achieve needed calories
Approximate total kcal	2500-3600
Approximate carbohydrate	65%-80%

*For 2 to 3 days before competition.

exhaustive exercise increases the risk of injury to the athlete, and the high-fat, low-carbohydrate diet is unpalatable and may result in nausea, fatigue, and irritability. Moreover, similar levels of muscle glycogen can be achieved if the individual simply ceases training for 2 to 3 days before competition, while consuming a high-carbohydrate diet (8 to 10 g carbohydrate/kg body weight), with emphasis on complex carbohydrates (Table 5-2). On the day of the event, the athlete should consume his or her usual diet, preferably one that is 55% or more carbohydrate.

Disadvantages

1. Carbohydrate loading offers no benefit during short-duration events (less than 1 to 2 hours).
2. It can be harmful in individuals with diabetes or hypertriglyceridemia. They should undertake carbohydrate loading only under a physician's supervision.
3. It is not recommended for preadolescent or young adolescent athletes.
4. Water stored with the glycogen in muscles can make the muscles feel stiff and swollen.

Pregame meal

The timing and composition of the pregame meal can influence performance. It is particularly important that the stomach not be full at the time of the event, since this diverts blood flow to the mesentery and may impede performance. See Intervention and Client Teaching later in this chapter for specifics of the pregame meal.

Fluid and electrolyte replacement

Losses from perspiration are primarily water; sweat electrolyte levels are lower than those in plasma. Therefore water makes the best replacement for perspiration losses. Salt tablets are unnecessary and may be hazardous, and sport drinks are not usually needed except in endurance events.

Nutritional Care

The objectives of care are for clients to (1) establish a lifelong habit of regular aerobic exercise and a nutritionally balanced diet to promote health and physical fitness, (2) avoid nutritional deficiencies, and (3) attain optimal athletic performance in a manner consistent with maintaining good health and nutritional status.

Assessment

Assessment is summarized in Table 5-3.

Intervention and Client Teaching

Encourage regular aerobic exercise

1. Emphasize benefits of exercise, which vary with age and physiologic state.

Age Group or Physiologic State	Benefits of Exercise
All age groups	Weight control; feeling of well-being
Childhood and adolescence	Establish habit of regular exercise
Adulthood	Potential for reducing the risk of obesity, heart disease, hypertension, non-insulin-dependent diabetes, gout, gallstones, and osteoporosis
Pregnancy	Possibly less constipation
Elderly	Same as Adulthood (above); decrease constipation; opportunity for social contact

2. Recommend exercises that use large muscle groups rhythmically and that can be maintained continuously.
   a. Examples of aerobic activities are running or jogging, walking, hiking, swimming, ice or roller skating, bicycling, cross-country skiing, rope skipping, or rowing.
   b. Certain activities, such as those requiring running or jumping and those associated with overuse (e.g., marathon training), have great potential for injury. The beginning exerciser and the elderly should be especially cautious if they choose these activities.

Prevent nutritional deficiencies

Kilocalories
Maintain sufficient kcal intake to prevent underweight.

Protein
Maintain intake of at least 1 g/kg (adults) or the RDA (for children and pregnant and lactating women).

Table 5-3   Assessment in physical fitness and athletic competition

Areas of Concern	Significant Findings
Inadequate Energy (kcal) Intake	*History* Energy intake by diet history or food record < 35-40 kcal/kg ideal body weight (adults) or < RDA for children or pregnant and lactating women; frequent dieting to achieve and maintain low "competitive" weight; physiologic state requiring ↑ kcal: childhood, adolescence, pregnancy, lactation; extremely strenuous exercise habits (e.g., distance running); possible eating disorder *Physical examination* ↓ Body fat, athletic performance; TSF < 5th percentile; weight for height < 90% of standard or BMI less than 19.1 (women) or 20.7 (men), (for children or adolescents, weight more than one percentile marking < that for height, i.e., if height is at 50th percentile, weight should be at least at the 25th); amenorrhea; delayed growth and development (children and adolescents)
Inadequate Protein Intake	*History* Frequent dieting, kcal intake so low that protein consumed is utilized for energy; physiologic state requiring ↑ protein: childhood, adolescence, pregnancy, lactation *Physical examination* Edema; delayed growth and development (children and adolescents); thinning of hair, changes in hair texture *Laboratory analysis* ↓ Serum albumin, transferrin, or prealbumin, lymphocyte count

Continued.

Table 5-3   Assessment in physical fitness and athletic competition — cont'd

Areas of Concern	Significant Findings
Inadequate Mineral Intake	
Fe	*History*
	Intake < RDA by diet history or food record
	Physical examination
	Pallor; ↓ athletic performance
	Laboratory analysis
	↓ Hct, Hgb, MCV, MCH, MCHC, serum Fe; ↑ serum transferrin or total iron-binding capacity
Volume Fluid Deficit	*History*
	Failure to replace fluid losses by drinking during and after athletic endeavors; fluid restriction in an attempt to achieve competitive weight; use of diuretics to achieve competitive weight or produce dilute urine in an effort to confound drug testing
	Physical examination
	Dry, sticky mucous membranes; poor skin turgor; thirst; disorientation; weakness; hypotension
	Laboratory analysis
	↑ serum sodium, Hct, BUN, serum osmolality
Serum Lipids	*History*
	Consumption of high-cholesterol, high-fat diet (common in athletes); use of anabolic steroids
	Laboratory analysis
	↑ serum cholesterol, ↑ LDL cholesterol, ↓ HDL cholesterol

Iron

Individuals participating regularly in vigorous physical exercise should be instructed in a diet that includes good sources of iron (see Appendix B), as well as vitamin C, which promotes iron absorption. Females, particularly, may have difficulty maintaining adequate iron nutriture, and the physician may prescribe an iron supplement if there is evidence of anemia or low iron stores. Absorption of iron from the supplement will be best if it is taken between meals or at bedtime and with fluids other than tea or milk.

Attain optimal athletic performance while maintaining good health and nutrition

Carbohydrate loading

The athlete desiring to follow a carbohydrate loading diet should be encouraged to avoid the traditional regimen (p. 90) and assisted in planning a nutritious diet high in carbohydrate (Table 5-2).

Carbohydrate during exercise

Carbohydrate taken regularly (approximately 25 to 50 g/hr) during prolonged exercise improves endurance and performance. Simple carbohydrates can be in either solid or liquid forms (e.g., sport drinks, fruit juice, or sweetened tea). Exceed Fluid Replacement (Ross Laboratories), which is 7% carbohydrate, and Gatorade (Quaker Oats), which is 6% carbohydrate, are examples of commercial sport drinks.

Fluid and electrolyte replacement

1. Plain, cold water is the best fluid replacement. Cold water is more rapidly emptied from the stomach than warm, and it does not cause cramps.
2. Thirst is not a reliable indicator of fluid needs during competition. About 10 to 15 minutes before the event, the athlete should drink 400 to 500 ml (13 to 17 oz) of water. This should be followed by 100 to 200 ml (3 to 7 oz) approximately every 15 minutes during prolonged exertion. The athlete needs 480 ml (16 oz) to replace each 0.45 kg (1 lb) lost during exercise.

3. Sport drinks containing glucose and electrolytes are unnecessary in most athletic events. However, with extreme exertion (greater than 1 hour duration) or environmental conditions, they may be warranted.

Pregame meal

1. Consume the last solids 2 to 4 hours before the event to allow time for gastric emptying. A light (150 to 500 kcal) high-carbohydrate meal is best.
2. Avoid high-fat foods because they delay gastric emptying.
3. Avoid simple sugars in the 30- to 45-minute period before vigorous exercise, because they stimulate insulin release, which may result in rebound hypoglycemia. Carbohydrate taken *immediately* before exercise may improve performance, however. (The immediate onset of exercise, and the concomitant release of glucagon and catecholamines, will prevent hypoglycemia.)

CASE STUDY

Ms. J., who is 32 years old and bicycles regularly, wants to determine her target heart rate for aerobic benefit.

Method A. Calculating Target Rate as Percentage of Maximum Heart Rate (HR_{max})

Step	Example
1. Determine maximum attainable heart rate (220 beats/min minus age in years)	$220 - 32 = 188$ beats/min
2. Multiply by 60% to 90% to obtain target heart rate*	$188 \times 75\% = 141$ beats/min

---

*The lower end of the range is for beginning exercisers, the upper end for highly trained athletes.

Method B. Calculating Target Rate Using Maximum Heart Rate Reserve (HR_{max} reserve)

Step	Example
1. Determine HR_{max} (see Method A)	$220 - 32 = 188$ beats/min
2. Find heart rate reserve (HR_{max} reserve)	$188 - 68† = 120$ beats/min
3. Multiply HR_{max} reserve by 50% to 85%*	$120 \times 65\% = 78$ beats/min
4. Add resting heart rate to the product of Step 3	$68 + 78 = 146$ beats/min

*The lower end of the range is for beginning exercisers, the upper end for highly trained athletes.

†Ms. J's resting heart rate.

Bibliography

American College of Sports Medicine: The recommended quantity and quality of exercise for developing and maintaining cardiorespiratory and muscular fitness in healthy adults, *Med Sci Sports Exerc* 22:265, 1990.

Burke LM, Read RS: Sports nutrition: approaching the nineties, *Sports Med* 8:80, 1989.

Costill DL: Carbohydrates for exercise: dietary demands for optimal performance, *Int J Sports Med* 9:1, 1988.

Hoffman CJ, Coleman E: An eating plan and update on recommended dietary practices for the endurance athlete, *J Am Diet Assoc* 91:325, 1991.

Kleiner SM: Performance-enhancing aids in sport: health consequences and nutritional alternatives, *J Am Coll Nutr* 10:163, 1991.

Leaf A, Frisa KB: Eating for health or for athletic performance? *Am J Clin Nutr* 49(suppl 5):1066, 1989.

Pavlou KN and others: Physical activity as a supplement to a weight-loss dietary regimen, *Am J Clin Nutr* 49(suppl 5), 1989.

PART II

NUTRITION AND CLINICAL CARE

Nutrition Support Techniques

6

Individuals who are unwilling or unable to consume an adequate diet by mouth and those with impaired ability to digest or absorb foods require specialized nutrition support. Nutrition support is the provision of specially formulated or delivered intravenous or enteral nutrients to prevent or treat malnutrition. There are three methods of delivering nutrition support: oral supplements, enteral tube feedings, and total parenteral nutrition (TPN). Whenever possible, oral or tube feedings should be used because they are safer, more physiologic, and less expensive than TPN. A good motto is "If the gut works, use it."

Administering Nutrition Support

Oral Supplements

Indications

Oral supplements are useful for clients who can digest and absorb nutrients. They are most effective when clients are consuming some foods but cannot take in enough because of anorexia or increased metabolic demands resulting from causes such as trauma, burns, and infection.

Types of supplements

Some individuals may prefer home-prepared foods such as shakes and eggnogs. Commercial formulas that contain protein, carbohydrates, fat, vitamins, and minerals may also be used (Table 6-1). Generally, products for oral consumption should provide at least 1.5 kcal/ml, since it is difficult for the client to take in adequate amounts of more dilute products.

Modular products (Table 6-2) can be added to such foods as cooked or dry cereals, mashed potatoes, applesauce, juices, tea,

Table 6-1 Formulas for enteral feeding

Formula	Indications	Examples of Commerical Formulas (Manufacturer)
Intact, or "Polymeric," Formulas Used When GI Tract Is Functional		
Standard formulas	Inability to ingest any food or inability to consume enough to meet nutrient needs, e.g., oral or esophageal cancer, anorexia or chronic illness, anorexia nervosa, coma	Tube or oral feeding Newtrition Isotonic (O'Brien) Isosource (Sandoz) Ensure (Ross)† Primarily tube feeding Osmolite (Ross) Isocal (Mead Johnson) Fortison (Sherwood) Primarily oral feeding Resource (Sandoz) Instant Breakfast (Clintec)†‡ Meritene (Sandoz)†‡
-Percentages of macronutrients approximately the same as in typical U.S. diet (approximately 50%-60% of kcal from CHO*, 10%-15% from protein, 25%-40% from fat) -Isosmolar to blood (≈ 300 mOsm/kg) unless marked† -Approximately 1 kcal/ml unless otherwise stated		

High-nitrogen formulas

->15% of kcal are protein

-Approximately 1 kcal/ml unless otherwise stated

Isotein HN (Sandoz), 1.2 kcal/ml
Osmolite HN (Ross)
Isosource HN (Sandoz)
Newtrition High Nitrogen (O'Brien)
Sustacal, Sustacal HC (Mead Johnson)†, 1 or 1.5 kcal/ml

Concentrated formulas

-Macronutrients in the same proportions as typical U.S. diet

-2 kcal/ml

TwoCal HN (Ross)†
Isocal HCN (Mead Johnson)†
Magnacal (Sherwood)†
Nutren 2.0 (Clintec)†

Fiber-containing or blenderized formulas

-Macronutrients in the same proportions as the typical U.S. diet

-Contain fiber from foods or from added soy or oat polysaccharide

-Approximately 1 kcal/ml

Enrich (Ross)†
Jevity (Ross)
Compleat Modified (Sandoz)
Newtrition Isofiber (O'Brien)
Ultracal (Mead Johnson)

Same as for standard formulas, plus catabolism and protein deficits, e.g., trauma, burns, sepsis

Same as for standard formulas, plus need for fluid restriction

Same as for standard formulas, plus need for fiber to maintain normal bowel function (i.e., control diarrhea or constipation)

---

*CHO, Carbohydrate.

†Osmolality greater than 450 mOsm/kg. Tube feedings of these hyperosmolar formulas may be better tolerated if administered continuously; oral feedings are best tolerated if sipped slowly.

‡Contain lactose; may cause diarrhea in stressed clients and those with known lactose intolerance.

Continued.

Table 6-1   Formulas for enteral feeding—cont'd

Formula	Indications	Examples of Commerical Formulas (Manufacturer)
Formulas Used When GI Function is Impaired		
Elemental, or "predigested," formulas -Protein is hydrolyzed into peptides or amino acids -Either low fat (<10% of kcal) or high in medium-chain triglycerides (MCT)	Impaired digestion or absorption of nutrients, e.g., short-bowel syndrome, severe radiation enteritis	Criticare HN (Mead Johnson)† Vital High Nitrogen (Ross)† Reabilan (O'Brien)† Vivonex T.E.N. (Norwich Eaton)† Peptamen (Clintec)
Specialized Formulas for Specific Disease States		
Disease-specific formulas -Modification of protein, carbohydrate, and/or fat content, as appropriate for disease -Some are concentrated to allow for fluid restriction	Diabetes mellitus Pulmonary disease Hepatic failure Renal failure Trauma Stimulate immune function	Glucerna (Ross) Pulmocare (Ross)† Hepatic Aid II (Kendall)† Travasorb Hepatic (Clintec)† Replena (Ross)† Travasorb Renal (Clintec)† Amin-Aid (Kendall)† TraumaCal (Mead Johnson)† Traum-Aid HBC (Kendall)† Impact (Sandoz)

Table 6-2   Modular components for enteral feeding

Nutrient Module	Examples of Commercial Products (Manufacturer)
Carbohydrate	Polycose (Ross)
	Moducal (Mead Johnson)
	Nutrisource Carbohydrate (Sandoz)
	Pro-Mix (Navaco)
Lipid (fat)	MCT Oil (Mead Johnson)
	Microlipid (Sherwood)
	Nutrisource Lipid (Sandoz)
Combined carbohydrate and lipid protein	Controlyte (Sandoz)
	Casec (Mead Johnson)
	Pro-Mix (Navaco)
	Propac (Sherwood)
	Nutrisource Protein (Sandoz)
	ProMod (Ross)

coffee, shakes, soups, salad dressings, and sandwich fillings. The modular carbohydrates are especially versatile since they can be added to most soft foods or liquids without altering flavor or texture.

Delivery of oral supplements

Liquid supplements contain readily digested carbohydrate. As a result, they may cause dumping syndrome, with abdominal cramping, weakness, tachycardia, and diarrhea, if they are consumed rapidly. Clients should be cautioned to sip these products slowly, taking 180 to 360 ml over 15 to 45 minutes. Liquid supplements taste best if they are chilled or served over ice.

Modular products may be added to any meal or snack.

Enteral Tube Feedings
Indications

There are at least three indications for enteral tube feedings:

1. Inability to ingest food or meet needs fully by the oral route. Mechanical or psychological problems limiting food intake, unconsciousness, and markedly increased nutritional requirements with inadequate oral intake may neces-

sitate tube feedings. *Examples:* Head and neck tumors, esophageal stricture or carcinoma, coma, anorexia or chronic illness, trauma, burns, congenital heart disease, anorexia nervosa, and neurologic disorders interfering with swallowing.

2. Maldigestion or malabsorption requiring unpalatable modified formulas or necessitating continuous feedings to maintain adequate nutritional status. *Examples:* Pancreatic or biliary insufficiency; cystic fibrosis; short-bowel syndrome; inflammatory bowel disease; and protracted diarrhea with malnutrition.

3. Organ failure or severe injury requiring unpalatable formulas. *Examples:* Renal or hepatic failure, major trauma. Specialized formulas for these conditions are discussed in Chapters 7, 9, and 11.

Types of tube feeding formulas

Unimpaired digestion and absorption

When the gastrointestinal (GI) tract is functional, nutritionally complete formulas containing proteins, complex carbohydrates or oligosaccharides, and long-chain triglycerides (LCTs) or fats are used (Table 6-1). For home tube feedings, formulas made of blended foods are often the most economical.

Impaired digestion or absorption

When maldigestion and malabsorption are present, *elemental* or predigested formulas containing protein hydrolysates, peptides, or amino acids; oligosaccharides or simple carbohydrates; and medium-chain triglycerides (MCTs), or minimal fat are used. Fat is among the most difficult of nutrients to digest and absorb because it requires adequate amounts of lipase and bile salts, adequate bowel surface area, and an optimal bowel pH. MCTs are less reliant on pancreatic lipase and bile salts for digestion and absorption than LCTs, and thus MCTs are preferred in treating bowel dysfunction. Commercial formulas are available to meet the needs of almost every individual (Table 6-1). Where they are inadequate, modular components (Table 6-2) permit preparation of formulas specially tailored to meet individual needs.

Tube feeding procedures

Routes for tube feedings

Table 6-3 describes the routes for tube feedings, along with their advantages and disadvantages, and Fig. 6-1 illustrates the tube locations. Nasogastric (NG) and nasoduodenal (ND)/nasojejunal (NJ) tubes are usually used for temporary feedings (arbitrarily defined as less than 3 months) and esophagostomy, gastrostomy, and jejunostomy for long-term feedings.

Table 6-3 Tube feeding routes

Location	Advantages	Disadvantages
Intragastric		
Nasogastric (NG) or orogastric (OG)*	Easily inserted; allows use of almost all of GI tract	Easily dislodged, especially with altered sensorium; potential for pulmonary aspiration; potential for development of sinusitis and otitis media
Gastrostomy	More difficult to dislodge than NG or OG; new methods allow percutaneous insertion without general anesthesia; usually has a larger diameter than NG; viscous formulas (e.g., home blenderized) will flow through; conventional gastrostomy can bypass esophageal obstruction (patent esophagus necessary for percutaneous insertion)	Potential for irritation of skin around insertion site caused by leakage of gastric juices

*OG tubes are used only in infants.

Continued.

Table 6-3   Tube feeding routes—cont'd

Location	Advantages	Disadvantages
Enteric		
Nasoduodenal (ND) or nasojejunal (NJ)	Decreases possibility of pulmonary aspiration; useful in individuals with delayed gastric emptying (e.g., diabetic gastroparesis)	More difficult to insert than NG; bypasses stomach, a barrier to infection; usually necessitates continuous feedings given with a pump; can cause dumping syndrome; easily dislodged; potential for development of sinusitis and otitis media
Jejunostomy	Same as for ND/NJ; can bypass upper GI obstruction	Except for insertion and dislodgement, same as for ND/NJ; requires surgical insertion

Types of feeding tubes

Nonreactive. Nonreactive tubes are soft, nonirritating tubes made of polyurethane, silicone rubber, or similar materials ranging in size from 5 to 12 French (Fr). (1 Fr ≈ 0.34 mm.) Because nonreactive tubes are soft, insertion is sometimes difficult, but stylets are available to facilitate insertion. Nonreactive tubes can be left in place for several weeks. No syringe smaller than 35 ml should be used to aspirate or irrigate these tubes because they can collapse or rupture with smaller syringes, which exert higher pressures. Some tubes have weighted tips, but the weights have been shown to have no benefit in promoting transpyloric passage of the tube or maintaining tube position within the GI tract.

Polyethylene and polyvinylchloride. Polyethylene (PE) and polyvinylchloride (PVC) tubes range from 5 to 18 Fr in size. They are stiffer than nonreactive tubes and require no stylets for

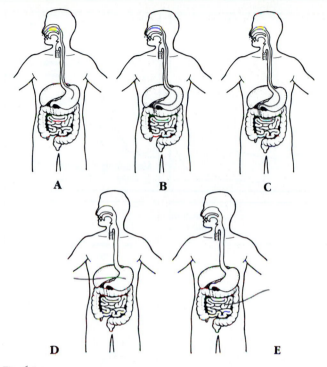

Fig. 6-1
Tube feeding routes. **A**, Nasogastric; **B**, nasoduodenal; **C**, nasojejunal; **D**, gastrostomy; **E**, jejunostomy. (From Moore MC: Alterations in nutrition. In Beare PG and Myers JL, eds: *Principles and practice of adult health nursing,* St Louis, 1990, Mosby–Year Book.)

insertion. These tubes harden during use. To avoid GI perforation, they should be replaced every 3 to 4 days. They tend to irritate the nose and throat more than nonreactive tubes. PE and PVC tubes are initially cheaper than nonreactive ones, but the need for frequent replacement may make them more expensive in the long run.

Procedure for insertion of NG and ND/NJ tubes (Fig. 6-2)

1. Select an appropriately sized tube. Generally, 8 Fr tubes, often called "small-bore" or "fine-bore," are suitable for

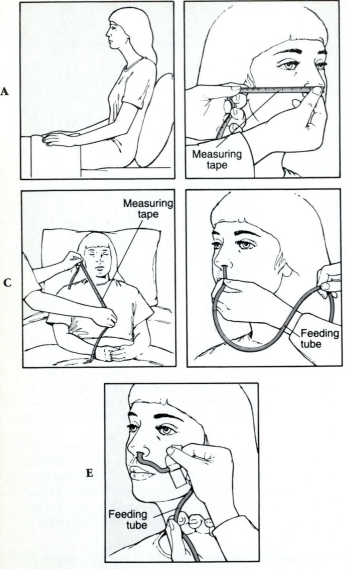

Fig. 6-2
For legend see opposite page.

Fig. 6-2

Insertion of a feeding tube. **A,** Place the client in the Fowler's position before tube insertion, if possible, so that gravity can facilitate passage of the tube. **B** and **C,** Measure the distance from nose to ear and then to xiphoid process and calculate length of tube needed. **D,** Encourage client to sip fluids or chew ice chips while the tube is gently advanced. **E,** Tape tube securely to clients' cheek. (From Moore MC: Alterations in nutrition. In Beare PG and Myers JL, eds: *Principles and practice of adult health nursing,* St Louis, 1990, Mosby—Year Book.)

---

adults and children. If blenderized tube feedings or other thick fluids are to be used, a 12 Fr tube may be needed. Most infants can use 6 or 8 Fr tubes, but premature infants may need a 5 Fr tube.

2. Explain the procedure to the client. Clients may be reassured by the information that tube insertion is not painful, although it may cause gagging. Have the client sit up, if possible, and lean the head forward.

3. If ND/NJ placement is desired, the physician may order oral or parenteral metoclopramide to be given *before* beginning tube insertion to stimulate passage of the tube through the pylorus. Metoclopramide seems to do little good if given when the tube tip is already in the stomach.

4. Determine the length of tube to be inserted. For adults:

$$\text{Length for NG insertion} = \frac{\begin{array}{c}\text{Nose to ear to}\\\text{xiphoid process}\\\text{measurement (cm)} - 50\text{ cm}\end{array}}{2} + 50\text{ cm}$$

Add at least 15 cm for placement beyond the pylorus. For children, one suggested method is:

Length for NG insertion = 6.7 + 0.226 (Height in cm) + 3 cm + Distance from distal tip to feeding pores on tube (cm)

5. Lubricate the tip of the tube with water-soluble lubricant. Gently advance the tube through the nostril parallel to the roof of the mouth and then down the esophagus. Inhalable nasal decongestants used before tube insertion can make the process more comfortable. The patient can help by sipping fluids, unless they are contraindicated, or swallowing while the tube is being advanced.

6. If the client begins to cough or choke during the insertion, the tube may be in the trachea. Remove it and try again.
7. When the proper length of tube has been inserted, secure the tube to the face with tape.
8. If ND/NJ placement is desired, instruct the client to lie on the right side for 2 to 3 hours after tube insertion to facilitate passage of the tube out of the stomach.
9. Confirm tube placement before administering feedings.

Methods of confirming tube placement

1. An abdominal radiograph is the most accurate method for confirming tube placement.
2. Aspiration of fluid that has a pH less than or equal to 4 in patients not receiving H_2-receptor antagonists, or 5.5 in patients who are receiving H_2-receptor antagonists, is highly correlated with gastric tube placement. (In contrast, intestinal and tracheo-bronchial fluid is usually, although not always, alkaline.)
3. Insufflation of air through the tube while auscultating the left upper quadrant of the abdomen with a stethoscope is a commonly used method, but it is possible to hear an inrush of air even when the tube tip is in the esophagus or pleural space. This method is consequently not recommended.

Delivery of tube feedings

Continuous feedings

Continuous feedings, feedings delivered over the entire day or some portion of the day (usually 10 to 12 hours), are preferred in many cases, such as:

1. Duodenal or jejunal feedings because continuous feedings reduce the risk of dumping syndrome.
2. Decreased absorptive area (chronic diarrhea, short-bowel syndrome, acute radiation enteritis, and severe malnutrition with atrophy of the villi) because continuous feedings may increase the total amount tolerated.
3. Some cases of severe stress with normal GI function. Burn patients, for instance, have been found to have less diarrhea and more adequate intake if given continuous, rather than intermittent, feedings.

Intermittent feedings

Feedings given every 2 to 4 hours are preferred for:

1. Confused clients who, if left unattended, are in danger of dislodging the tube.
2. Stable long-term clients, especially outpatients, where continuous feedings interfere with normalization of life-style.

Intermittent feedings are usually better tolerated if given by slow drip rather than by rapid bolus infusion. Healthy adults can tolerate a feeding as large as 750 ml, as long as it flows no faster than 30 ml/minute. Sick adults may not tolerate a volume that large, but they, too, will benefit from the slow flow rate. Abdominal discomfort, diarrhea, tachycardia, and nausea during or shortly after feedings signal that the flow is too rapid or the volume too large.

Promoting comfort

The most common complaints of tube-fed clients are thirst, being deprived of tasting food, sore nose or throat, and dry mouth. Comfort can be increased by:

1. Encouraging intake of food and fluids if not contraindicated (many individuals are initially afraid that they cannot eat while the tube is in place).
2. Providing adequate fluid. Most formulas for adults provide 1 kcal/ml. This may not provide adequate fluid for some patients. If the individual cannot drink fluid and is not fluid-restricted, provide extra water by tube. For example, irrigate the tube after each feeding or every 4 to 6 hours with 30 to 60 ml or more of water.
3. Providing regular mouth care and stimulation of saliva flow. Important comfort measures include rinsing the mouth with water or mouthwash; brushing the teeth; sucking lemon drops or chewing gum in moderation, if not contraindicated; and gargling with warm salt water to relieve sore throat.
4. Using nonreactive tubes and using the tube with the smallest possible size.
5. Taping the tube in place securely so that it does not move back and forth.

Total Parenteral Nutrition
Indications

Generally, total parenteral nutrition (TPN) should be used only when oral or tube feedings are expected to be inadequate or inappropriate for at least 7 to 10 days. The following are specific indications for TPN:

1. GI tract unable to digest or absorb adequate nutrients. *Examples:* Intractable vomiting, such as that occurring with chemotherapy, radiation, and bone marrow transplantation; severe diarrhea; prematurity; severe burns and trauma with inability to tolerate enough enteral feedings to meet increased metabolic demands; prolonged ileus; and massive small bowel resection.

2. Need for bowel rest. *Examples:* Moderate to severe pancreatitis, where enteral feedings stimulate pancreatic secretion; enteral fistulae, inflammatory adhesions, or obstruction, where TPN may allow for healing and resolution of the problem; and acute inflammatory bowel disease.

Feeding with TPN alone is associated with atrophy of the intestinal villi, and subsequent impaired absorption and increased risk of translocation, or movement of bacteria through the GI mucosal barrier. Where the patient can tolerate them, small amounts of food or enteral feedings with intact macronutrients help to prevent villous atrophy. Fiber, dietary fat, and glutamine are factors that are being explored in relation to maintaining mucosal integrity.

Routes for parenteral nutrition

TPN may be delivered via peripheral or central veins. Central venous catheters are usually inserted into the superior or inferior vena cava via the subclavian, internal or external jugular, or femoral veins. Table 6-4 compares peripheral and central TPN. Fig. 6-3 shows a central venous catheter inserted via the subclavian vein, the most common site.

Table 6-4   Peripheral and central TPN

Route	Advantages	Disadvantages
Peripheral	Few mechanical complications; daily use of lipid emulsions allows adequate kcal delivery	Requires good peripheral venous access; not appropriate for home TPN; dextrose concentrations are limited to approximately 10%, since peripheral veins do not tolerate concentrations >900 mOsm/kg
Central	Appropriate for long-term use, including home TPN; allows use of extremely hypertonic solutions ($\geq$1800 mOsm/kg)	Associated with several potentially serious complications, including pneumothorax, air embolism, central vein thrombosis, superior vena cava syndrome, and catheter-related sepsis

Composition of TPN solutions

Composition of sample TPN solutions is shown in Table 6-5. Specialized amino acid solutions are available for use in renal and hepatic failure and severe injury. These are discussed in Chapters 7, 9, and 11.

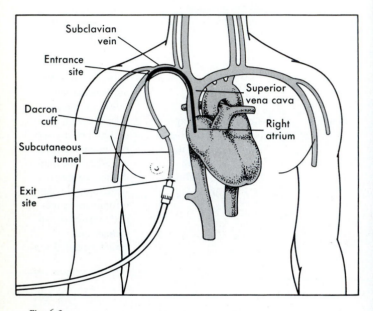

Fig. 6-3
The Hickman central venous catheter. The proximal end is tunneled under the subcutaneous tissue to increase stability. A Dacron cuff on the catheter provides a roughened surface, which encourages subcutaneous tissue to adhere to the catheter and further secure it. (From Moore MC: Alterations in nutrition. In Beare PG and Myers JL, eds: *Principles and practice of adult health nursing,* St Louis, 1990, Mosby–Year Book.)

Table 6-5   Usual components of TPN solution[a]

Component	Adults (per L)	Term infants (per kg per day)	Children over 1 yr (per kg per day)
Amino acids (g)[b]	42.5	2-3	2.5-3
Glucose (dextrose) (g)[c]	250	20-30	20-30

	Usual Daily Needs		
	Total	Per kg	Per kg
Electrolytes and minerals			
Sodium (mEq)	≥60	2-3	3-4
K (mEq)	≥60	1-2	2-4
Mg (mEq)	8-20	0.3-0.7	0.2-0.3
Calcium (mg)	200-300	60-70[d]	20-60
Phosphate (mg)	600-1200	50-55[d]	40-45
Zinc (mg)	4	0.25 <3 mo 0.10 > 3 mo	0.05 (max. 5/day)
Copper (mg)	0.8-1	0.02	0.02 (max. 0.3/day)
Chromium (μg)[e]	10-12.5	0.20	0.20 (max. 5 /day)
Manganese (μg)[f]	150-800	1.0	1.0 (max. 50/day)

[a]Amounts of constituents must be individualized; the levels listed are "usual" ranges.

[b]Usually 500 ml of 8.5% amino acids and 500 ml of 50% dextrose are used as the base for adult TPN. The percentage of a substance in solution refers to the number of g/100 ml. Thus an 8.5% solution = 8.5 g/100 ml. 500 ml of this solution yields 42.5 g.

[c]Glucose monohydrate, used in IV solutions, contains 3.4 kcal/g.

[d]Calcium and phosphate not to exceed 500-600 mg/L and 400-450 mg/L, respectively, to prevent precipitation.

[e]Omit in patients with renal dysfunction.

[f]Excreted in bile; omit in patients with obstructive jaundice.

Continued.

Table 6-5   Usual components of TPN solution[a]—cont'd

Component	Adults (per L)	Term infants (per kg per day)	Children over 1 yr (per kg per day)
Vitamins (per day)			
A (IU)	3300	2300	2300
D (IU)	200	400	400
E (IU)	10	7	7
K (μg)	200	200	200
C (mg)	100	80	80
Thiamin (mg)	3	1.2	1.2
Riboflavin (mg)	3.6	1.4	1.4
Niacin (mg)	40	17	17
Pyridoxine (B$_6$) (mg)	4	1	1
Pantothenic acid (mg)	15	5	5
Folate (μg)	400	140	140
Vitamin B$_{12}$ (μg)	5	1	1
Biotin (μg)	60	20	20

From American Medical Association Department of Foods and Nutrition: Multivitamin preparations for parenteral use: a statement by the Nutrition Advisory Group, *J Parenter Enteral Nutr* 3:258, 1979; Greene HL and others: Guidelines for the use of vitamins, trace elements, calcium, magnesium, and phosphorus in infants and children receiving total parenteral nutrition: report of the Subcommittee on Pediatric Parenteral Nutrient Requirements from the Committee on Clinical Practice Issues of the American Society for Clinical Nutrition, *Am J Clin Nutr* 48:1324, 1988.

Assessing Response to Nutrition Support

Anthropometric measurements, physical assessment, and hematologic and biochemical measurements are used in assessing response to nutrition support. See Table 6-6.

Table 6-6   Assessing response to nutrition support

Parameter	Frequency of Measurement*	Purpose/Comments
Anthropometric Measurements		
Weight	Daily	Indicator of efficacy, client should have steady gain; use usual or IBW for guide to desirable wt; a gain of >0.1-0.2 kg (0.25-0.5 lb) a day usually indicates fluid retention
Skinfolds, AMC	Weekly	Indicator of efficacy
Length or height (pediatrics only)	Monthly	Indicator of efficacy; see growth charts (Appendix F) for expected growth pattern
Physical Assessment		
State of hydration	Daily	Overhydration: check for edema of dependent body parts, shortness of breath, rales in lungs, fluid intake consistently >output; dehydration: look for poor skin turgor, dry mucous membranes, complaints of thirst, output >intake (measure stool volumes if liquid), >10% difference between blood pressure when lying and standing

*These are suggested frequencies only. Individual clients may need more or less frequent assessment.
IBW, Ideal body weight; *BUN,* blood urea nitrogen; *Ca,* calcium; *P,* phosphorus; *Mg,* magnesium; *Fe,* iron.

Continued.

Table 6-6   Assessing response to nutrition support—cont'd

Parameter	Frequency of Measurement*	Purpose/Comments
Physical Assessment—cont'd		
Gastric emptying (tube-fed clients)	Every 4-8 hr or as ordered	Aspirate gastric residual volumes via feeding tube; volumes >half the previous feeding or twice the hourly rate are often thought to be excessive
Bowel motility	Daily	Auscultate bowel sounds to be sure that peristalsis is present during enteral feeding; hard, dry stools, decreased stool frequency, or <3 stools/wk may indicate constipation in the enterally fed client; infrequent stools are expected in the client lacking enteral intake; loose or liquid stools, increased frequency, or >3 stools/day may indicate diarrhea

Preventing and Correcting Complications of Nutrition Support

Tables 6-7 and 6-8 summarize complications of nutrition support and list measures for their prevention or correction.

Malnourished clients receiving either enteral or parenteral feedings are at risk of developing the "refeeding syndrome." One major factor in the refeeding syndrome is hypophosphatemia,

Table 6-6   Assessing response to nutrition support—cont'd

Parameter	Frequency of Measurement*	Purpose/Comments
Hematologic and Biochemical Measurements		
Serum glucose and electrolytes	Daily until stable, then 2-3/wk	Indicates whether intake is adequate or excessive
BUN	1-2/wk	Increased: inadequate fluid intake, renal impairment, or excessive protein intake; decreased: inadequate protein intake is possible
Serum Ca, P, Mg	1-2/wk	Measure of adequacy of intake
Complete blood count	1/wk	Indicator of adequacy of Fe, protein, folic acid, and vitamin B_{12}; see Chapter 1 for more information
Serum triglycerides	After each ↑ in lipid dosage; 2-3/wk when stable	Elevated levels indicate inadequate lipid clearance and possibly a need for reduction in lipid dosage
Serum albumin, transferrin, or prealbumin	1/wk	Indicator of efficacy in maintaining or improving protein nutriture

which arises in the following way. As muscle and fat are lost in starvation, fluid and minerals, including phosphorus, are also lost. With refeeding, especially with high-carbohydrate feedings, insulin levels rise, and cellular uptake of glucose, water, phosphorus, potassium, and other nutrients is enhanced. Serum levels of phosphorus subsequently fall, and this can lead to cardiac arrhythmias, congestive heart failure, hemolysis of red blood cells,

Text continued on p. 127.

Table 6-7 Management of tube feeding complications

Complication	Possible Cause	Intervention
Pulmonary aspiration*	Feeding tube in esophagus or respiratory tract	Confirm proper placement of tube before administering any feeding; check placement (e.g., check pH of fluid aspirated from tube) at least every 4-8 hr during continuous feedings
	Regurgitation of formula	Aspiration is thought by some authorities to be less likely if feedings are administered below the pylorus; keep head elevated 30 degrees during feedings; stop feedings temporarily during treatments such as chest physiotherapy; formula can be tinted with food coloring to make detection of formula in the respiratory tract easier
Diarrhea	Antibiotic therapy	Physician may order pectin (e.g., banana flakes) or kaolin and pectin (e.g., Kaopectate [Upjohn]); lactobacillus-containing medications or dairy products (e.g., yogurt) are sometimes used in an effort to establish benign gut flora but are often ineffective

Hypertonic formula or medications (e.g., KCl)	Deliver formula continuously, decrease volume; dilute enteral medications well
Malnutrition/hypoalbuminemia	Physician may order parenteral nutrition or IV albumin to help restore plasma oncotic pressure; physician may order antidiarrheals (e.g., diphenoxylate hydrochloride with atropine sulfate [Lomotil] or loperamide hydrochloride [Imodium]) if all other causes of diarrhea are ruled out
	It has been suggested that peptide formulas may be tolerated better than intact protein, but newer evidence indicates that this may not be true
Bacterial contamination	Use scrupulously clean formula preparation and administration techniques; hang formula no longer than 4–8 hr and rinse feeding container and tubing before adding fresh formula; refrigerate home-prepared, reconstituted, or opened cans of formula until ready to use, and use all such products within 24 hr

*Signs and symptoms of pulmonary aspiration include tachypnea, shortness of breath, hypoxia, and infiltrate on chest x-ray films.

†Some nurses recommend fluids such as cranberry juice or Coca-Cola as an irrigant, but research has shown cranberry juice to be inferior to and Coca-Cola no better than water.

‡In one report commercial fiber-containing formulas were most likely to be associated with tube occlusion; tubes through which these formulas are delivered should be irrigated often.

Continued.

Table 6-7 Management of tube feeding complications—cont'd

Complication	Possible Cause	Intervention
Constipation	Lack of fiber	Use fiber-containing formula, unless contraindicated; increase fluid intake; physician may order stool softeners if problem is severe
Tube occlusion	Giving medications via tube	Irrigate feeding tube with water before and after giving medications; avoid crushed tablets and administer medications in elixir or suspension form whenever possible
	Sedimentation of formula	Irrigate tube with water† every 4-8 hr during continuous feedings and after every intermittent feeding‡; one study found less clogging of polyurethane than silicone rubber tubes; checking residuals from nasogastric tubes may cause precipitation of formula by gastric juices in the tube, so NG tubes should be irrigated well after residuals are measured; pancreatic enzyme has been reported effective in clearing some occlusions
Delayed gastric emptying	Serious illness, diabetic gastroparesis, prematurity	Physician may order temporary reduction in feeding volume, administration of feedings into small bowel, or metoclopramide (Reglan [A.M. Robins]) to stimulate gastric emptying

Table 6-8   TPN complications

Complication	Signs/Symptoms	Intervention
Catheter-related sepsis	Fever, chills, glucose intolerance, positive blood culture	Maintain an intact dressing, change if contaminated by vomitus, sputum, etc; use aseptic technique whenever handling catheter, IV tubing, and TPN solutions; hang a single bottle of TPN no longer than 24 hr, lipid emulsion no longer than 12 hr; use an in-line 0.22 μ filter with TPN to remove bacteria
Air embolism	Dyspnea, cyanosis, tachycardia, hypotension, possibly death	Use "Luer-lok" system or secure all connections well; Groshong catheter, which has valve at tip, may reduce risk of air embolism; use an in-line 0.22 μ air-eliminating filter; have patient perform Valsalva's maneuver during tubing changes; if air embolism is suggested, place patient in left lateral decubitus position and administer oxygen; immediately notify physician, who will attempt to aspirate air from the heart
Central venous thrombosis	Unilateral edema of neck, shoulder, and arm; development of collateral circulation on chest; pain in insertion site	Follow measures to prevent sepsis; repeated or traumatic catheterizations are most likely to result in thrombosis

Continued.

Table 6-8   TPN complications—cont'd

Complication	Signs/Symptoms	Intervention
Catheter occlusion or semi-occlusion	No flow or sluggish flow through the catheter	Flush catheter with heparinized saline if infusion is stopped temporarily; if catheter appears to be occluded, attempt to aspirate the clot; if ineffective, physician may order thrombolytic agent such as streptokinase or urokinase instilled in the catheter
Hypoglycemia	Diaphoresis, shakiness, confusion, loss of consciousness	Do not discontinue TPN abruptly, taper rate over several hours; use pump to regulate infusion so that it remains ±10% of ordered rate; if hypoglycemia is suggested, administer oral carbohydrate; if oral intake is contraindicated or patient is unconscious, physician may order a bolus of IV dextrose
Hyperglycemia	Thirst, headache, lethargy, increased urination	Monitor blood glucose at least daily until stable; TPN is usually initiated at a slow rate or with a low dextrose concentration and increased over 2-3 days to avoid hyperglycemia; the patient may require insulin added to the TPN if the problem is severe

muscular weakness, seizures, acute respiratory failure, and a variety of other complications, including sudden death. Hypokalemia, hypomagnesemia, and vitamin (thiamin) deficiency may occur for similar reasons. Glucose intolerance and fluid overload may also be a concomitant with the refeeding syndrome. Caregivers should be aware of clients who are at risk for refeeding syndrome (especially those with kwashiorkor or marasmus [see Chapter 1], anorexia nervosa, morbid obesity with recent massive weight loss, and prolonged fasting). In these clients it is especially important to monitor blood levels of electrolytes, phosphorus, glucose, and magnesium carefully, particularly during the first week of refeeding, keep careful records of fluid intake and output, record weight daily, and monitor heart rate frequently. (Severely malnourished patients are often bradycardic. With overfeeding and an increase in the intravascular volume, heart rate often increases; a rate of 80 to 100 beats/min in a previously bradycardic patient may be a sign of significant cardiac stress.)

Preparing the Client and Family for Home Nutritional Support

For a growing number of clients, enteral or parenteral feedings are continued at home. Preparation for home nutritional support is a multidisciplinary process, usually involving the physician, nurse, and dietitian. In many instances, the pharmacist and social worker will also be involved. Topics which must be covered in patient teaching include clean or sterile technique (as appropriate); caring for the access device (feeding tube or central venous catheter) including irrigation of the device, checking for residual volumes (if applicable), and dressing changes (if applicable); preparation of the TPN or enteral feeding solutions (if necessary); signs and symptoms of complications and management of those complications; and self-monitoring (e.g., monitoring of blood glucose, especially in TPN patients, regular weighing, checking body temperature as needed, evaluating state of hydration, etc.).

CASE STUDY

The following 24-hour recall illustrates the use of supplements to improve the intake of Johnny S., a 6-year-old child with neuroblastoma. *Breakfast:* cereal served with strawberry instant breakfast; biscuit, butter and honey; and orange juice with 1 tbsp. Polycose; *Snack:* Kool-Aid sweetened with corn syrup*; *Lunch:* chicken noodle soup with added chopped chicken; peanut butter, jam, and Polycose sandwich; hot chocolate made with half-and-half; *Snack:* Sustacal HC and ice cream shake; *Dinner:* meat loaf, mashed potatoes with gravy, broccoli in cheese sauce, and milk with 1 tbsp Polycose.

*Corn syrup is less sweet than sucrose (table sugar); thus more kcal are required to reach the desired sweetness.

Bibliography

Barclay BA, Litchford MD: Incidence of nasoduodenal tube occlusion and patient removal of tubes: a prospective study, *J Am Diet Assoc* 91:220, 1991.

Beckstrand J and others: The distance to the stomach for feeding tube placement in children predicted from regression on height, *Res Nurs Health* 13:411, 1990.

Gottschlich MM and others: Diarrhea in tube-fed burn patients: incidence, etiology, nutritional impact, and prevention, *J Parenter Enteral Nutr* 12:338, 1988.

Guidelines for use of total parenteral nutrition in the hospitalized adult patient: a statement by the ASPEN Board of Directors, *J Parenter Enteral Nutr* 10:441, 1986.

Hanson R: Predictive criteria for length of nasogastric tube insertion for tube feeding. *J Parenter Enteral Nutr* 3:160, 1979.

Marcuard SP, Stegall KS: Unclogging feeding tubes with pancreatic enzyme, *J Parenter Enteral Nutr* 14:198, 1990.

Metheny N, Eisenberg P, and McSweeney M: Effect of feeding tube properties and three irrigants on clogging rates, *Nurs Res* 37:165, 1988.

Metheny N and others: Effectiveness of pH measurements in predicting feeding tube placement, *Nurs Res* 38:280, 1989.

Metheny N and others: Effectiveness of the auscultatory method in predicting feeding tube location, *Nurs Res* 39:262, 1990.

Monturo C: Enteral access device selection, *Nutr Clin Prac* 5:207, 1990.

Mowatt-Larssen CA and others: Comparison of tolerance and nutritional outcome between a peptide and a standard enteral formula in critically ill, hypoalbuminemic patients, *J Parenter Enteral Nutr* 16:20, 1992.

Patterson ML and others: Enteral feeding in the hypoalbuminemic patient, *J Parenter Enteral Nutr* 14:362, 1990.

Smith CE and others: Diarrhea associated with tube feeding in mechanically ventilated critically ill patients, *Nurs Res* 39:148, 1990.

Solomon SM and Kirby DF: The refeeding syndrome: a review, *J Parenter Enteral Nutr* 14:90, 1990.

Srp F and others: Psychosocial issues of nutritional support: a multidisciplinary interpretation, *Nurs Clin North Am* 24:447, 1989.

Whatley K and others: When does metoclopramide facilitate transpyloric intubation? *J Parenter Enteral Nutr* 8:679, 1984.

Whitney RG: Comparing long-term central venous catheters, *Nursing* 21:70, 1991.

Worthington PH and Wagner BA: Total parenteral nutrition, *Nurs Clin North Am* 24:355, 1989.

Surgery, Trauma, and Burns 7

Surgery, trauma, and burns are physiologic stressors that result in hypermetabolism. Nutritional care is a priority to minimize nutritional deficits during the period of hypermetabolism and to promote repair during convalescence.

Pathophysiology

Major surgery, trauma, and burns are accompanied by a stress response. The stress response is designed to:

1. Produce adequate kcal to meet increased metabolic needs from surgery and injury. Increased secretion of epinephrine, norepinephrine, and corticosteroids results in breakdown of glycogen, fat stores, and body proteins, especially skeletal muscles (Fig. 7-1). The net effect in severe injury is increased urinary nitrogen loss, muscle wasting, and weight loss.
2. Maintain the blood volume. Antidiuretic hormone (ADH) secretion increases during the stress response, with decreased urine output and retention of fluid. In hypovolemia, increased aldosterone secretion occurs, and sodium and fluid are retained.

Fig. 7-1
Immediate neuroendocrine response to trauma, which results in increased gluconeogenesis (formation of glucose from noncarbohydrates, such as amino acids and lipids) and hyperglycemia. *ACTH,* Adrenocorticotropic hormone; *NE,* norepinephrine; *EPI,* epinephrine. (Redrawn from Popp MB, and Brennan MF: Metabolic response to trauma and infection. In Fischer JE, ed: *Surgical nutrition,* Boston, 1983, Little, Brown & Company. Used with permission.)

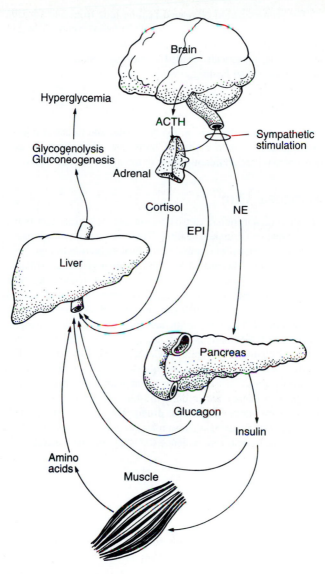

Fig. 7-1
For legend see opposite page.

The primary period of wound healing lasts from 5 to 15 days in minor surgery to more than a month in major trauma or burns. During this time the wound has priority needs for kcal, amino acids, and other nutrients needed in healing. Nutritional deficits may impair wound healing.

Treatment

Wound treatment depends on the type, site, and extent of injury. Skin grafting is often a part of burn care. Corticosteroids and phenobarbital are commonly used in treatment of head injury.

Nutritional Care

The goal of nutritional care is to prevent or correct nutritional deficits that could impair healing. There is currently much ongoing research related to optimal nutritional support in trauma, sepsis, and burns. The use of medium-chain triglycerides (MCTs, see Chapter 6) and "structured" triglycerides (containing both medium- and long-chain fatty acids) as energy sources; the effect of supplementation with fish oil; and the influence of increasing the amount of the amino acid, arginine, given to these patients are some of the interventions being studied. The role of the branched chain amino acids (BCAAs) is also of interest. The BCAAs (leucine, isoleucine, and valine) have been postulated to be advantageous in treating the client with stress because they can provide energy and reduce muscle catabolism. While they appear to be more effective in producing positive nitrogen balance in stressed patients than standard amino acid solutions, there is as yet no conclusive evidence that they are more effective in improving outcome.

Assessment

Assessment is summarized in Table 7-1.

Intervention

Provide adequate nutrients to meet the individual's needs for maintenance and anabolism

Text continued on p. 138.

Table 7-1   Assessment in surgery, trauma, and burns

Area of Concern	Significant Findings
Protein calorie malnutrition (PCM)*	*History* Increased needs caused by hypermetabolism from trauma, burns, surgery, fever, sepsis, pneumonia, or other infection; and catabolic effects of corticosteroid therapy (used in head injury); weight loss before surgery, especially if >2% in 1 wk, >5% in 1 mo, >7.5% in 3 mo, or >10% in 6 mo; poor intake caused by anorexia (can be caused by pain, malignancy, psychologic factors), intestinal obstruction or ileus, nausea or vomiting, and alcoholism; increased losses caused by resection of small intestine, especially ileum, gastrectomy, fistula, burns (loss of serum proteins through damaged capillaries) *Physical examination* Muscle wasting; triceps skinfold or arm muscle circumference <5th percentile (see Appendix G); edema; weight <90th percentile or BMI < 19.1 (women) or 20.7 (men)

*Surgical morbidity (e.g., sepsis, wound dehiscence, abscess or fistula formation) and mortality is greater in individuals with PCM. The Prognostic Nutritional Index (PNI) devised by Mullen and others (*Ann Surg* 192:604, 1980) provides a systematic way of estimating the likelihood of surgical complications.

PNI (%) = 158 − 16.6 (albumin) − 0.78 (TSF) − 0.2 (transferrin) − 5.8 (ST),

Where albumin is expressed in g/dl, triceps skinfold (TSF) in mm, transferrin in mg/dl, and response to skin testing (ST) graded as: 0 = nonreactive, 1 = <5 mm reaction, and 2 = ≥5 mm reaction.

An example of the PNI in a poorly nourished patient is:

PNI = 158 − 16.6 (2.3) − 0.78 (7) − 0.2 (123) − 5.8 (1) = 84% likelihood of complications

Continued.

Table 7-1   Assessment in surgery, trauma, and burns—cont'd

Area of Concern	Significant Findings
Protein calorie malnutrition (PCM)*—cont'd	*Laboratory analysis* ↓ Serum albumin, transferrin, or prealbumin (serum albumin levels may be ≥0.5 g/dl lower than usual because of the hemodilution that occurs during bed rest, the effects of fluid resuscitation, blood loss, etc.); ↓ lymphocyte count; negative nitrogen balance; ↓ creatinine height index (see Table 1-4); nonreactive skin tests
Altered carbohydrate metabolism	*History* Catabolism caused by trauma or corticosteroid therapy *Physical examination* Polyuria; muscle wasting (over weeks or months) *Laboratory analysis* ↑ Blood glucose; presence of glucosuria
Vitamin Deficiencies	
C	*History* Increased needs caused by trauma, burns, or major surgery; poor intake caused by anorexia *Physical examination* Gingivitis; petechiae, ecchymoses; delayed wound healing *Laboratory analysis* ↓ Serum or leukocyte vitamin C
B complex	*History* Increased needs caused by fever or hypermetabolism; poor intake (same reasons as for PCM) *Physical examination* Glossitis; cheilosis; peripheral neuropathy; dermatitis

Table 7-1   Assessment in surgery, trauma, and burns—cont'd

Area of Concern	Significant Findings
B complex —cont'd	*Laboratory analysis* ↑ Enzyme activity coefficients (e.g., thiamin pyrophosphate [vitamin B_1], and glutathione reductase [vitamin B_2]): see Laboratory Reference Values in Appendix H for relevant analyses; ↓ urinary niacin; NOTE: The above tests are rarely done; because of the low toxicity of B vitamins, clients exhibiting signs of deficiency are usually empirically supplemented with the vitamins and observed for a response
K	*History* Antibiotic usage *Physical examination* Petechiae, ecchymoses *Laboratory analysis* ↑ Prothrombin time
Mineral Deficiencies	
Iron (Fe)	*History* Blood loss, acute or chronic, as in stress ulcer, trauma, long bone fracture; poor intake (same causes as PCM); impaired absorption, especially after gastrectomy *Physical examination* Pallor; koilonychia; tachycardia *Laboratory analysis* ↓ Hct, Hgb, MCV, MCH, MCHC; ↓ serum Fe and ferritin; ↑ serum transferrin or total iron-binding capacity
Zinc (Zn)	*History* Increased losses from burns (loss of albumin to which Zn is bound), fistula drainage, diarrhea or steatorrhea; increased needs for healing of surgical wounds, burns, trauma; poor intake (same reasons as for PCM)

Continued.

Table 7-1 Assessment in surgery, trauma, and burns—cont'd

Area of Concern	Significant Findings
Zinc (Zn) —cont'd	*Physical examination* Hypogeusia, dysgeusia; ↓ tensile strength of wounds; dermatitis *Laboratory analysis* ↓ Serum Zn
Phosphorus (P)	*History* Aggressive refeeding (especially high-carbohydrate feedings, as in TPN) in malnourished individuals; alcoholism; increased losses or impaired absorption caused by use of antacids (Phosphate-binders) as prophylaxis/treatment for stress ulcer, severe diarrhea, or vomiting *Physical examination* Tremor, ataxia; irritability progressing to stupor, coma, and death *Laboratory analysis* ↓ Serum P; respiratory alkalosis (↑ blood pH, ↓ blood P_{CO_2})
Magnesium (Mg)	*History* Increased losses caused by prolonged vomiting, diarrhea, steatorrhea, fistula drainage; poor intake caused by alcoholism *Physical examination* Tremor; disorientation; hyperactive deep reflexes *Laboratory analysis* ↓ Serum Mg
Fluid and Electrolyte Imbalances	
Potassium (K^+) excess	*History* Loss of K^+ from damaged cells into extracellular fluid caused by burns (early, usually within first 3 days) or crushing injuries

Table 7-1   Assessment in surgery, trauma, and burns—cont'd

Area of Concern	Significant Findings
Potassium (K^+) excess —cont'd	*Physical examination* Irritability; nausea, diarrhea; weakness *Laboratory analysis* ↑ Serum K^+
K^+ deficit	*History* Increased losses caused by burns (after the fifth day), diarrhea or vomiting *Physical examination* Weakness, ↓ reflexes, intestinal ileus *Laboratory analysis* ↓ Serum K^+
Fluid deficit	*History* Increased losses from burns, persistent vomiting or diarrhea, gastric suction without adequate replacement, fever, tachypnea, fistula drainage, transient diabetes insipidus following head injury, use of radiant warmers or phototherapy (infants); poor intake caused by intestinal obstruction, coma, or confusion, causing failure to recognize or communicate thirst, use of tube feedings (especially in obtunded individual) without adequate fluid (formulas providing 1 kcal/ml may not provide enough fluid for patients with increased losses; more concentrated formulas require especially close monitoring of client hydration) *Physical examination* Poor skin turgor; acute weight loss (can be 5%-10% of usual weight within 3-7 days); oliguria (adult: <20 ml/hr; infant or child: <2-4 ml/kg/hr; infant <6 days: <1-3 ml/kg/hr); hypotension; dry skin and mucous membranes; sunken fontanel (infants)

Continued.

Table 7-1 Assessment in surgery, trauma, and burns—cont'd

Area of Concern	Significant Findings
Fluid deficit —cont'd	*Laboratory analysis* Serum Na >150 mEq/L; ↑ serum osmolality, urine specific gravity, Hct, BUN
Fluid volume excess	*History* Head injury *Physical examination* Decreased urine output because of temporary syndrome of inappropriate antidiuretic hormone secretion *Laboratory analysis* Serum Na < 126 mEq/L

Fluid and electrolyte needs

Daily maintenance requirements for fluid and electrolytes during stress response are presented in Table 7-2. Needs for fluids and electrolytes may be much higher in severe stress. In burns, for instance, the following formulas may be used in estimating fluid needs.

First 24 hours: 2 to 4 ml lactated Ringer's solution × wt (kg) × %BSA burned. Give half in first 8 hours and half in remaining 16 hours (Parkland-Baxter formula).

Second 24 hours: 0.5 ml colloids (plasma, plasmanate, or dextran) × wt (kg) × %BSA burned plus maintenance fluids (approximately 2000 ml dextrose in water for adults) (Brooke Army formula).

Kilocalorie needs

Table 7-3 summarizes calculation of kcal needs in the injured individual. For paraplegic and quadriplegic individuals, the figures for fractures, head injury, or soft tissue trauma (whichever is most appropriate) can be used in the first few weeks after injury. Once they are stable and rehabilitating, adult paraplegics need 27.9 kcal/kg and quadriplegics need 22.7 kcal/kg. IBW of paraplegics and quadriplegics is 4.5 kg and 9 kg, respectively, less than that of healthy adults of the same height.

Table 7-2 Fluid and electrolyte requirements

Infants, Children, and Adults	Water (ml)	Na$^+$ (mEq/kg)*	K$^+$ (mEq/kg)*
Infants/Children		2-4	1-3
≤10 kg	100/kg		
11-20 kg	1000 + 50/kg over 10 kg		
>20 kg	1500 + 20/kg over 20 kg		
Adults	35-55/kg	2-3	2-3

*1 mEq Na$^+$ (sodium) = 23 mg; 1 mEq K$^+$ (potassium) = 39 mg.

Table 7-3 Estimating kcal needs in sick or injured patients*

Clinical Condition	Injury Factor†
Fever	1+0.13/° C above normal (or 0.07/° F)
Elective surgery	1-1.2
Peritonitis	1.2-1.5
Soft tissue trauma	1.14-1.37
Multiple fractures	1.2-1.35
Major sepsis	1.4-1.8
Major head injury	
With steroids	1.4-2.0
Without steroids	1.4
Burns (%BSA‡)	
0%-20%	1.0-1.5
20%-40%	1.5-1.85
40%-100%	1.85-2.05
Starvation (adults)	0.70

Modified from Silberman H: Parenteral and enteral nutrition, ed 2, Norwalk, Conn, 1989, Appleton & Lange.

*Total energy expenditure = (basal energy expenditure, or BEE) × (activity factor) × (injury factor). If W = actual weight in kg, H = ht in cm, and A = age in yr,
  BEE (males) = 66 + (13.7 × W) + (5 × H) − (6.8 × A)
  BEE (females) = 665 + (9.6 × W) + (1.7 × H) − (4.7 × A)
  Activity factors = 1.2 for bed rest and 1.3 for ambulatory clients.

†These are maximum increases; they must be tapered as recovery progresses.
‡Percent of body surface area burned.

Protein needs

Needs for trauma and postoperative clients are approximately 1.2 to 2 g/kg/day for adults and 2 to 3 g/kg/day for children. One method for calculating protein needs in burns is:

Adults 1 g/kg + (3 g × % body surface area burned);

Children 3 g/kg + (1 g × % body surface area burned)

BCAA-enriched products are available for nutrition support of injured clients. Enteral formulas include Stresstein (Sandoz), TraumaCal (Mead Johnson), and Traum-Aid HBC (Kendall McGaw). FreAmine HBC (Kendall McGaw), Aminosyn-HBC (Abbott), and Branchamine (Travenol) are amino acid mixtures used in total parenteral nutrition (TPN).

Vitamin and mineral needs

Needs for most vitamins and minerals increase following trauma. However, with increased caloric intake, these needs are usually met. An exception is two micronutrients that are especially important in healing, vitamin C and zinc. Vitamin C is needed for collagen formation for optimal wound healing. Supplements of 500 to 1000 mg/day should provide adequate vitamin C. Zinc increases the tensile strength (the force required to separate the edges) of the healing wound, commonly-used supplementation dosages are 6 mg/day IV during acute stress; 4 mg/day IV or 50 to 75 mg/day orally when stable. Additional zinc is needed when there are unusually large intestinal losses; estimated needs are 12.2 mg zinc/L of small bowel fistula drainage and 17.1 mg zinc/kg of stool or ileostomy drainage.

Deliver nutrition support in a safe and effective manner

A. Intravenous (IV) fluids, glucose, and electrolytes
   1. Indications: Maintenance of fluid and electrolyte balance in the initial postinjury or postsurgical period. Should be used as the sole source of nutrition for no more than 7 to 10 days, since IV glucose/electrolyte solutions are inadequate in kcal and most nutrients.
   2. Example of use: Immediately after a burn or gastrointestinal (GI) surgery.
B. Oral diet
   1. Indications: Preferred method of feeding for all individuals. Requires GI motility (presence of bowel sounds), fe-

cal output <10 ml/kg/day, unobstructed GI tract.

2. Example of use: Many burn clients; gastric, gallbladder, or colon surgery.

3. Comments: Feedings often start with clear liquids (tea, broth, gelatin, SLD [Ross], Citrotein [Sandoz]), advance to full liquids (cream soups, shakes, puddings, custards, commercial liquid supplements), and then progress according to patient tolerance.

C. Enteral tube feedings

1. Indications: Same as for oral feedings, except that oral intake is precluded or inadequate as a result of upper GI injury or surgery, anorexia, unconsciousness.

2. Example of use: Burn clients who cannot consume enough orally; esophageal, mouth, or jaw surgery; coma.

3. Comments: Ileus and gastric atony are common after head or abdominal injury. If bowel sounds return but large gastric residuals persist, nasoduodenal feedings may be possible. Cardiopulmonary stability is essential before the administration of enteral feedings; intestinal ischemia from low cardiac output or poor oxygen saturation results in deepithelization of the villi with impaired absorption of all nutrients and secretion of fluid and electrolytes into the intestine.

D. TPN

1. Indications: Enteral intake unlikely for 7 to 10 days or longer as a result of ileus, bowel obstruction, diarrhea, or vomiting. May be indicated for periods shorter than 7 to 10 days in severe injury (e.g., major burns) or preexisting malnutrition. May be used as an adjunct to enteral feedings in clients where vomiting or diarrhea limits enteral intake.

2. Example of use: Extensive small intestinal resection, high output intestinal fistula, multiple organ system failure.

3. Comments: Special care should be taken to prevent catheter infection in burn clients, whose wounds are likely to be colonized with microorganisms.

Prevention of renal lithiasis (stones)

Some recuperating individuals, particularly those with head or spinal injuries, are relatively immobile. These individuals are highly susceptible to developing kidney and bladder stones. Individuals requiring bed rest for several weeks or longer are often given a calcium-restricted diet, with one serving or less of dairy products daily, until mobility has increased. Acid ash diets (see Chapter 11) are sometimes used to prevent precipitation of calcium stones in the urinary tract. A fluid intake of at least 50 ml/ kg will produce a dilute urine in which stones are less likely to precipitate.

Alleviation of constipation

Immobility following injury or surgery contributes to constipation. The individual who has no dietary restrictions can be encouraged to choose foods rich in fiber (whole grains, legumes, fresh fruits and vegetables). For tube feedings, formulas containing fiber—Compleat (Sandoz), Enrich (Ross), or blenderized foods—can be used. A fluid intake of 50 ml/kg or more will also help produce softer stools.

Client Teaching
Instruct the client/family in the principles of a nutritious diet

Encourage a diet high in protein (1.2 to 1.5 g/kg) and adequate in kcal. This diet should be maintained through the period of convalescence, usually 6 to 12 weeks for major surgeries. Individuals with severe impairment of nutrition as a result of surgery (e.g., massive small bowel resection) or preexisting malnutrition will need to continue this diet until their weight is at the desirable level and serum proteins are within the reference range. The health care team can help by:

1. Teaching client to choose foods such as those from Table 7-4 to meet protein requirements.
2. Recommending supplements (see Tables 6-1 and 6-2) if intake of regular foods is inadequate.
3. Providing specialized supplements for individuals with pancreatic or intestinal resection. Medium-chain triglycerides (MCTs) are generally better absorbed than long-chain triglycerides (LCTs). Complete liquid supplements containing MCTs, such as Portagen (Mead Johnson), can be used, or MCTs can be substituted for LCTs in cooking. Supplements of calcium, zinc, and magnesium may be required, also.

Table 7-4   Protein sources

Food	Serving Size	Protein (g)
Beef, cooked	1 oz ($\sim$3″ × 3″ × ¼″)	7
Poultry, cooked	1 oz (1 small chicken drumstick)	7
Canned fish	¼ cup	7
Milk	1 cup	8
Powdered milk, instant	⅓ cup	8
Cheese	1 oz	7
Cottage cheese	¼ cup	7
Egg	1 large	7
Dried beans or peas (kidney, garbanzo, lentils)	½ cup	7
Peanut butter	2 tbsp	8

Teach the client/family to monitor the clients' nutritional status regularly

The client should be weighed at least weekly after hospital discharge until weight is stable. Weight loss or declining intake should be reported to the health care team so that appropriate interventions can be planned.

Instruct the client/family in home tube feeding or TPN, if necessary

Individuals with short-bowel syndrome as a consequence of bowel resection are especially likely to require home tube feeding or TPN. Some of these individuals can maintain adequate nutritional status with the use of an elemental enteral formula. However, elemental formulas taste very bad, and tube feedings are usually necessary to maintain an adequate intake. Other individuals have too little absorptive surface to sustain their nutrition and hydration with enteral feedings and require TPN to meet at least part of their needs.

CASE STUDY

Mr. T, a 35-year-old man, sustained a broken pelvis, femur, and humerus and a ruptured spleen in a motor vehicle accident 3 days ago. He underwent splenectomy and insertion of a jejunostomy tube on his first hospital day. Although an ileus was present initially, it has now resolved. Facial trauma limits oral intake.

Nutrition Assessment

Height: 183 cm (6′)   Usual weight (unable to weigh presently):

83 kg (183 lb)   Ideal weight: 81 kg (178 lb)

Serum albumin   3.2 g/dl

Mr. T's wife reports that he had a "good diet" before the accident

Kilocalorie and Protein Needs

Kcal needs = BEE × activity factor × injury factor = [66 + (13.7 × 83) + (5 × 183) − (6.8 × 35)] × 1.2 × 1.35 = 3046

Protein needs = 81 kg × 2 g = 162 g

Nutritional Plan

Continuous feedings of a high-nitrogen formula providing 1.2 kcal/ml and 52 g protein/1000 kcal were begun at 50 ml/hr via the jejunostomy tube. Since the feedings were well tolerated, the infusion rate was advanced every 8 to 12 hours until it reached 110 ml/hr, which provided 3120 kcal and 162 g protein.

Bibliography

Bell SJ and others: Alternative lipid sources for enteral and parenteral nutrition: long- and medium-chain trilgycerides, structured triglycerides, and fish oils, *J Am Diet Assoc* 91:74, 1991.

Brennan MF and others: Report of a research workshop: branched-chain amino acids in stress and injury, *J Parenter Enteral Nutr* 10:446, 1986.

Cox SAR and others: Energy expenditure after spinal cord injury: an evaluation of stable rehabilitating patients, *J Trauma* 25:419, 1985.

Meguid MM, Campos AC, and Hammond WG: Nutritional support in medical practice: part I, *Am J Surg* 159:345, 1990.

Nelson KM, Long CL: Physiologic basis for nutrition in sepsis, *Nutr Clin Prac* 4:6, 1989.

Pasulka PS, Wachtel TL: Nutritional considerations for the burned patient, *Surg Clin North Am* 67:109, 1987.

Perkin RM, Levin DL: Common fluid and electrolyte problems in the pediatric intensive care unit, *Pediatr Clin North Am* 27:567, 1980.

Rolandelli RH and others: Critical illness and sepsis. In Rombeau JL, Caldwell, MD, eds, *Clinical nutrition: enteral and tube feeding,* ed 2, Philadelphia, 1990, WB Saunders.

Sandstead HH and others: Zinc and wound healing, *Am J Clin Nutr* 23:514, 1970.

Varella LD: Nutritional support and head trauma, *Crit Care Nurse* 9(6):28, 1989.

Cancer

8

Cancer can have severe adverse effects on nutritional status. Not only does the cancerous tumor draw nutrients from the host, but the treatment modalities and the psychologic impact of cancer can further interfere with maintenance of adequate nutrition.

Pathophysiology

Cancerous tumors differ according to their site, size, cellular types, and metabolic effects. Some of the potential effects of cancer on nutrition include:

A. Weight loss caused by:
1. Reduced intake, perhaps induced by altered neurotransmitter (serotonin) levels in the central nervous system; elevated levels of lactate produced by anaerobic metabolism, a method of metabolism favored by tumors; psychologic stress; dysgeusia (distorted taste); and aversions to specific foods. About 70% of individuals with cancer experience food aversions, apparently because of altered taste thresholds to certain flavor components.
2. Increased basal metabolic rate.
3. Increased gluconeogenesis (production of glucose by breakdown of glycogen, fat, and body proteins) caused by the tumor's reliance on anaerobic metabolism.
B. Decreased synthesis of body proteins.

"Cancer cachexia" is a severe form of malnutrition characterized by anorexia, early satiety, weight loss, anemia, weakness, and muscle wasting. Even though adequate nutritional support can help prevent marked wasting and weight loss, only successful cancer therapy can fully reverse the syndrome of cancer cachexia.

Treatment of Cancer

Surgery, radiation therapy, and chemotherapy are used alone or in combination in cancer treatment. Table 8-1 demonstrates some of the nutritional effects of cancer therapies. Poor nutritional status can interfere with cancer treatment. For example, a malnourished client will often require reduced drug dosages or a shortened radiotherapy schedule. Although surgery may be successful in removing the cancer, a poorly nourished client is more likely to develop pneumonia or wound dehiscence postoperatively.

Nutritional Care

The goals of nutritional care are: (1) to identify and prevent or correct nutritional deficiencies resulting from cancer or its therapies, and (2) to maintain or improve functional capacity and quality of life.

Assessment

Assessment is summarized in Table 8-2.

Intervention

Provide adequate nutrients to meet the individual's needs for maintenance and anabolism

Kilocalorie needs

Individuals with good nutritional status may need no more than 30 to 35 kcal/kg/day to maintain their weight. Undernourished individuals may need as much as 45 to 50 kcal/kg/day.

Protein needs

Intake of 1.5 to 2 g/kg/day is usually sufficient.

Vitamin and mineral needs

Needs for most vitamins increase as kcal intake increases. However, increased food consumption usually provides the increased vitamins needed. A single daily multivitamin supplement may be given to ensure adequate intake. Adequate intake of the following minerals should be ensured.

Iron. Anemia often occurs as a result of blood loss or aversions to iron-containing foods. Poultry and fish may be accept-

Text continued on p. 153.

Table 8-1 Nutritional effects of cancer therapy

	Surgery	
Site of Resection	Effect on Nutrition
Tongue, mouth, jaw	Oral intake precluded
Esophagus	Oral intake precluded (temporary); gastric stasis and fat malabsorption as a result of vagotomy
Stomach	Dumping syndrome; impaired absorption of vitamin B_{12} and iron
Pancreas (pancreatoduodenectomy or Whipple's operation)	Diabetes mellitus; impaired absorption of fat and fat-soluble vitamins, calcium, zinc, magnesium, and protein
Small bowel	Depends on extent of resection and portion of bowel involved (see Fig. 9-1); lactose intolerance possible; ileal resection: impaired absorption of fat and fat-soluble vitamins, calcium, zinc, magnesium, and vitamin B_{12}, impaired absorption of bile salts with resulting diarrhea and loss of fluid and electrolytes. With massive resection, loss of all nutrients, weight loss, and dehydration occur unless adequate nutritional support is given promptly
Colon	Impaired absorption of water and electrolytes

	Radiation Therapy	
	Effect on Nutrition	
Site	Acute	Long Term*
Central nervous system	Anorexia, nausea, vomiting (occasionally)	
Head and neck	Xerostomia (dry mouth), mucositis, anorexia, hypogeusia ("mouth blindness")	Xerostomia, bony necrosis, dental caries, altered taste

*Long-term effects may occur within a few months after therapy or may appear years later.

Table 8-1   Nutritional effects of cancer therapy—cont'd

| | Radiation Therapy | |
| | Effect on Nutrition | |
Site	Acute	Long Term*
Esophagus, lung	Dysphagia, sore throat	Esophageal stenosis
Upper abdomen	Anorexia; nausea, vomiting	Gastrointestinal (GI) ulcer
Whole abdomen	Nausea, vomiting; diarrhea; cramping	GI ulcer; diarrhea, malabsorption; chronic enteritis or colitis
Pelvis	Diarrhea	Diarrhea; chronic enteritis or colitis

| | Chemotherapy |
Effect on Nutrition	Chemotherapeutic Agent
Anorexia, nausea, vomiting	BCNU, bleomycin, CCNU, carboplatin, cisplatin, cyclophosphamide, cytarabine (ara-C), dacarbazine (DTIC), doxorubicin, estramustine phosphate sodium, etoposide (VP-16), floxuridine, fluorouracil, ifosfamide, mechlorethamine, mesna, methotrexate, mitotane, mitoxantrone, octreotide, plicamycin, procarbazine, vinblastine
Mucositis (stomatitis, esophagitis, intestinal ulcerations)	Bleomycin, cytarabine (ara-C), doxorubicin, floxuridine, fluorouracil, methotrexate, mitoxantrone, plicamycin, vinblastine
Diarrhea	Cytarabine (ara-C), estramustine phosphate sodium, fluorouracil, mesna, mitotane, mitoxantrone, octreotide, plicamycine, vinblastine
Constipation/ paralytic ileus	Vinblastine, vincristine
Hyperglycemia	Asparaginase, streptozocin

Table 8-2 Assessment in cancer

Area of Concern	Significant Findings
Protein calorie malnutrition (PCM)	*History* Poor intake of protein and kcal as a result of food aversions, anorexia, nausea, vomiting, dysgeusia, difficulty chewing or swallowing (especially meats), inadequate financial resources; increased needs as a result of infection or drainage from an abscess or fistula; impaired absorption caused by dumping syndrome, ileal or pancreatic resection, or lactose intolerance; weight loss, especially if >2% in 1 wk, >5% in 1 mo, >7.5% in 3 mo, >10% in 6 mo *Physical examination* Muscle wasting; edema; delayed wound healing; diarrhea (↓ oncotic pressure in the gut); triceps skinfold or arm muscle circumference <5th percentile (see Appendix G); weight <90% standard for height or BMI <19.1 (women) or 20.7 (men), or decline of weight and/or height by one or more percentile change (children) (see Appendix F) *Laboratory analysis* ↓ Serum albumin, transferrin, or prealbumin; nonreactive skin tests; ↓ BUN; ↓ creatinine-height index (CHI); ↓ lymphocyte count
Vitamin Deficiencies	
A	*History* Poor intake (same reasons as listed for PCM); steatorrhea (greasy stools, difficult to flush away); ileal or pancreatic resection *Physical examination* Dry, scaly skin; dry cornea; ↓ night vision *Laboratory analysis* ↓ Serum retinol

Table 8-2 Assessment in cancer—cont'd

Area of Concern	Significant Findings
Vitamin Deficiencies—cont'd	
K	*History* Antibiotic usage *Physical examination* Petechiae, ecchymoses *Laboratory Analysis* ↓ Prothrombin time
C	*History* Poor intake of citrus and other fruits as a result of stomatitis, esophagitis, or anorexia *Physical examination* Petechiae, ecchymoses; delayed wound healing *Laboratory analysis* ↓ Serum or lymphocyte ascorbic acid
Folate	*History* Poor intake of fruits, vegetables, and liver caused by anorexia, nausea, vomiting, stomatitis, or esophagitis; methotrexate (a folate antagonist) treatment; alcohol abuse *Physical examination* Pallor, glossitis *Laboratory analysis* ↓ Hgb, ↑ MCV, ↓ serum folate
Mineral/Electrolyte Deficiencies	
Iron (Fe)	*History* Poor intake as a result of aversions to or difficulty chewing/swallowing meats, poultry or fish; anorexia; nausea; vomiting; dysgeusia; increased losses from acute or chronic blood loss; decreased absorption caused by gastric resection *Physical examination* Pallor, blue sclerae; koilonychia *Laboratory analysis* ↓ Hgb, Hct, MCV, MCH, MCHC; ↓ serum Fe or ferritin; ↑ serum transferrin or TIBC

Continued.

Table 8-2 Assessment in cancer—cont'd

Area of Concern	Significant Findings
Mineral/Electrolyte Deficiencies—cont'd	
Zinc (Zn)	*History*
	Poor intake caused by same factors as listed for Fe; increased losses caused by diarrhea or fistula drainage; impaired absorption as a result of pancreatic or small bowel resection
	Physical examination
	Dysgeusia, hypogeusia; delayed wound healing; dermatitis
	Laboratory analysis
	↓ Serum Zn
Calcium (Ca)	*History*
	Poor intake caused by lactose intolerance; decreased absorption caused by steatorrhea, pancreatic or small bowel resection
	Physical examination
	Tingling of the ends of the fingers; muscle cramps
	Laboratory analysis
	↓ Serum Ca (possible, but not common)
Potassium (K^+)	*History*
	Increased losses from vomiting or diarrhea
	Physical examination
	Malaise, weakness
	Laboratory analysis
	↓ Serum K^+
Magnesium (Mg)	*History*
	Poor intake as a result of alcoholism; increased losses/decreased absorption caused by prolonged vomiting, diarrhea, steatorrhea, fistula drainage, pancreatic or small bowel resection
	Physical examination
	Tremor, hyperactive deep reflexes; disorientation
	Laboratory analysis
	↓ Serum Mg

able to the individual with aversion to red meat, and green leafy vegetables and whole grain or enriched breads and cereals can provide additional iron. Cast iron cookware can be used to increase iron content of food.

A supplement of 20 to 50 mg/day may be needed. To increase iron absorption, tea or coffee should not be consumed with the supplement. The supplements should be taken with meat, fish, poultry, or citrus fruits and juices when possible.

Calcium. Lactose intolerance is a common result of the intestinal damage caused by radiation or chemotherapy. Calcium intake may be low when dairy products are avoided. Lactose-intolerant individuals may be able to use yogurt, cheese, cottage cheese, buttermilk, or milk treated with enzymes (Lact-Aid or Lactrase). A supplement of 800 mg of calcium per day can be used to replace milk products.

Zinc. Zinc is found in many of the same foods as iron, and food aversions may limit intake. Client needs during healing and anabolism are high. A zinc supplement of 20 to 50 mg/day may be used.

Promote comfort and alleviate problems associated with cancer therapy

Table 8-3 summarizes common problems during cancer therapy and approaches that may help alleviate them.

Nausea and vomiting are common problems during chemotherapy and radiation therapy. Medications to relieve nausea and vomiting promote comfort and help make adequate nutritional intake possible.

Food aversions can develop as a conditioned response in individuals suffering from nausea and vomiting caused by radiation or chemotherapy. For example, aversions to red gelatin have occurred in individuals receiving doxorubicin (Adriamycin), a red drug. Individualization of the diet through a process of trial and error appears to be the most successful way of dealing with food aversions.

Use appropriate nutrition support methods
Oral feedings
Indications. Method of choice whenever feasible. Requires bowel motility (presence of bowel sounds), ability to ingest food orally.

Text continued on p. 160.

Table 8-3   Common nutritional problems in individuals with cancer

Problem	Dietary Recommendations/Other Interventions	"Problem" Foods
Nausea and vomiting	*Diet:* Liquids and soft foods served cold: juices, carbonated beverages, gelatin, fruits; dry, bland foods: toast, crackers, plain bagels; serve small amounts frequently *Supplements:* Glucose oligosaccharides, clear liquids such as Citrotein (Sandoz) and SLD (Ross) *Suggestions:* Keep environment cool, well ventilated, free of cooking odors; dry starchy foods (crackers, toast) before rising can help prevent vomiting; liquids should be sipped slowly; help the individual to use distraction, imagery, and relaxation techniques; premedicate with antiemetics if appropriate; plan the medication schedule so that drugs with high emetic potential are not given close to mealtime, if possible;	Hot foods, fatty foods, foods with strong odors, spicy foods

| Anorexia | avoid serving favorite foods during nausea to reduce the risk of developing aversions to them; avoid coaxing or pressure to increase intake
Diet: Regular foods served attractively, with variety in texture and color; small, frequent feedings
Supplements: Glucose oligosaccharides and other modular products (Table 6-2); complete liquid supplements; milk powder added to liquid milk, cereals, mashed potatoes (if lactose tolerance not a problem); Lipomul (Upjohn); tube feedings if necessary; if liquid supplements are used, allow the individual to taste several and select the one(s) preferred.
Suggestions: Avoid offering beverages until individual has finished eating, since fluids can be filling; encourage activity; children may eat more if they are involved in food preparation or if decorating candies and chocolate chips are used to decorate foods | Large meals can overwhelm the person and suppress the appetite |

Text continued on p. 160.

Table 8-3 Common nutritional problems in individuals with cancer—cont'd

Problem	Dietary Recommendations/Other Interventions	"Problem" Foods
Stomatitis, esophagitis	*Diet:* Nonabrasive, soft foods served cold or at room temperature: sherbet, frozen fruits, fruit ices, popsicles, custard, gelatin, ice cream, yogurt, cottage cheese, puddings, canned or cooked vegetables and fruits, boiled or poached egg, sandwiches *Supplements:* Glucose oligosaccharides, complete liquid supplements *Suggestions:* Rinse mouth often with saline, plain water, sodium bicarbonate solution (1 tsp baking soda/ 500 ml water), or hydrogen peroxide diluted to one-sixth strength; viscous lidocaine provides topical analgesia, but the client	Acidic juices such as citrus (evaluate vitamin C intake when citrus fruits are avoided); salty or spicy foods; hard or abrasive foods such as chips, pretzels, nuts, seeds; foods served hot

	must be careful in eating after using it because numbed tissues may inadvertently be bitten or burned by hot foods or beverages	Thin liquids such as water, tea, coffee; foods that are not uniform in consistency (e.g., stews); dry foods (e.g., overcooked meats, hard rolls, nuts); foods such as peanut butter or white bread, which stick to the palate; slippery foods such as gelatin
Dysphagia	*Diet:* Emphasize foods that form a semisolid bolus in the mouth (e.g., macaroni and cheese)	
	Supplements: Carbohydrate or protein modules added to foods (Table 6-2); thickened liquid supplements (see suggestions)	
	Suggestions: Thicken liquids with dry infant cereals, mashed potatoes, potato flakes, or cornstarch; use gravies and sauces to moisten meats and vegetables; if dysphagia is severe, keep suction equipment available	
Xerostomia (reduced saliva production)	*Diet:* Regular, moist foods: casseroles, gravies, sauces; encourage fluids; tea, juice, carbonated beverages, popsicles, fruit ices, gelatin	Breads, dry foods

Continued.

Table 8-3   Common nutritional problems in individuals with cancer—cont'd

Problem	Dietary Recommendations/Other Interventions	"Problem" Foods
	Suggestions: Dental caries is common because saliva production is insufficient to buffer acids produced by mouth bacteria; encourage good oral hygiene; rinse mouth often with saline or mouthwash; offer sugarfree candies (mints, lemon drops) and gum between meals to promote saliva flow; artificial saliva can be used in severe cases	Sweet, sticky foods, sugar-containing gum and candy
Hypogeusia ("mouth blindness")	*Diet:* Regular foods with strong flavors or seasonings and interesting textures	Bland foods
	Supplements: Complete liquid supplements with added flavors if necessary	
Dysgeusia (altered taste)	*Diet:* Regular foods; use trial and error to determine the most suitable foods	Coffee, chocolate, red meats, others (varies with the individual)
	Supplements: Fruit-flavored supplements, glucose oligosaccharides	

		Foods and supplements low in fiber
Diarrhea	*Diet:* Low lactose, low fiber, low fat; encourage fluids *Supplements:* Glucose oligosaccharides, lactose-free liquid supplements	Milk and milk products, raw fruits, whole grain breads and cereals, fatty or fried foods
Constipation	*Diet:* High fiber; encourage large amounts of fluids *Supplements:* Bran, 2 tbsp/day	Foods and supplements low in fiber
Neutropenia with potential for infection	*Diet:* Regular with eggs, meats, poultry, and fish thoroughly cooked *Suggestions:* Thoroughly wash fruits and vegetables to be eaten raw (in severe neutropenia, it is sometimes necessary to avoid raw foods altogether); avoid cross-contamination (e.g., thoroughly clean cutting boards used for trimming raw meat before using them to prepare raw vegetables for salad); refrigerate cooked foods immediately after the meal, and discard any leftovers within 3 days* *Supplements:* Glucose oligosaccharides, canned supplements	Raw eggs, meats, poultry, fish and shellfish; unpasteurized milk or cheese made with unpasteurized milk

*For further food safety measures, see Hecht A: The unwelcome dinner guest: preventing food-borne illness, *FDA Consumer* 25(1):19, 1991.

Example of use. Mild to moderate anorexia related to any type of tumor.

Comments. Supplements may be used where regular foods are insufficient. See Tables 6-1 and 6-2 for suitable supplements.

Enteral tube feedings: nasogastric (NG), nasoduodenal or nasojejunal (ND/NJ), gastrostomy, or jejunostomy

Indications. Inadequate oral intake, impaired digestion or absorption requiring an elemental or "predigested" diet. Requires adequate bowel motility, unobstructed lower gastrointestinal (GI) tract.

Example of use. Severe anorexia, oral or upper GI tumor preventing oral intake, short-bowel syndrome, pancreatic resection.

Comments. ND/NJ feedings may be tolerated by the nauseated patient who cannot tolerate feedings into the stomach, but the tubes are unlikely to stay in place during active vomiting.

Total parenteral nutrition (TPN)

Indications. GI obstruction preventing tube feeding; severely impaired digestion or absorption that prevents adequate enteral intake or causes dehydration, uncontrollable vomiting; need for "bowel rest" to promote healing or regeneration of the bowel.

Example of use. Severe short-bowel syndrome; jejunal or ileal obstruction; enterocutaneous fistula, where bowel rest may promote healing.

Comments. TPN should generally be reserved for malnourished individuals, or those likely to become malnourished as a result of treatment, for whom an effective cancer therapy is available. In general, the risk-benefit ratio associated with TPN is unacceptably high for those individuals who are terminally ill and for whom no further treatment is contemplated.

Client Teaching

Instruct the client/family in the principles of a nutritious diet

Encourage a high-kcal, high-protein intake. Protein sources are listed in Table 7-4. Kcal intake can be increased by following guidelines in the accompanying box. Where regular foods are inadequate, commercial supplements may be needed. See Tables 6-1 and 6-2 for suggestions.

Suggestions for Increasing Kcal Intake

Fat is an especially concentrated source of kcal.*

Salad dressings, cooking oils, mayonnaise, nuts, cream, sour cream, sauces, and gravies are some fat sources.

Butter or margarine provide 35 kcal/tsp. Add them to hot foods such as soup, vegetables, mashed potatoes, cooked cereals, and rice. Serve hot bread because more butter is used when it melts into the bread.

Peanut butter is high in fat, providing 90 kcal/tbsp. It can be served on crackers, apple or pear slices, bananas, or celery.

Snacks should be available at all times.

Nuts, dried fruits, popcorn with lots of butter, cookies, crackers and cheese, granola, ice cream or sherbet, yogurt or frozen yogurt, milkshakes made with ice cream, and puddings are good kcal sources.

Foods should be prepared in a manner that will make them as kcal-dense as possible.

Soups, hot cereals, cocoa from a mix, and instant puddings can be prepared with whole milk or half and half, rather than water.

Meat, chicken, and fish that are breaded and fried are higher in kcal than when broiled or roasted.

Foods of low caloric density should not be allowed to displace more concentrated kcal sources.

Beverage consumption is best delayed until after, rather than before or during, meals.

Low-calorie or no-calorie beverages (artificially sweetened drinks, unsweetened tea or coffee, water) should be avoided as much as possible.

Raw vegetables and salads should be served only at the end of the meal, or kcal-dense foods (cheese, egg, poultry, meat, beans, salad dressing) should be added liberally.

---

*Clients with malabsorption and steatorrhea may not tolerate increased fat intake. MCT oil (see Chapter 6) is one potential source of kcal.

Sweets and sugar are often distasteful to the individual with cancer, yet they are useful in increasing caloric intake. Glucose oligosaccharides (Modular [Mead Johnson], Polycose [Ross], L.C. or P.C. [Navaco]) or corn syrup are less sweet than sugar and are not objectionable to most individuals. They can be added to beverages (except carbonated beverages) and foods such as cereals and applesauce.

Help the client/family learn methods of promoting comfort and alleviating side effects of therapy

Table 8-3 provides suggestions for coping with side effects of therapy. Relevant interventions should be shared with the family.

Teach the client/family to monitor the client's nutritional status regularly

The client should be weighed at least weekly while at home. Progressive weight loss should be reported to the health care team so that appropriate interventions can be planned.

The client or family may need to keep daily records of intake. They can be provided with lists showing the nutritional contributions of common foods to ensure that the daily intake meets the goal.

Instruct the client/family in home tube feeding or TPN, if necessary

Many individuals find it impossible to maintain their weight and nutritional status without aggressive nutrition support. Because of the long-term nature of many cancer treatments, these clients are well-suited to home tube feeding or TPN. Chapter 6 describes procedures for safe delivery of nutrition support.

CASE STUDY

Mr. L., a 55-year-old man, was seen in the clinic with complaints of anorexia, weight loss, and a persistent cough. Diagnostic tests indicated that he had small cell carcinoma of the lung. Laboratory tests revealed a serum albumin of 3.6 g/dl and serum transferrin of 175 mg/dl (low normal) and normal Hgb, Hct, and lymphocyte count. Diet history showed no food aversions; recent intake was about 2000 kcal and 70 g of protein per day. Chemotherapy consisting of cyclophosphamide, doxorubicin, and vincristine was begun, with treatments being given on an outpatient basis once every 3 weeks.

Anthropometric Measurements

Height: 185 cm (6'1")

Current weight: 84.1 kg (185 lb)

Desirable weight: 83.6 kg (184 lb)

Weight 6 months ago (before loss began): 95.4 kg (210 lb)

AMC and TSF are between the 5th and 95th percentiles.

Nutritional Diagnoses

1. *Marasmus*: Even though weight and TSF are at desirable levels, this formerly obese individual has sustained a loss of 12% of his body weight in the past 6 months.
2. *Potential for kwashiorkor*: Laboratory indicators of protein nutriture are low normal, and the client suffers from anorexia.

Nutrition Plan

This chemotherapy regimen usually causes nausea and vomiting for about 48 hours after each treatment. During the period of nausea, small amounts of fluids should be taken frequently. Mr. and Mrs. L. should be instructed about choosing high-kcal, high-protein foods to provide about 2800 kcal and 125 g of protein per day during the nausea-free periods. Mr. L. should weigh himself 1 to 2 times a week as a guide to adequacy of intake.

Mr. L.'s nutritional status should be reevaluated in the clinic at the time of each treatment. If his nutritional status continues to deteriorate, home tube feedings should be considered. These are usually tolerated well if they are discontinued before each treatment and reinstituted 24 to 48 hours later.

Bibliography

American College of Physicians: Parenteral nutrition in patients receiving cancer chemotherapy, *Ann Intern Med* 110:734, 1989.

Bendorf K, Meehan J: Home parenteral nutrition for the child with cancer, *Issues Compr Pediatr Nurs* 12:171, 1989.

Bernstein IL, Bernstein ID: Learned food aversions and cancer anorexia, *Cancer Treat Rep* 65(suppl 5):43, 1981.

Camp-Sorrell D: Controlling adverse effects of chemotherapy, *Nursing* 21:34, 1991.

Chernoff R, Ropka M: The unique nutritional needs of the elderly patient with cancer, *Semin Oncol Nurs* 4:189, 1988.

D'Agostino NS: Managing nutrition problems in advanced cancer, *Am J Nurs* 89:50, 1989.

Daly JM and others: Nutrition support in the cancer patient, *J Parenter Enteral Nutr* 14:244S, 1990.

Mauer AM and others: Special nutritional needs of children with malignancies: a review, *J Parenter Enteral Nutr* 14:315, 1990.

Padilla GV: Psychological aspects of nutrition and cancer, *Surg Clin North Am* 66:1121, 1986.

Rhodes VA: Nausea, vomiting, and retching, *Nurs Clin North Am* 25:885, 1990.

Ulander K and others: Needs and care of patients undergoing subtotal pancreatectomy for cancer, *Cancer Nurs* 14:27, 1991.

Wilson PR, Herman J, and Chubon SJ: Eating strategies used by persons with head and neck cancer during and after radiotherapy, *Cancer Nurs* 14:98, 1991.

Gastrointestinal Disorders

9

A variety of disorders that affect the gastrointestinal (GI) tract and its accessory organs, the liver, gallbladder, and pancreas, can impair nutritional status. Effects of these disorders include malabsorption, discomfort associated with eating, anorexia, impaired intake, and food intolerances. The most common disorders affecting the GI system will be discussed in this chapter.

Esophageal Disorders

Pathophysiology

Among the problems that can interfere with normal esophageal function are gastroesophageal reflux, esophageal obstruction, and motor dysfunction. Reduced lower esophageal sphincter (LES) pressure contributes to gastroesophageal reflux disease (GERD). Other contributing factors include impaired gastric emptying and impaired esophageal peristalsis. The disorder results in reflux of stomach contents into the esophagus, with esophagitis and heartburn. Ulcer and stricture formation are two possible complications, and long-term GERD can predispose the individual to adenocarcinoma of the esophagus.

Mechanical obstructions of the esophagus can result from strictures (e.g., from caustic injury caused by ingestion of lye or from GERD) or tumors. Dysphagia is a common symptom.

Two motor disorders affecting the esophagus are achalasia, or incomplete relaxation of the LES after swallowing, and scleroderma, a collagen-vascular disease, resulting in proliferation of connective tissue and fibrosis in many organs. Achalasia obstructs the passage of food into the stomach, and dysphagia and regurgitation of food are common symptoms. Carcinoma of the

165

esophagus is a potential long-term sequela. Scleroderma impairs peristalsis and LES closure; symptoms are those of GERD.

Esophageal dysfunction places the patient at risk for pulmonary aspiration, dyspnea, and pneumonia.

Treatment

Antireflux measures include the following: elevation of the head of the bed; cessation of smoking, which reduces LES pressure; avoiding medications that reduce LES pressure (e.g., anticholinergics, α-adrenergic antagonists, β-adrenergic agonists, calcium channel blockers, opiates, progesterone and theophylline) if possible; use of antacids; and dietary modification (see the following discussion on nutritional care). If these measures are ineffective, the following additional medications are available: histamine H_2 receptor-blocking agents to reduce gastric acidity, bethanechol to increase LES pressure, and metoclopramide to increase LES pressure and promote gastric emptying. Antireflux surgery is a consideration for the patient who does not benefit from medical therapy.

Mechanical dilatation may be used in treatment of strictures and achalasia, and surgery, or a combination of surgery and radiation therapy, is usually used in the treatment of esophageal tumors.

Nutritional Care

Assessment

Assessment is summarized in Table 9-1.

Intervention and client teaching

Prevent or reduce reflux

Alcohol, fatty foods, and chocolate reduce LES pressure and should be avoided. The client should eat the last meal of the day several hours before bedtime, avoid late-night snacking, and avoid lying flat after eating. Small, frequent meals may reduce reflux.

Cope with dysphagia

Solid foods and thin liquids usually cause the most difficulty. Foods that create a semisolid bolus when chewed are generally best tolerated. Liquids can be thickened with dry infant cereals,

Text continued on p. 171.

Table 9-1 Assessment in gastrointestinal disorders

Areas of Concern	Significant Findings
Protein calorie malnutrition (PCM)	*History*
	Decreased intake of kcal- or protein-containing foods caused by a desire to prevent pain associated with eating (e.g., GER,* gastric ulcer, cholecystitis, pancreatitis), alcohol abuse, nausea and vomiting, anorexia, dysphagia, anticipation of dumping syndrome; increased losses (malabsorption) related to severe diarrhea or steatorrhea (stools greasy or difficult to flush away), pancreatic insufficiency (pancreatitis, cystic fibrosis), short-bowel syndrome, dumping syndrome; increased kcal/protein needs in healing, infection, fever; increased work of breathing (cystic fibrosis); catabolism resulting from corticosteroids.
	Physical examination
	Muscle wasting; edema; alopecia; triceps skinfold < 5th percentile (see Appendix G); weight < 90% of that expected for height or BMI < 19.1 (females) or 20.7 (males); failure to follow individual established pattern on growth charts (children)
	Laboratory analysis
	↓ Serum albumin, transferrin, or prealbumin; ↓ lymphocyte count, ↓ creatinine-height index (see Table 1-4); nonreactive skin tests
Inadequate fluid balance	*History*
	Excessive losses caused by severe vomiting or diarrhea (especially short-bowel syndrome and dumping syndrome); when diarrhea is severe, stools should be weighed or measured to determine output accurately

*Gastroesophageal reflux.

Continued.

Table 9-1 Assessment in gastrointestinal disorders—cont'd

Areas of Concern	Significant Findings
Inadequate fluid balance —cont'd	*Physical examination* Poor skin turgor; dry, sticky mucous membranes; feeling of thirst; loss of ≥ 0.23 kg (0.5 lb) in 24 hr; hypotension *Laboratory analysis* ↑ BUN; ↑ Hct; ↑ serum Na
Vitamin Deficiencies	
A	*History* Decreased absorption as a result of steatorrhea, pancreatic insufficiency; or cholestyramine use *Physical examination* Drying of skin and cornea; papular eruption around hair follicles (follicular hyperkeratosis) *Laboratory analysis* ↓ Serum retinol; ↓ retinol-binding protein (indicating PCM, with inadequate protein to manufacture carrier for vitamin A)
E	*History* Decreased absorption as a result of steatorrhea, pancreatic insufficiency or cholestyramine use *Physical examination* Neuromuscular dysfunction (causing extreme weakness)
K	*Laboratory analysis* ↓ Serum tocopherol *History* Decreased absorption as a result of steatorrhea or pancreatic insufficiency; decreased production caused by destruction of intestinal bacteria by antibiotic usage (e.g., in hepatic encephalopathy or cystic fibrosis) *Physical examination* Petechiae, ecchymoses *Laboratory analysis* Prolonged prothrombin time (PT)

Table 9-1   Assessment in gastrointestinal disorders—cont'd

Areas of Concern	Significant Findings
B_{12}	*History*
	Decreased absorption as a result of gastrectomy (loss of intrinsic factor necessary for absorption), distal ileal disease (e.g., Crohn's disease), or resection (loss of absorptive sites); bacterial overgrowth in the bowel competing for B_{12} (seen in short-bowel syndrome or gastric resection)
	Physical examination
	Pallor; sore, inflamed tongue; neuropathy
	Laboratory analysis
	$\downarrow$ Serum vitamin B_{12}; $\downarrow$ Hct, $\uparrow$ MCV

Mineral/Electrolyte Deficiencies

Calcium (Ca)	*History*
	Decreased intake of milk products, caused by lactose intolerance; increased losses as a result of steatorrhea or corticosteroid use
	Physical examination
	Tingling of fingers; muscular tetany and cramps, carpopedal spasm; convulsions
	Laboratory analysis
	$\downarrow$ Serum Ca (severe deficits only); $\downarrow$ bone density on radiograph (chronic Ca deficit)
Magnesium (Mg)	*History*
	Inadequate intake as a result of alcoholism; increased losses as a result of steatorrhea or diarrhea, vomiting (e.g., pancreatitis, hepatitis), loss of small bowel fluid (e.g., short-bowel syndrome, fistula formation in inflammatory bowel disease)
	Physical examination
	Tremor, hyperactive deep reflexes; convulsions
	Laboratory analysis
	$\downarrow$ Serum Mg

Continued.

Table 9-1 Assessment in gastrointestinal disorders—cont'd

Areas of Concern	Significant Findings
Mineral/Electrolyte Deficiencies —cont'd	
Iron (Fe)	*History*
	Blood loss (e.g., inflammatory bowel disease, ulcer); impaired absorption caused by decreased acid within upper GI tract, resulting from gastrectomy or chronic antacid or cimetidine use (as in peptic ulcer); decreased intake (e.g., restriction of protein foods in liver disease)
	Physical examination
	Koilonychia; pallor, blue sclerae; fatigue
	Laboratory analysis
	↓ Hct, Hgb, MCV, MCH, MCHC; ↓ serum Fe and ferritin; ↑ serum transferrin
Zinc (Zn)	*History*
	Increased losses as a result of diarrhea/ steatorrhea, loss of intestinal fluid (e.g., short-bowel syndrome, high output ileostomy, fistula drainage); decreased intake caused by protein restriction
	Physical examination
	Anorexia; hypogeusia, dysgeusia; diarrhea; dermatitis
	Laboratory analysis
	↓ Serum Zn
Potassium (K^+)	*History*
	Increased losses caused by diarrhea
	Physical examination
	Muscle weakness, ileus; diminished reflexes
	Laboratory analysis
	↓ Serum K^+; inverted T wave on ECG

mashed potatoes or potato flakes, cornstarch, or yogurt. Fluids can also be served in frozen form, for example, sherbet or fruit ices. Speech therapists may be able to assist dysphagic individuals in improving their swallowing techniques. In achalasia the risk of pulmonary aspiration is so great that it is usually better to wait until dilatation or surgical therapy has been performed before trying to increase oral intake.

Provide nutrition support as indicated

Where esophageal obstruction exists or reflux or dysphagia is very severe, impairing intake so much that there is weight loss or placing the individual at high risk of pulmonary aspiration, tube feedings (via gastrostomy or jejunostomy, if esophageal obstruction is present) may be needed. Special care must be taken to reduce the risk of pulmonary aspiration, for example, frequent monitoring of gastric residual volumes and elevation of the head of the bed. Nasoenteric feedings are generally not used before definitive therapy of achalasia.

Gastric Disorders

Peptic Ulcer (Gastric and Duodenal Ulcer)

Pathophysiology

Excess acid secretion or disruption of the GI mucosal barrier predisposes the individual to ulcer formation. *Helicobacter pylori* (formerly known as *Campylobacter pylori*), a bacillus found only on gastric epithelium, is currently believed to be a major factor in the pathogenesis of peptic ulcers, although cigarette smoking; regular use of nonsteroidal antiinflammatory drugs (NSAIDs), such as aspirin; genetic predisposition; and emotional stress may be contributory factors. Gastric ulcers are often associated with pain exacerbated by eating, and duodenal ulcers are associated with pain relieved by eating.

Treatment

Medications that reduce gastric acidity, such as antacids and the histamine H_2 receptor antagonists, cimetidine and ranitidine, are often prescribed. Sucralfate (Carafate) and bismuth are specific antiulcer agents. Bismuth and antibiotics are sometimes used in attempts to eradicate *H. pylori,* but recurrence is common. In addition, the client is usually advised to avoid smoking, alcohol, and NSAIDs, which increase gastric acid production or impair the mucosal barrier that protects the GI tract from damage. Stress reduction techniques may also be of benefit. Endoscopic thermal therapy or injection of a sclerosing agent is increasingly common for treatment of bleeding ulcers, and partial gastrectomy and vagotomy are usually performed only when perforation or uncontrollable bleeding occurs.

Nutritional Care

Assessment

Assessment is summarized in Table 9-1.

Intervention

Dietary practices that promote comfort

Current practice is to liberalize the ulcer diet, restricting only those foods that cause the individual patient discomfort. For some patients these include caffeine-containing foods (see Appendix D), decaffeinated coffee, alcohol, and red or black pepper or other spicy foods.

Client teaching

Recognition of symptoms and modification of the diet to maximize comfort

Work with the client and the family to individualize the diet and limit only those foods that cause pain. Small, frequent meals and snacks may reduce pain in some individuals.

Relaxation and stress reduction techniques

It is especially important to keep mealtimes calm and relaxed, to avoid excessive gastric acid secretion.

Gastrectomy

Pathophysiology

Partial or total resection of the stomach is sometimes required for treatment of peptic ulcer or gastric cancer. Two problems are likely after gastrectomy: fat malabsorption and dumping syndrome. Fat malabsorption results from the bypass of the duodenum by the Roux-en-Y esophagojejunostomy and other common gastrectomy procedures. Bacteria multiply within the bypassed duodenum, and the bacteria deconjugate bile salts, making micelle formation and fat absorption inadequate. Dumping syndrome results from the accelerated influx of nutrients into the small bowel, caused by the loss or bypass of the pyloric sphincter. Rapid hydrolysis of nutrients increases the osmolality within the upper small bowel. Fluid from the plasma and extracellular space is drawn into the bowel to dilute the hypertonic intestinal contents. Symptoms include nausea, abdominal pain, weakness, diaphoresis, diarrhea, and weight loss.

Nutritional Care

Assessment

Assessment is summarized in Table 9-1.

Intervention

Prevent protein calorie malnutrition

Diet should be high in protein (1.5 to 2 g/kg/day) and kcal and moderate in fat to maintain weight. The likelihood of dumping syndrome is reduced if the diet consists of small, frequent feedings; simple carbohydrates are avoided; and beverages are not drunk with meals.

Supplementation

Since they are best absorbed in an acid environment, calcium and iron may be poorly absorbed postoperatively. Supplements of calcium and iron may be prescribed.

Intrinsic factor and hydrochloric acid, both produced in the stomach, are required for absorption of vitamin B_{12}. Therefore supplemental vitamin B_{12} is usually required for the remainder of the client's life. This is most often given as a monthly injection.

Client teaching

Dietary principles and their rationale

The client needs to know how to select a high-protein and moderate-fat diet. This can be done by emphasizing the use of skinned poultry, lean meats, low-fat milk or cheeses, and vegetables, such as dried beans and peas, and by avoiding fried or fatty foods.

Prevention of dumping syndrome

Client instruction should include:

1. Planning a nutritious diet that incorporates small meals and snacks. Six or more small meals a day may be needed.
2. Avoiding beverages at mealtime. Fluids should be drunk at least one hour before or after meals.
3. Avoiding concentrated sweets (e.g., candy, cookies, pies, cakes, jam, jelly, soft drinks, sugared beverages or foods). Although they are high in simple carbohydrates, fresh fruits are often well tolerated because of their fiber and pectin content. They can be used as desserts and snacks.
4. Maintaining nonstressful eating practices. The client should eat slowly in a relaxed setting. Lying down for about an hour after meals can also help prevent dumping syndrome.
5. In severe cases, the physician may recommend use of pectin or guar gum with meals and snacks. These fibers delay gastric emptying and absorption of carbohydrates.

Intestinal Disorders

Nutrients are absorbed at specific sites in the small intestine (Fig. 9-1); therefore the location and the extent of small intestinal disease or resection determines which nutrients will be affected.

Short-Bowel Syndrome

Pathophysiology

Massive resection of the small bowel severely reduces the area available for the absorption of nutrients. It is sometimes required in Crohn's disease, necrotizing enterocolitis, congenital atresias, acute volvulus, strangulated hernias, and mesenteric artery occlusion. Malabsorption and diarrhea are greater if: (1) more than 80% of the small bowel is resected, (2) the ileum is resected (the ileum can absorb most nutrients normally absorbed in the duodenum and jejunum, but these portions of the bowel cannot assume all of the roles of the ileum), (3) the ileocecal valve is removed, or (4) the unresected bowel is damaged.

For at least the first 2 years after massive bowel resection, ad-

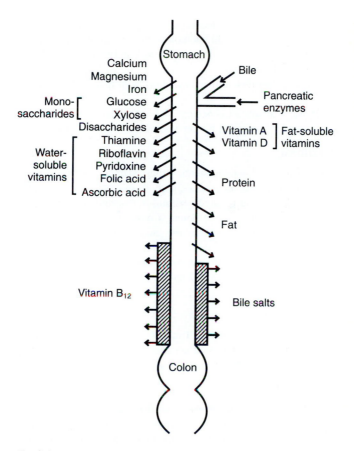

Fig. 9-1
Sites of nutrient absorption in the small intestine. (From Booth CC: Effect of location along the small intestine on absorption of nutrients. In Code CF, ed: *Handbook of physiology*, section 6: Alimentary canal, Vol III: Intestinal absorption, Washington, 1968, American Physiological Society. Used with permission.)

aptation occurs via bowel hyperplasia and hypertrophy. This response takes place in phases:

Phase 1: Immediate postoperative period with enormous losses of fluids, electrolytes, magnesium, calcium, zinc, and amino acids. In addition to the loss of absorptive area, temporary gastric hypersecretion contributes to fluid and electrolyte losses.

Phase 2: Diarrhea diminishes, along with fluid and electrolyte problems.

Phase 3: Stabilization occurs. The individual achieves a stable weight determined by the amount of bowel remaining.

Treatment

Antidiarrheal and anticholinergic drugs, such as codeine, loperamide (Imodium), diphenoxylate with atropine (Lomotil), or glycopyrrolate (Robinul), may be helpful in controlling diarrhea during Phases 1 and 2. If the ileum is removed, large amounts of bile salts may enter the colon and cause diarrhea by stimulating colonic water secretion. At least 100 cm of ileum is required for complete absorption of bile salts. Cholestyramine is sometimes used to bind the bile salts and reduce diarrhea.

Nutritional Care

Assessment

Assessment is summarized in Table 9-1. Massive small bowel resection can be expected to affect absorption of almost every nutrient and to have great potential for causing malnutrition.

Intervention

Replace losses and prevent malnutrition

Phase 1: Intravenous (IV) support is essential to replace fluids, electrolytes, and other nutrient losses. Most individuals require total parenteral nutrition (TPN) for at least a few weeks after surgery. It is especially important to replace zinc losses (12 to 17 mg of zinc are lost per kilogram of feces or ileostomy drainage), since wound healing is impaired without zinc, and standard TPN solutions do not contain enough to replace diarrheal losses.

Phase 2: The presence of nutrients within the GI tract is necessary for bowel adaptation to occur; enteral feedings are generally started as soon as the volume of fecal losses decreases to less than 1 L/day. Typically, TPN continues as continuous tube feedings are begun. Elemental formulas were previously favored, but evidence suggests that polymeric formulas may be as effective, while costing less (see Table 6-1). Small oral feedings may also be started. They are generally low in fat (less than 10 g/day) and fiber and high in starch. White rice, enriched white bread and toast, noodles, macaroni, and peeled boiled or baked potato (all without added milk, cheese, margarine, butter, or other fat) are examples.

Phase 3: Oral feedings can be advanced. They should be small and frequent. Fat intake can be increased unless steatorrhea worsens. Concentrated sugars, excessive fat, or alcohol consumption may exacerbate malabsorption. MCTs (medium-chain triglycerides) may be used for caloric supplementation, but excessive amounts often worsen diarrhea. They can be used in cooking or added to juice to increase caloric intake. Lactose, the sugar found in milk products, may cause diarrhea and cramping and should be limited in the diet.

TPN will continue to be required if the individual is unable to maintain adequate nutriture with oral or oral plus enteral tube feedings.

Supplementation

Individuals not receiving TPN often need daily supplements, particularly vitamins A and E, and iron, calcium, magnesium, and zinc. Water miscible forms of vitamins A and E are available and may be useful for those patients with severe steatorrhea. Individuals who have undergone resection of the terminal ileum should have vitamin B_{12} absorption monitored; they may need monthly injections.

Emotional support

The effects of massive bowel resection are catastrophic and may continue for the rest of the client's life. The client and family need encouragement and reinforcement, particularly if home TPN or tube feedings are required.

Client teaching

Dietary modifications and their rationale

The client will need instruction in a high-kcal diet with small frequent feedings. The need for a low-fat diet (Table 9-2) is controversial; some physicians recommend it in short-bowel syn-

Table 9-2   Fat-restricted diet

Type of Food	Foods to Include	Foods to Avoid
Milk products	Milk products made with skim milk	Milk products made with 2% or whole milk
Meat and meat substitutes	Lean meat, fish (water packed, if canned), poultry without skin, egg whites	Fried meats, sausage, frankfurters, poultry skins, duck, goose, salt pork, luncheon meats, peanut butter, egg yolk except as allowed*
Breads and cereals	Plain pasta, cereals, whole-grain or enriched bread or rolls	Biscuits, doughnuts, pancakes, sweet rolls, waffles, muffins, high-fat rolls such as croissants
Fruits	All except avocado	Avocado except as allowed*
Vegetables	All if plainly prepared	Fried, au gratin, creamed, or buttered
Desserts	Sherbet made with skim milk, angel food cake, gelatin, pudding made with skim milk, fruit ice	Cake, pie, pastry, ice cream, or any dessert containing fat or chocolate
Sweets	Jelly, jam, syrup, sugar, hard sugar candies, jelly beans, gum drops	Any candy made with chocolate, nuts, butter, or cream

*The following contain 5 g of fat per serving and usually no more than 5 to 6 per day are included in a low-fat diet: 1 tsp butter, margarine, oil, shortening, or mayonnaise; 1 tbsp salad dressing or heavy cream; 1 strip crisp bacon; 1/8 avocado; 6 small nuts; 10 peanuts; 5 small olives; 1/2 cup ice milk; 1 egg yolk or whole egg.

drome. Individuals with severe steatorrhea are often more comfortable when they restrict fat intake.

Individuals who do not tolerate lactose may be able to consume yogurt, hard cheeses, and milk treated with Lact-Aid or Lactrase, lactase products that hydrolyze lactose.

Clients should be discouraged from using alcohol and caffeine for at least a year after surgery, since these products stimulate GI activity.

Oxalate restriction may be of benefit in individuals found to have hyperoxaluria, or excessive urinary excretion of oxalates, which may be a factor in stone formation. Hyperoxaluria occurs in some individuals with steatorrhea because they lose unusually large amounts of calcium, as a result of formation of soaps with fat in the stool. Normally calcium complexes with oxalate in the gut to prevent oxalate absorption, but excessive fecal calcium losses allow oxalate to be absorbed. Foods high in oxalate are nuts, coffee, chocolate, green beans, green leafy vegetables, beets, rhubarb, eggplant, celery, carrots, artichokes, plums, blackberries, and whole wheat. Dietary restriction is not effective in reducing oxalate levels in some individuals. A calcium supplement may be useful in reducing oxalate absorption.

Administration of home nutritional support, if necessary

Some individuals will need instruction in home TPN or tube feedings, since these may need to continue at least until maximal adaptation occurs. (See Chapter 6.) TPN is tapered as bowel adaptation progresses.

Celiac Disease (Nontropical Sprue or Gluten-Sensitive Enteropathy)

Pathophysiology

The exact mechanism of celiac disease is unknown, but intestinal villi atrophy because of intolerance of gluten (a protein found in wheat and several other grains). The surface area of the bowel is markedly decreased, and there is loss of disaccharidase and peptidase activity, since both of these enzymes are found in the intestinal mucosal cells. Diarrhea, steatorrhea, impaired absorption of all macronutrients (carbohydrate, protein, and fat), muscle wasting, weight loss or failure to gain weight (in children), and anemia often occur.

Diagnosis of celiac disease is made through small-bowel biopsy, with microscopic evidence of blunting of the villi, and trial of a gluten-restricted diet.

Nutritional Care

Assessment

Assessment is summarized in Table 9-1.

Intervention

Deletion of gluten from the diet

Removal of gluten from the diet for the client's entire life is the only treatment. Eliminate wheat, barley, rye, oats, and all products made with these grains. Table 9-3 lists foods to include and to avoid in gluten sensitivity.

Emotional support

This diet is difficult to follow because of the widespread use of grain products in processed foods. The client and family need extensive encouragement and reinforcement. Adherence to the diet is especially important because GI carcinoma appears to be more common in individuals who fail to do so.

Client teaching

Dietary restriction and rationale

Careful instruction is needed since removal of gluten from the diet is permanent and is the only treatment. It is especially important for the client and family to read labels carefully, since gluten-containing grains are added to many products. Where it is unclear whether a product contains gluten, the client can use the address on the label to obtain further information. In restaurants, it may be necessary to ask whether unfamiliar foods contain restricted grains.

Inflammatory Bowel Disease (Crohn's Disease and Ulcerative Colitis)

Pathophysiology

In Crohn's disease, inflammation extends through all layers of the bowel wall. It can affect any part of the GI tract but most

Table 9-3   Diet for gluten intolerance

Type of Food	Foods to Include	Foods to Avoid
Milk products	Fresh, dry, evaporated, or condensed milk; whipping cream; sour cream (check vegetable gum used)	Malted milk, some commercial chocolate milk, some non-dairy creamers
Meat products	All fresh meats, poultry, and fish	Breaded products; some sausages, frankfurters, luncheon meats, and sandwich spreads
Cheeses	All natural cheeses	Any cheese containing oat gum, some pasteurized processed cheese
Breads and starches	Potatoes, potato flour, rice, rice flour, wild rice, corn, cornstarch, tapioca, arrowroot starch, soy flour, millet, special gluten-free pasta	Regular pasta products, all products containing wheat, rye, oats, barley, buckwheat, or triticale (wheat-rye hybrid)
Vegetables	All plain or buttered	Creamed, au gratin, breaded (unless made with gluten-free starch)
Fruits	All fresh, canned, or frozen	Canned fruit pie fillings
Beverages	Wine, instant and ground coffee, tea, distilled spirits	Beer and ale, roasted grain beverages such as Postum
Miscellaneous	Most spices, cider and wine vinegar, all nuts and seeds	Some dry seasoning mixes, some curry powder, some catsup and mustard, some soy sauce, distilled white vinegar

often affects the terminal ileum. In acute exacerbations, abdominal pain, fever, nausea, and diarrhea occur. In chronic disease, weight loss, anorexia, anemia, and steatorrhea are common.

In ulcerative colitis, congestion, edema, and ulcerations affect the mucosal and submucosal layer of the bowel. It usually involves the rectum and colon, and sometimes extends to the ileum. Bloody diarrhea, abdominal pain, weight loss, anorexia, and rectal pain are common.

Diagnosis is made by barium enema, endoscopy (sigmoidoscopy, colonoscopy, or esophagoscopy), and intestinal biopsy.

Treatment

Drugs that are often used include corticosteroids, to decrease inflammation; antidiarrheals, such as diphenoxylate (Lomotil); and antispasmodics, such as tincture of belladonna, to decrease discomfort. Sulfasalazine is used in ulcerative colitis for its antiinflammatory and antimicrobial effects. (See Chapter 18 for drug-nutrient interactions.)

Surgery may be necessary if fistulas, hemorrhage, perforation, or intestinal obstruction occur. Resection of the colon is often performed after several acute exacerbations of ulcerative colitis, because of the risk of development of colon cancer.

Nutritional Care

Assessment

Assessment is summarized in Table 9-1.

Intervention

Use dietary modifications as necessary to control symptoms

Acute disease. Supportive therapy with intravenous (IV) fluids and a clear liquid diet is often provided. In severe disease, or where a fistula is present, TPN without any oral intake may be used for several weeks in an effort to rest the bowel and promote healing. Enteral tube feedings may also be effective.

Chronic disease. A low-fat diet (Table 9-2) may be prescribed to decrease steatorrhea, which is common with ileal involvement. A high-protein diet (1.5 to 2 g/kg/day) helps promote bowel regeneration and replace losses.

If areas of intestinal stenosis are present, a restricted fiber diet that eliminates berries; raw fruits, except banana or avocado; raw vegetables; whole grains; and dried legumes is recommended to reduce the potential for bowel obstruction.

Lactose intolerance is common in Crohn's disease. Some lactose-intolerant individuals can tolerate yogurt, buttermilk, and hard cheeses. Lact-Aid or Lactrase can be added to milk to hydrolyze the lactose.

Supplementation

If there is involvement of the terminal ileum, injections of vitamin B_{12} may be needed monthly.

If steatorrhea occurs, there are likely to be increased losses of vitamins A and E and calcium, magnesium, and zinc, and appropriate supplements (e.g., water miscible vitamin preparations) will be needed. Iron supplementation may be needed if blood loss is sufficient to cause anemia.

Client teaching

Dietary modifications and rationale

The client may need instruction regarding restriction of fat, fiber, and lactose (see Intervention).

Stress reduction

Stress can exacerbate inflammatory bowel disease (IBD). Furthermore, chronic disease imposes its own stresses on the client. The client needs continued support, as well as assistance in developing coping and stress reduction skills.

Pancreatic Dysfunction

Pancreatitis (Acute or Chronic)

Pathophysiology

Pancreatitis refers to inflammation, edema, and necrosis of the pancreas as a result of autodigestion of the pancreas by enzymes normally secreted by the pancreas. Alcoholism, biliary tract disease, trauma, peptic ulcer disease, hyperlipidemia, and the use of certain drugs (glucocorticoids, sulfonamides, chlorothiazides, and azathioprine) may cause pancreatitis. Symptoms include pain in the epigastric region, persistent vomiting, abdominal rigidity, and elevated serum amylase. Malabsorption and decreased glucose tolerance are common in chronic pancreatitis.

Treatment

Anticholinergic agents, such as atropine, may be used to decrease pancreatic secretion. Meperidine is used for pain relief.

Nutritional Care

Assessment

Assessment is summarized in Table 9-1.

Intervention

Avoid stimulating pancreatic secretion and causing pain during acute pancreatitis

During severe attacks, all oral feedings are generally withheld. IV fluids and electrolytes are given to replace the massive losses that occur during inflammation. TPN may be needed if attacks are prolonged.

Once pain has subsided, clear liquids are usually introduced. If they are tolerated, low-fat, high-carbohydrate foods are often added, and the diet is then gradually liberalized.

Promote healing and modify diet to compensate for decrease in pancreatic secretion in chronic pancreatitis

The diet is usually a high-protein, high-carbohydrate diet with as much fat as can be tolerated without an increase in steatorrhea or pain. MCT oil can be used to promote weight gain. Pancreatic enzyme replacement is sometimes prescribed to be administered with each meal to improve digestion of fat, carbohydrates, and protein.

Insulin secretion is commonly impaired. If glucose intolerance is present, the patient should be treated as a diabetic, with a modified diet and insulin if indicated. (See Chapter 12.)

Supplementation

If fat malabsorption is severe, water miscible forms of vitamins A and E, as well as supplements of zinc and calcium may be needed.

Client teaching

Dietary restrictions and their rationale
The client may need to restrict fat in the diet if it causes steatorrhea or pain. MCT oil can be used in frying or baking, combined into a shake with milk and ice milk, or served in tomato or grape juice. A high-protein intake is necessary. Skinned, baked or broiled poultry, lean meats, low-fat cheeses, and vegetable proteins, such as dried beans and peas, provide protein with a low to moderate fat intake.

Eliminate alcohol intake
Alcohol increases pancreatic damage and pain.

Cystic Fibrosis

Pathophysiology
Cystic fibrosis (CF) is an abnormality of exocrine gland secretion that results in thick, viscous secretions. Involvement of the pancreas results in malabsorption, with fat being the nutrient most affected. Large, bulky stools and growth failure occur. Because the disease affects the mucus-producing glands of the respiratory tract, thick secretions accumulate. Progressive respiratory disease and susceptibility to infection result. Diagnosis is made when the sweat chloride concentration is found to be more than 60 mEq/L.

Treatment
Prevention of atelectasis and respiratory infections is a primary goal of treatment. Daily chest physiotherapy including percussion and postural drainage is done. Antibiotics are given as necessary to treat or prevent pneumonia.

Nutritional Care

Assessment
Assessment is summarized in Table 9-1.

Intervention

Promote optimum growth and prevent malnutrition
A high-kcal diet is needed to compensate for malabsorption, increased work of breathing, and increased needs imposed by infection. Each day, healthy children need about 1000 kcal + 100

kcal per year of life. Children with CF need 120% to 150% of this amount and at least 2 to 2.5 g protein per day. Carbohydrates, especially starch, are a good source of readily digested kcal. Fat helps to make the diet more palatable and to increase kcal intake. However, some children experience abdominal pain and severe steatorrhea with unrestricted fat intake and benefit from limitation of dietary fat (Table 9-2). MCT oil may be used to increase caloric intake.

Pancreatic enzyme replacement with each meal or snack helps promote more adequate absorption.

If severe malabsorption and malnutrition are present, an elemental diet containing protein hydrolysates and little or no fat, either as the sole feeding (in infants) or as a nocturnal tube feeding to supplement oral intake (in children) has been found to be beneficial.

Supplementation
Zinc and calcium supplements and water miscible forms of vitamins A and E may be necessary in clients with steatorrhea.

Emotional support
Cystic fibrosis is a chronic, invariably fatal disease. The client and family need much support to cope with the illness. The disease can be mild to severe, making it difficult to foresee exactly what the individual's functional level and length of survival will be. The median age of survival is continually increasing with improved treatment, with the current median being in the early 20s. Clients should be encouraged to participate in all activities compatible with their functional abilities.

Client teaching
Dietary modifications and rationale
Dietary instruction should be individualized for each client. Most clients experience less steatorrhea and abdominal discomfort if fat is at least moderately restricted (Table 9-2). However, it is important that they be able to participate in peer group activities, including eating experiences. Occasional high-fat meals, such as hamburgers, french fries, fried chicken and fish, and pizza, served at fast food restaurants, can be balanced by lower fat, home-prepared meals.

Replace electrolyte losses

Food should be generously salted, especially in hot weather, to replace abnormal electrolyte losses in sweat.

Hepatic Diseases

Hepatitis

Pathophysiology

Hepatitis is an inflammation of the liver caused by a virus, toxin, obstruction, parasite, or drug (alcohol, chloroform, or carbon tetrachloride). Symptoms include jaundice, abdominal pain, hepatomegaly, nausea, vomiting, and anorexia. Elevated serum levels of bilirubin, aspartate aminotransferase (AST, or SGOT), alanine aminotransferase (ALT, or SGPT), and lactic dehydrogenase (LDH) are commonly present.

Treatment

If the cause of hepatitis is known, it should be removed. Rest and nutritional therapy are the primary treatments.

Nutritional Care

Assessment

Assessment is summarized in Table 9-1.

Intervention

Promotion of liver regeneration

The diet should be high in kcal, high in protein (70 to 100 g) and moderate in fat. Carbohydrates should supply most of the kcal. Frequent, small feedings are better tolerated than large feedings.

Supplementation

If steatorrhea is present, supplemental water miscible vitamins A and E, calcium, and zinc may be needed.

Client teaching

Dietary modifications and rationale

High-protein foods, such as cheese, cottage cheese, lean meats, poultry, and legumes, should be encouraged. Starches, such as pasta, rice, potatoes, cereals, and breads, are good calorie sources.

Eliminate alcohol

Alcohol is toxic to the liver and should be avoided for at least a year.

Cirrhosis and Hepatic Encephalopathy or Coma

Pathophysiology

Cirrhosis occurs following hepatic damage. Causes of damage include alcoholism, biliary tract obstruction, and viral infection. Although the liver is able to regenerate much of the damaged tissue, some fibrous tissue develops, impairing the normal flow of blood, bile, and hepatic metabolites. Portal vein hypertension occurs, with esophageal and gastric varices, GI bleeding, hypoalbuminemia, ascites, and jaundice. Severe liver dysfunction results in intolerance to protein and encephalopathy. Signs of encephalopathy include confusion, increased serum ammonia levels (worsened by high-protein intake), and a flapping hand tremor, with progression to somnolence and coma. Aromatic amino acids (phenylalanine and tyrosine) and methionine appear to contribute to the problem, perhaps by formation of false neurotransmitters in the central nervous system.

Treatment

Drug therapy includes use of lactulose (Cephulac), which reduces serum ammonia by trapping the ammonium ion, replacing it as a bacterial substrate, or decreasing the colonic transit time. Poorly absorbed antibiotics such as neomycin are given orally to destroy gut bacteria that produce ammonia.

Nutritional Care

Assessment

Assessment is summarized in Table 9-1.

Intervention

Avoid inducing or worsening encephalopathy, while providing as nutritious a diet as possible

Kilocalories. A high-kcal diet (45 to 50 kcal/kg) is generally prescribed. Carbohydrates should provide most of these kcal.

Moderate fat (70 to 100 g) should be provided unless steatorrhea is present. If steatorrhea occurs, fat can be reduced. MCTs can be used to increase kcal intake.

Protein. Protein intake should be limited to 1 to 1.5 g/kg desirable weight per day unless hepatic encephalopathy is impending. In encephalopathy, protein is limited to 0.5 g/kg or less. With improvement, intake can be gradually liberalized, with the eventual goal being 1 g/kg/day. Vegetable protein appears to be better tolerated than meat protein by some patients with chronic hepatic encephalopathy.

Branched chain amino acids (BCAAs). BCAAs appear to be beneficial for selected patients with encephalopathy. Enteral formulas high in BCAAs (Hepatic-Aid II [Kendall McGaw] and Travasorb Hepatic [Clintec]) can be taken orally or delivered by tube. Parenteral mixtures (Hepatamine [Kendall McGaw]) are available for use in TPN. These BCAA products provide 37% to 50% BCAA, in contrast to the 22% found in standard products.

Sodium. 500 to 1500 mg (20 to 65 mEq)/day of sodium are needed. (See the box on p. 261 for sodium-restricted diets.)

Promote comfort and tolerance of feedings
Small, frequent feedings are better tolerated than larger, less frequent ones.

Prevent bleeding from esophageal varices
Soft foods that are low in fiber help prevent bleeding, which may result in shock and ultimately in elevated ammonia levels as the blood proteins are absorbed.

Supplementation
Supplements providing at least 2 to 3 times the RDA of B complex vitamins, especially folic acid, are usually required.

Client teaching
Dietary restrictions and rationale
Usually the client is not capable of understanding and remembering dietary instruction, so instruction should focus on the family or other home caregivers.

Servings of high-protein foods should be limited. In general, no more than 2 cups of milk and 6 oz of meat, fish, or poultry (or the equivalent: 1 oz cheese, 1 egg, or ¾ cup of legumes is approximately equal in protein content to 1 oz of meat) should be consumed daily, although this is individualized based on client tolerance. Starchy foods such as pasta, rice, potatoes, and breads provide needed calories. Fat can be used to increase palatability and caloric intake unless steatorrhea occurs.

Sodium is moderately limited to 1000 to 2000 mg/day in the maintenance diet. No salt should be added in cooking, and obviously salty foods should be avoided. See the box on p. 261.

Eliminate alcohol
Continuing alcohol intake further damages the liver.

Gallbladder Disease

Pathophysiology

Inflammation of the gallbladder, or cholecystitis, is usually caused by obstruction of the bile duct by gallstones. Pain in the right upper quadrant of the abdomen, nausea, vomiting, flatulence, and jaundice may occur. Diagnosis is made when there is nonvisualization of the gallbladder on cholecystogram or evidence of stones or occluded bile ducts on ultrasound.

Treatment

During the acute phase, analgesics and antiemetics are administered. Cholecystectomy and drainage of the biliary tree are necessary for permanent resolution of cholecystitis.

Nutritional Care

Assessment

Assessment is summarized in Table 9-1.

Intervention

Reduce stimulation of the gallbladder
A low-fat or fat-free diet (Table 9-2) should be followed during acute attacks. In severe attacks, the diet may be limited to clear liquids and IV fluids.

Supplementation
Because of poor fat absorption, supplementation with water miscible forms of the fat-soluble vitamins A and E may be needed.

Client teaching

Dietary restrictions and rationale

Clients who do not have a cholecystectomy are usually more comfortable if they follow a low-fat diet on a permanent basis. Since pain usually follows fat intake, clients tend to reduce fat intake spontaneously. Some individuals may find that gas-forming vegetables and highly spiced foods cause discomfort.

Those who undergo cholecystectomy should follow a low-fat diet for several weeks after surgery until inflammation decreases and adaptation occurs.

CASE STUDY

Paul C., a 12-year-old boy with cystic fibrosis, was growth retarded, with both height and weight well below the 5th percentile for age and sex. He was so weak that he had to stop attending school. A diet history showed that he ate about 1300 kcal daily. Intake of fatty foods was associated with abdominal pain and steatorrhea.

Dietary counseling was given in order to increase kcal intake. A subsequent 24-hour recall revealed an intake of about 2250 kcal/day as follows:

Breakfast: Cornflakes with skim milk,* sliced bananas, and sugar; toast with honey; grape juice with Moducal glucose oligosaccharides (Mead Johnson)

Lunch: Turkey sandwich, pretzels, dried apricots, skim milk

Snack: Toasted bagel with jam, instant breakfast made with skim milk*

Dinner: Lean roast beef, carrots and potatoes cooked with the roast, apple crisp, iced tea

Snack: Fruit yogurt

However, Paul's growth was still poor. He was taught to give himself tube feedings of an elemental formula containing protein hydrolysate, glucose oligosaccharides, and almost no fat for 9 hours every night. The tube feeding, combined with his food intake, resulted in marked growth in height and weight. His strength and endurance increased, and he was able to return to school.

---

*⅓ cup skim milk powder added per cup of skim milk.

Bibliography

Cashman MD: Principles of digestive physiology for clinical nutrition, *Nutr Clin Prac* 1:241, 1986.

Cole SG, Kagnoff MF: Celiac disease, *Annu Rev Nutr* 5:241, 1985.

Freston JW: Overview of medical therapy of peptic ulcer disease, *Gastroenterol Clin North Am* 19:121, 1990.

Marotta RB, Floch MH: Dietary therapy of steatorrhea, *Gastroenterol Clin North Am* 18:485, 1989.

Marsano L, McClain CJ: Nutrition and alcoholic liver disease, *J Parenter Enteral Nutr* 15:337, 1991.

McCullough AJ and others: Nutritional therapy and liver disease, *Gastroenterol Clin North Am* 18:619, 1989.

Meguid MM, Campos AC, and Hammond WG: Nutritional support in surgical practice: part II, *Am J Surg* 159:427, 1990.

Moore MC and others: Enteral-tube feeding as adjunct therapy in malnourished patients with cystic fibrosis: a clinical study and literature review, *Am J Clin Nutr* 44:33, 1986.

Perkal MR, Seashore JH: Nutrition and inflammatory bowel disease, *Gastroenterol Clin North Am* 18:567, 1989.

Peterson WL: *Helicobacter pylori* and peptic ulcer disease, *N Engl J Med* 24:1043, 1991.

Purdum PP III, Kirby DF: Short-bowel syndrome: a review of the role of nutrition support, *J Parenter Enteral Nutr* 15:93, 1991.

Sleisenger MH, Fordtran JS, editors: Gastrointestinal disease: pathophysiology, diagnosis, management, ed. 4, Philadelphia, 1989, WB Saunders.

AIDS

10

Malnutrition is a common finding among patients with acquired immunodeficiency syndrome (AIDS). Malnutrition can decrease functional capacity, contribute to immune dysfunction, and increase the morbidity and mortality of these individuals, as it does in others.

Pathophysiology

The human immunodeficiency virus (HIV), the causative organisms of AIDS, selectively infects helper T-lymphocytes, leaving the individual susceptible to opportunistic infections and cancers such as Kaposi's sarcoma and non-Hodgkin's lymphoma. Weight loss and malabsorption are common in AIDS, even in the early stages of the disease, with 80% or more of clients reporting unintentional weight loss. Multiple factors are responsible for the malnutrition associated with AIDS. Respiratory infections, such as *Pneumocystis carinii* pneumonia, which frequently occurs in individuals with AIDS, cause anorexia, dyspnea, fever, and increased needs for protein, kcal, and vitamins. Diarrhea is a common finding, occurring secondary to gastrointestinal (GI) pathogens, including fungi, viruses, bacteria, and protozoans, or resulting from enteropathy caused by HIV itself. Central nervous sytem (CNS) infections caused by HIV or by opportunistic organisms cause confusion, dementia, and impaired coordination, which interfere with food intake.

Treatment

The antiviral agent, zidovudine (AZT), is used in treating some patients with AIDS. Patients with secondary infections receive a wide variety of antibiotic agents, and, where applicable, they also receive cancer therapy (see Chapter 8). The side effects of commonly used medications include anorexia, nausea and vomiting, mucosal lesions, and diarrhea (Table 10-1).

Because there is no cure for AIDS at present, some clients seek help from unconventional therapies, which include dietary modifications and nutrient supplements. Representative therapies that are most likely to have an impact on nutritional status are summarized in Table 10-2. Other alternative therapies include coenzyme Q and the amino acids cysteine and ornithine, which

Table 10-1   Nutritional impacts of some drugs commonly prescribed for clients with AIDS

	Side Effect				
Drug	Nausea/ vomiting	Diarrhea	Sore mouth/ throat*	Unpleasant taste in mouth	Anorexia
Antivirals					
Acyclovir		x	x	x	
Dihydroxyphenoxy- methylguanine (DHPG)	x				x
Zidovudine (AZT)	x	x		x	x
Antifungals					
Amphotericin B	x	x		x	
Clotrimazole	x				
Ketoconazole	x	x			x
Nystatin	x	x			
Spiramycin	x	x			
Antibacterials/antiprotozoals					
Clindamycin	x	x	x	x	
Dapsone			x		x
Pentamidine isethionate (IV)	x	x	x	x	x
Trimethoprim- sulfamethoxaxole	x	x	x		x

*Esophagitis, glossitis, and/or oral mucosal lesions.

are used as immune stimulators and modulators; a homemade version of AL 721 (a drug approved for investigation by the FDA, which is prepared from egg yolk), reputed to reduce the infectivity of HIV; BHT (butylated hydroxytoluene, a food additive), to destroy HIV; and physical and psychologic therapies such as massage, acupuncture, and meditation. None of the unconventional or alternative therapies have been proven effective.

Table 10-2   Unconventional and unproven therapies sometimes used by AIDS clients

Therapy	Comments/Nutritional Implications
Treatments Purported to Bolster Immune Function	
Megadoses of vitamins, especially A, C, E	Toxicity is associated with chronic vitamin A intakes >50,000 IU/day; "rebound" scurvy can occur if megadose vitamin C is stopped
Immune power diet*	Attributes much poor health to hypersensitivity to common foods (milk products, soy, wheat, corn, sugar, yeast); 21-day initial diet eliminates these foods, then reintroduction is begun; diet is highly restrictive (low in kcal and calcium, limited in protein), making adequate intake difficult
Herbal remedies	Purported to regenerate the immune system; garlic is also reported to have antiviral properties (odor-free capsules are purchased in health food stores by some clients); the purity and safety of some preparations are questionable, and trace quantities of lead and other heavy metals have been found in some

*Berger M: *Dr. Berger's immune power diet,* New York, 1985, Avon Books.
†Crook WG: *The yeast connection,* New York, 1986, Random House.

Continued.

Table 10-2 Unconventional and unproven therapies sometimes used by AIDS clients — cont'd

Therapy	Comments/Nutritional Implications
Therapies Purported to Have Antiviral or Other Antiinfective Properties	
Yeast-free diet†	Advocated to prevent opportunistic yeast infection such as candidiasis; eliminates yeast-containing and simple carbohydrate foods, as well as mushrooms, melons, cheese, peanuts, coffee and tea, smoked meats, condiments; client may have difficulty obtaining enough kcal because of the many restrictions
Macrobiotic diet	Claimed to restore balance and harmony between yin and yang forces and therefore to promote health; consists of whole grains, vegetables, beans, seaweed, miso (fermented soy paste); very low-fat, high-bulk diet could make it difficult for the client to consume enough kcal; potential for deficiencies of protein, riboflavin, niacin, vitamins B_{12} and D, calcium, iron

Nutritional Care

Nutritional care of the client with AIDS focuses on identifying and correcting, if possible, nutritional deficits that might weaken the patient, exacerbate immune dysfunctions, and/or impair quality of life.

Assessment

Nutrition assessment is summarized in Table 10-3.

Intervention

Encourage adequate intake to meet nutrient requirements
Energy (kcal) needs can be estimated using Table 7-3. Protein needs are usually at least 2 g/kg/day. There is no evidence that

Table 10-3   Nutrition assessment of the client
with AIDS

Area of Concern	Significant Findings
Protein Calorie Malnutrition (PCM)	*History*
	Nutrient losses caused by diarrhea and malabsorption (from AIDS enteropathy, GI infections, medications), vomiting; increased needs because of infection and fever; poor intake caused by anorexia (related to respiratory or other infections, depression, medications), oral and esophageal pain (e.g., *Candida* or herpes esophagitis, endotracheal Kaposi's sarcoma), dyspnea, dysphagia, dysgeusia related to medication use or zinc deficiency, dementia or CNS infections
	Physical examination
	Recent weight loss; weight <90% of desirable or BMI <19.1 (women) or <20.7 (men), or decline in percentiles for height and/or weight on growth chart for children (see Appendix F); wasting of muscle and subcutaneous tissue; triceps skinfold or AMC <5th percentile
	Laboratory analysis
	↓ Serum albumin, transferrin, or prealbumin; negative nitrogen balance; ↓ creatinine-height index (see Table 1-4). NOTE: lymphocyte count and skin tests are likely to be of little value in nutrition assessment.
Mineral Deficiencies	
Iron (Fe)	*History*
	Poor intake (same causes as PCM); increased losses or impaired utilization caused by medications such as pentamidine, amphotericin B, DHPG
	Physical examination
	Pallor, koilonychia, fatigue, tachycardia
	Laboratory analysis
	↓ Hct, hgb, MCV, MCH, MCHC, ferritin

Continued.

Table 10-3   Nutrition assessment of the client
with AIDS—cont'd

Area of Concern	Significant Findings
Mineral Deficiencies—cont'd	
Zinc (Zn)	*History* Poor intake (same reasons as PCM); impaired absorption in diarrhea *Physical examination* Hypogeusia, dysgeusia, alopecia, dermatitis, diarrhea *Laboratory analysis* ↓ Serum Zn
Selenium (Se)	*History* Poor intake of meats, fish, poultry (same reasons as PCM); impaired absorption in diarrhea *Physical examination* Congestive cardiomyopathy, muscle weakness, pallor, fatigue, tachycardia *Laboratory analysis* ↓ Serum Se; ↓ hct, ↑ nucleated RBC, Howell-Jolly bodies, Heinz bodies (hemolytic anemia resulting from fragility of the RBC membrane)

megadoses of any vitamin or mineral will affect the course of the disease. However, where the oral diet is inadequate, the individual with AIDS may benefit from a daily multivitamin and mineral supplement, which supplies 100% of the RDA for each nutrient.

Promote comfort and alleviate symptoms that interfere with adequate intake

Nutritional care is tailored to the individual's needs, taking into account his or her symptoms. Many of the disease- and drug-related symptoms having an impact on nutrient intake (anorexia, nausea and vomiting, stomatitis and esophagitis, dysphagia, neutropenia, diarrhea) are similar to those in the client with cancer. Interventions for these problems are summarized in Table 8-3. In addition, dyspnea is a common finding in individuals with pulmonary infections secondary to AIDS. For these clients, small, frequent meals are usually best, and foods of high nutrient density, for example, cheese, meats, and quick breads, such as biscuits or muffins, are preferred over foods with low nutrient density, such as green, leafy vegetables and no- or low-calorie beverages. If clients are receiving oxygen, a nasal cannula used during meals may improve eating ability.

Clients with dementia or neurologic dysfunction may need to be reminded and encouraged to eat. Occupational therapists can assist in evaluating patients with motor problems and selecting special eating utensils that can improve their ability to feed themselves. Clients who cannot feed themselves should be fed in a calm, unhurried manner, with family members or friends being involved whenever possible.

Provide enteral and parenteral feedings in a safe and conscientious manner

For some patients who cannot consume or absorb enough nutrients administered orally, enteral or parenteral (TPN) feedings will be necessary. The enteral route is preferred whenever possible. Continuous enteral feedings may be better absorbed than intermittent ones in clients with malabsorption. Formulas that are low in total fat or those in which medium-chain triglycerides (MCT) provide a substantial portion of the fat kcal are likely to be better absorbed than formulas that are rich in long-chain triglycerides. Where oral or esophageal infections are present, the patient may be unable to tolerate a nasogastric, nasoduodenal, or nasojejunal tube. Gastrostomy or jejunostomy feedings are often utilized when the nasal route is unavailable or when long-term feedings are necessary. Indications for TPN include a nonfunctional GI tract and extraordinary caloric requirements that cannot be totally met via the enteral route. Careful attention to infection control measures is important during both enteral and parenteral feedings. Contamination of enteral feedings can be reduced by using commercially sterile products, adhering to aseptic technique during formula preparation and administration, and limiting hang time for the formula to 8 hours. For TPN, preparation in the pharmacy under sterile conditions, careful attention to aseptic technique during administration, and limiting the hang time to 24 hours (12 hours for intravenous lipid) will reduce the risk of contamination.

Teaching
Principles of a good diet

Clients need an understanding of what a good diet entails, since optimal nutrition will help to maintain functional capacity, improve quality of life, and improve tolerance of treatment. The Food Group Plan in Appendix A can be used as a guide. Many individuals infected with HIV are extremely interested in nutrition and in its potential benefits in controlling disease, and it is possible to build on this interest in teaching about diet.

Unconventional and unproven therapies for AIDS

The client with AIDS who is using or interested in unproven therapies should be provided with factual information regarding these therapies, presented in a nonjudgmental fashion. At the very least, these therapies should be expected to include no substances that are actually harmful, allow for intake of a varied and nutritionally balanced diet that will not cause any nutritional deficiencies, not be unduly expensive, and not take the place of health care that is generally accepted as appropriate and effective. By establishing a relationship of trust, it may be possible to influence the patient to alter some of the regimens to make them nutritionally adequate. For example, the addition of seafood to the macrobiotic diet provides complete protein and vitamin B_{12}, as well as increasing dietary iron and niacin.

Safe handling practices for food

Surveys have shown that individuals with AIDS have a twenty-fold increase in incidence of salmonellosis, compared with individuals without AIDS, and that the infection, which often results from contaminated food, is apt to be more serious in HIV-infected individuals, with 45% developing *Salmonella* bacteremia. Infection with Listeriosis, caused by *Listeria monocytogenes,* another pathogen spread via food, is 200- to 300-fold more likely to affect patients with AIDS than it is to affect the general public. A multitude of other pathogens are also potentially food-borne. To prevent unnecessary morbidity, it is therefore essential that the individual and caregivers choose, prepare, and store foods carefully. Table 8-3 provides general guidelines for food safety for the immunosuppressed patient. An inexpensive and highly instructive videotape, *Eating Defensively: Food Safety Advice for Persons with AIDS,* prepared by the Food and

Drug Administration, the Centers for Disease Control, and the Whitman-Walker Clinic, may be obtained from the National AIDS Information Clearinghouse, P.O. Box 6003, Rockville, MD 20850.

CASE STUDY

Ms. L., a 25-year-old woman with AIDS, had had diarrhea for 3 months. During this time, she lost 5 kg (11 lb). She received dietary counseling and for 6 months was able to maintain her weight with five low-fat, low-lactose meals daily. At that time, however, she developed *Candida* esophagitis. Because of the pain, her oral intake declined drastically, and she rapidly lost 4 kg (8.8 lb). After discussing the options with the nutrition support team, Ms. L. underwent a percutaneous endoscopic gastrostomy (PEG), and she and her mother, with whom she lived, were taught to administer gastrostomy feedings of a low-fat, lactose-free defined formula diet at home. She tolerated six intermittent daily feedings well, along with small amounts of food, and gradually began to regain the weight she had lost.

Bibliography

Archer DL: Food counseling for persons infected with HIV: strategy for defensive living, *Public Health Rep* 104:196, 1989.

Crocker KS: Gastrointestinal manifestations of the acquired immunodeficiency syndrome, *Nurs Clin North Am* 24:395, 1989.

Dwyer JT and others: Unproven nutrition therapies for AIDS: What is the evidence? *Nutr Today* 23(2):25, 1988.

Keithley JK, Kohn CL: Managing nutritional problems in people with AIDS, *Oncol Nurs Forum* 17:23, 1990.

Kotler DP and others: Enteral alimentation and repletion of body cell mass in malnourished patients with acquired immunodeficiency syndrome, *Am J Clin Nutr* 53:149, 1991.

Resler SS: Nutrition care of AIDS patients, *J Am Diet Assoc* 88:828, 1988.

Taber J: Nutrition in HIV infection, *Am J Nurs* 89:1446, 1989.

Task Force on Nutrition Support in AIDS: Guidelines for nutrition support in AIDS, *Nutrition* 5(1):39, 1989.

Renal Disease   11

The kidneys are responsible for maintaining the optimal chemical composition of all body fluids. A variety of diseases can affect the kidneys. When renal failure occurs, there is difficulty in controlling the body content of sodium, potassium, and nitrogenous by-products of metabolism. In nephrotic syndrome, large amounts of protein are lost in the urine. Nephrolithiasis, or renal calculi formation, refers to the precipitation of stones in the urinary tract.

Acute or Chronic Renal Failure

Pathophysiology

In acute renal failure (ARF), a sudden reduction in glomerular filtration rate occurs, with impairment in excretion of wastes. Causes for this sudden reduction include inadequate renal perfusion (e.g., hemorrhage); acute tubular necrosis following trauma, surgery, or sepsis; nephrotoxic drugs or chemicals; acute glomerulonephritis; and obstruction (e.g., ureterovesical stricture). There are two phases:

1. Oliguric phase—creatinine and blood urea nitrogen (BUN) rise, with urinary output usually less than 400 ml/day (less than 0.5 to 1 ml/kg/hr in children). This lasts about 8 to 15 days.
2. Diuretic phase—urine output increases. Creatinine and BUN levels gradually decrease. This phase usually lasts 2 to 3 weeks.

If renal disease progresses, rather than resolves, most of the functional nephrons can be lost. Chronic renal failure (CRF) results. BUN and creatinine levels are high, and retention of fluid, potassium, sodium, phosphorus, and other constituents occurs.

Treatment

Treatment involves removal or, if possible, correction of the cause of renal failure. The major complications during the oliguric phase include acidosis, hyperkalemia, infection, hyperphosphatemia, hypertension, and anemia. Alkalinizing agents (e.g., sodium bicarbonate or Shohl's solution), cation-exchange resins to bind potassium, antibiotics, aluminum hydroxide or aluminum carbonate antacids to bind phosphorus, antihypertensive agents, and diuretics are the most commonly used treatment measures.

Dialysis is needed if these measures, combined with dietary restrictions, are insufficient to prevent or control hyperkalemia, fluid overload, symptomatic uremia (drowsiness, nausea, vomiting, and tremors), or rapidly rising BUN and creatinine levels. Although hemodialysis is widely used, a growing number of clients use chronic ambulatory peritoneal dialysis (CAPD) or continuous cycling peritoneal dialysis (CCPD), which is usually done daily and is especially popular because either can readily be done on an outpatient basis. In CRF, the ultimate goal is transplantation.

Nutritional Care

The goal of nutritional care is to reduce the production of wastes that must be excreted by the kidney and to avoid fluid and electrolyte imbalance. In the undialyzed individual, dietary measures are usually aimed at delaying the need for dialysis.

Assessment

Assessment is summarized in Table 11-1.

Intervention

Dietary restrictions to reduce the fluid, electrolytes, and wastes that must be excreted by the kidney
Fluid
Undialyzed clients. When oliguria is present, the daily allowance of fluid is usually 400 to 500 ml (to account for insensible losses) plus the volume lost from sources such as urine, diarrhea, and vomitus during the previous 24 hours. During the diuretic phase of ARF, it is not necessary to replace all losses, although enough fluid should be supplied to prevent dehydration.

Dialyzed clients. Fluid intake is limited to an amount that re-
Text continued on p. 208.

Table 11-1 Assessment in renal disease

Areas of Concern	Significant Findings
Protein Calorie Malnutrition (PCM)	*History* Poor intake of protein-containing and kcal-containing foods as a result of dietary restrictions or anorexia from zinc deficiency or depression; losses of amino acids or serum proteins caused by dialysis (hemodialysis losses $\approx$ 14 g/session, CAPD losses $\approx$ 5 to 15 g/day), steroid-induced tissue catabolism, and proteinuria; increased needs during infection *Physical examination* Muscle wasting; thinning of hair; dry weight <90% of ideal for height, BMI <19.1 (females) or 20.7 (males), or decline in growth percentile for height or weight (children) (see Appendix F); triceps skinfold <5th percentile (see Appendix G); NOTE: Loss of weight or decrease in subcutaneous fat may be masked by edema *Laboratory analysis* ↓ Serum albumin, transferrin, or prealbumin; ↓ lymphocyte count; nonreactive skin tests (NOTE: This may occur in the well-nourished uremic individual); nitrogen (N_2) losses in urine and dialysate greater than intake (negative N_2 balance)
Altered Lipid Metabolism	*History* Nephrotic syndrome, excessive consumption of carbohydrates (CHO) caused by dietary emphasis on CHO as a source of kcal or use of glucose as an osmotic agent in dialysis *Laboratory analysis* ↑ Serum cholesterol, LDL- and VLDL-cholesterol, serum triglycerides

Table 11-1   Assessment in renal disease—cont'd

Areas of Concern	Significant Findings
Potential for Fluid Excess	*History* Oliguria or anuria *Physical examination* Edema; hypertension; acute weight gain ($\geq$1%-2% of body weight) *Laboratory analysis* $\downarrow$ Hct

Potential for Mineral/Electrolyte Imbalance

Areas of Concern	Significant Findings
Phosphorus (P) excess	*History* Oliguria or anuria *Physical examination* Tetany *Laboratory analysis* $\uparrow$ Serum P; Ca $\times$ P product (Ca in mg/dl $\times$ P in mg/dl) > 70; renal calcification on radiographs
Calcium (Ca) deficit	*History* Metabolic acidosis (serum pH <7.35, bicarbonate <22 mEq/L); hyperphosphatemia *Physical examination* Renal osteodystrophy with bone pain and deformities; tetany *Laboratory analysis* $\downarrow$ Serum Ca (NOTE: $\approx$45% of Ca is bound to albumin, if the client is hypoalbuminemic, the Ca level will be misleading; it can be "corrected" by adding 0.8 mg/dl to the total Ca level for each 1 g/dl decrease in albumin below 3.5 g/dl)
Zinc (Zn) deficit	*History* $\downarrow$ Intake caused by restriction of protein-containing foods; loss during dialysis *Physical examination* Hypogeusia, dysgeusia; alopecia; seborrheic dermatitis *Laboratory analysis* $\downarrow$ Serum Zn

Continued.

Table 11-1 Assessment in renal disease — cont'd

Areas of Concern	Significant Findings
Iron (Fe) deficit	*History*
	Decreased production of erythropoietic factor by diseased kidney; decreased intake as a result of dietary restrictions
	Physical examination
	Fatigue; pallor
	Laboratory analysis
	↓ Hct, Hgb, MCV, MCH, MCHC
Sodium (Na) excess	*History*
	Oliguria or anuria
	Physical examination
	Edema; hypertension
Potassium (K^+) excess	*History*
	Oliguria or anuria
	Physical examination
	Weakness, flaccid muscles
	Laboratory analysis
	↑ Serum K^+; electrocardiogram: elevated T wave, depressed ST segment
Aluminum (Al) excess	*History*
	Use of Al-containing phosphate binders, especially if Al dosages are >30 mg/kg/day
	Physical examination
	Ataxia, seizures, dementia; renal osteodystrophy with bone pain and deformities
	Laboratory analysis
	Plasma Al >100 μg/L
Potential for Vitamin Imbalance	
A excess	*History*
	Oliguria or anuria
	Physical examination
	Anorexia, fatigue; alopecia, dry skin; hepatomegaly; irritability (progressing to hydrocephalus and vomiting in infants and children)
	Laboratory analysis
	↑ Serum retinol

Table 11-1 Assessment in renal disease—cont'd

Areas of Concern	Significant Findings
C deficit	*History*
	Losses in dialysis; ↓ intake caused by restriction of K^+-containing fruits and vegetables
	Physical examination
	Gingivitis; petechiae, ecchymoses
	Laboratory analysis
	↓ Serum or leukocyte ascorbic acid
B_6 deficit	*History*
	Failure of the diseased kidney to phosphorylate (activate) B_6; loss in dialysis
	Physical examination
	Dermatitis; ataxia, irritability, seizures
	Laboratory analysis
	Plasma pyridoxal phosphate (PLP) <34 nmol*
Folic acid	*History*
	Loss of folate during dialysis, ↓ intake caused by restriction of K^+-containing fruits, vegetables, and meats
	Physical examination
	Glossitis (inflamed tongue); pallor
	Laboratory analysis
	↓ Hct, ↑ MCV; ↓ serum folate
D deficit	*Physical examination*
	Rickets (children), osteomalacia
	Laboratory analysis
	↓ 1,25-OH_2 vitamin D

*Normal values are not well established.

sults in a gain of no more than 0.45 kg (1 lb)/day on the days between dialyses. This usually results in a daily intake of 500 ml plus the volume lost in urine, diarrhea, and vomitus.

Electrolytes

Undialyzed clients. Sodium intake should be restricted to 2 to 2.5 g (87 to 109 mEq)/day or less in adults and 50 mg (2.2 mEq)/kg/day in children. See the box on p. 261. Potassium intake should be restricted to 1.5 to 2.5 g (38.5 to 64 mEq)/day in adults and about 50 mg (1.3 mEq)/kg/day in children.

Dialyzed clients. More liberal allowances are often needed to maintain normal serum sodium and potassium levels in dialyzed clients. During chronic ambulatory peritoneal dialysis (CAPD), potassium allowances are usually about 2.7 to 3.1 g (70 to 80 mEq)/day for adults and 75 mg (1.9 mEq)/kg/day in children.

Sodium in medications. Antibiotics, sulfonamides, and barbiturates contain sodium. Some, especially the penicillins, contain large amounts. These sources should be deducted from the total sodium allowance when clients are on low-sodium diets. Consult a pharmacist for the sodium content of drugs.

Protein

Undialyzed clients. Adults should restrict their protein intake to 0.6 g/kg of desirable weight per day. Children should consume no more than the RDA for protein (see Appendix I). The protein should be at least 75% high biologic value (HBV), since HBV protein contains more essential than nonessential amino acids. HBV protein is found mainly in eggs, meat, poultry, fish, and milk products. By restricting the amount of total protein and of nonessential amino acids, the diet causes the individual to manufacture nonessential amino acids, thus decreasing the amount of nitrogen that must be excreted as urea.

Essential amino acids. Supplements of essential amino acids (EAAs) are sometimes used. The usual dose is 10 to 20 g/day. Intake of other proteins should be reduced to less than or equal to 0.4 g/kg/day when EAAs are used. EAA formulations are available as tablets (Aminess [Kabivitrum]) or in formulas for oral or tube feeding (Amin-Aid [Kendall McGaw] or Travasorb Renal [Clintec]). The macronutrients in these formulas are shown in Table 11-2. EAA products (RenAmin [Travenol], Nephramine [Kendall McGaw], or Aminosyn RF [Abbott]) are also available for use in TPN.

Advantage of EAAs. The primary advantage of EAAs is that the

Table 11-2   Formulas for use in renal failure (composition per 1000 kcal)

Composition	Amin-Aid (Kendall McGaw)	Travasorb Renal (Clintec)
Amino acids (g)	9.9	17.1
Carbohydrates (g)	186.4	202.6
Fat (g)	23.6	13.3
Sodium (mg)	172	0
Potassium (mg)	0	0
Volume (ml)	375	578
Osmolality (mOsm/kg)	850	590

diet can be liberalized, since the supplements make it unnecessary to emphasize HBV protein.

Disadvantages of EAAs. Among the disadvantages of EAAs is the fact that many tablets (approximately 30 per day) are required; the osmolalities of the formulas are high and may promote diarrhea; and the formulas lack important minerals and should not be used for prolonged periods without mineral supplements.

Dialyzed clients. Dialyzed clients should receive protein on the following bases: adult hemodialysis—1.2 g/kg/day; adult peritoneal dialysis—1.2 to 1.5 g/kg/day with 50% HBV; pediatric hemodialysis—1.5 to 2 g/kg/day; pediatric peritoneal dialysis—3 g/kg/day for children up to age 5, 2 to 2.5 g/kg/day from age 5 through puberty, 1.5 g/kg/day after puberty.

Kilocalories. Adult allowances of kcal are 35 to 40 kcal/kg/day. Children's allowances are 75 to 100 kcal/kg/day. It is important that enough kcal be consumed to prevent catabolism, since this not only reduces the amount of functional tissue but also releases nitrogen, which must be excreted by the kidney. Caloric supplements may be necessary to achieve an adequate kcal intake while adhering to the dietary restrictions. These supplements usually contain glucose oligosaccharides or vegetable oils. Some of the more common ones are listed in the Exchange Lists for Renal Diets (Tables 11-3 and 11-4).

During CAPD and CCPD, 1.5% to 4.25% glucose solutions (containing 1.5 or 4.25 g glucose/dL) are utilized in the dialysate as an osmotic agent to draw fluid out of the body. About 70% of the glucose instilled is absorbed by the peritoneum. The glucose

Text continued on p. 222.

Table 11-3 Exchange lists for renal diets

Milk Exchanges			
Average Analysis			
Protein	4.0 g	Phosphorus	110.00 mg
Sodium	60.0 mg	Calcium	140.0 mg
Potassium	170.0 mg	Calories	varies
Chocolate milk (whole milk)	½ cup	Ice milk, hard	¾ cup
Cream, half-and-half	½ cup	Skim milk	½ cup
Evaporated whole milk, canned	¼ cup	Whole milk	½ cup

Seafood/Meat Exchanges			
Average Analysis			
Protein	6.9 g	Phosphorus	75.0 mg
Sodium	30.0 mg	Calcium	15.0 mg
Potassium	95.0 mg	Calories	75
Seafood		*Meat*	
Bluefish, cooked	1 oz	Beef, lean, cooked, rump	1 oz
Clams, soft, raw, fresh	¼ cup	Chicken, cooked	1 oz
Cod, fresh, cooked	1 oz	Lamb, lean, cooked, shoulder	1 oz
Flounder, cooked	1 oz	Liver (chicken), cooked	1 oz
Haddock, cooked	1 oz	Pork, lean, cooked, loin	1 oz
Halibut, cooked	1 oz	Turkey, cooked	1 oz

Lobster, cooked	1 oz
Ocean perch, cooked	1 oz
Oysters, raw	1 oz
Salmon, canned, cooked	1 oz
Shrimp, cooked	1 oz
Tuna, canned, low sodium	1 oz
Veal, cooked, loin	1 oz
Egg	2 oz (1 large)

Fruit Exchanges

GROUP A
Average Analysis

Protein	0.5 g	Phosphorus	12.0 mg
Sodium	1.5 mg	Calcium	15.0 mg
Potassium	115.0 mg	Calories	40-80

Apple, fresh (2½″ diameter)	1	Pears, canned, sweetened	½ cup
Applesauce, sweetened	½ cup	Pineapple, fresh or canned, sweetened	½ cup
Apricot, fresh	1 cup	Plum, fresh, prune type	2 cups
Blackberries, fresh or frozen	½ cup	Raspberries, red, fresh, canned or frozen	½ cup
Blueberries, fresh or frozen	½ cup	Strawberries, fresh, canned, unsweetened	½ cup
Cherries, fresh	½ cup	Strawberries, frozen, whole, sweetened	½ cup
Figs, fresh, medium	1 cup	Tangerine, fresh, medium	1
Grapefruit, fresh, sections	½ cup	Watermelon, diced	½ cup
Mandarin orange, sections	½ cup		

Text continued on p 222.

Table 11-3   Exchange lists for renal diets—cont'd

Fruit Exchanges—cont'd

Juices

Apple juice	½ cup
Birdseye Awake	½ cup
Grape juice	½ cup
Peach nectar	½ cup
Pear nectar	½ cup

Phosphorus	18.0 mg
Calcium	18.0 mg
Calories	40-80

GROUP B

Average Analysis

Protein	0.7 g
Sodium	3.5 mg
Potassium	215.0 mg

Honeydew, cubed, fresh	½ cup
Melon balls, frozen	½ cup
Orange sections	½ cup
Papaya, fresh, cubed	½ cup

Apricots, canned, halves, sweetened	½ cup
Banana, sliced	½ cup
Cantaloupe, cubed, fresh	½ cup
Casaba, cubed, fresh	½ cup

Cherries, red, canned	½ cup	Peach, fresh	1 medium
Figs, canned, sweetened	½ cup	Peach, canned, sweetened	½ cup
Fruit cocktail, canned, sweetened	½ cup	Pear, fresh, Bartlett	1 medium
Grapefruit sections, canned, unsweetened	½ cup	Plums, canned, sweetened	½ cup
Grapes, fresh	1 cup	Rhubarb, cooked, sweetened	½ cup
Juices			
Apricot nectar	½ cup		
Blackberry juice	½ cup		
Grapefruit juice	½ cup		
Orange juice	½ cup		
Pineapple juice	½ cup		
Prune juice	½ cup		
Tomato juice, low sodium	½ cup		

Bread/Cereal Exchanges			

GROUP A
Average Analysis

Protein	2.0 g	Phosphorus	27.0 mg
Sodium	1.0 mg	Calcium	5.0 mg
Potassium	38.0 mg	Calories	70

Continued

Table 11-3   Exchange lists for renal diets—cont'd

Bread/Cereal Exchanges—cont'd

Bread

Bread, salt-free	1 slice
Flour, wheat	2 tbsp
Grits	½ cup
Matzo	1 piece
Pasta: macaroni, spaghetti, noodles, etc.	½ cup
Popcorn, popped in oil	1 cup
Rice, white enriched, cooked	½ cup

Cereal

Cornflakes, salt-free	1 cup
Cream of wheat, regular, enriched	½ cup
Oatmeal, regular, cooked	½ cup
Puffed rice (Quaker Oats)	1 cup
Puffed wheat (Quaker Oats)	1 cup
Shredded wheat, spoon size (Kellogg's)	½ cup

GROUP B

Average Analysis

Protein	2.0 g	Phosphorus	31.0 mg
Sodium	125.0 mg	Calcium	16.0 mg
Potassium	35.0 mg	Calories	70 or more

Biscuit, homemade (2" diameter—¼" high)	1	Bran flakes, 40% (Kellogg's)	¾ cup
Bread, white, whole wheat, rye, or raisin	1 slice	Captain Crunch (Quaker Oats)	¾ cup

Bread, French	¾ slice
Cracker, graham, plain (5" × 2½")	1
Crackers, unsalted (Nabisco)	4
Doughnut, raised	1 small
Muffin, plain	1
English muffin (Thomas)	½
Pancake, homemade 1-4" diameter	1
Roll, dinner 1-2½" diameter	1
Roll, hamburger, hotdog, or kaiser	1 or ½

Cocoa Krispies (Kellogg's)	¾ cup
Rice Chex (Ralston)	¾ cup
Special K (Kellogg's)	¾ cup
Sugar Corn Pops (Kellogg's)	1½ cup
Sugar Smacks (Kellogg's)	1 cup
Crackers, animal	10

Fat Exchanges

Average Analysis

Protein	trace	Phosphorus	1.0 mg
Sodium	50.0 mg	Calcium	1.0 mg
Potassium	1.0 mg	Calories	45

Butter	1 tsp
Margarine	1 tsp
Mayonnaise	1 tsp
Salad dressing (mayonnaise type)	1 tsp

Continued.

Table 11-3 Exchange lists for renal diets—cont'd

Vegetable Exchanges

GROUP A
Average Analysis

Protein	1.0 g		Phosphorus	25.0 mg
Sodium	9.0 mg		Calcium	29.0 mg
Potassium	113.0 mg		Calories	25

Beans, cooked, green, fresh or frozen, low sodium, canned	½ cup	Eggplant, cooked, diced	½ cup
Beans, cooked wax, fresh; low sodium, canned	½ cup	Endive/Escarole, fresh, cut	½ cup
		Kale, fresh or frozen, cooked	½ cup
Beans, French cut, frozen, cooked	½ cup	Lettuce, iceberg, chopped	½ cup
Beets, canned, low sodium	½ cup	Mushrooms, fresh	½ cup
Cabbage, fresh, cooked	½ cup	Mustard greens, frozen, cooked	½ cup
Carrots, raw	½ cup	Okra, fresh, cooked, sliced	½ cup
Carrots, canned, low sodium	½ cup	Onions, fresh, raw or cooked	½ cup
Cauliflower, fresh, raw or cooked	½ cup	Peppers, green, fresh, cooked	½ cup
Celery, raw or cooked	¼ cup	Spinach, fresh, chopped, raw	½ cup
Corn, kernels, fresh, cooked	½ cup	Squash, summer, fresh, cooked	½ cup
Corn on the cob, fresh, cooked	5" cob	Tomato, medium, fresh	1 slice
		Turnips, fresh, cooked, diced	½ cup

Corn, canned, low sodium	½ cup
Cucumber, fresh peeled	½ cup
Turnip greens, frozen, cooked	½ cup

GROUP B

Average Analysis

Protein	1.7 g
Sodium	18.0 mg
Potassium	196.0 mg
Phosphorus	34.0 mg
Calcium	35.0 mg
Calories	35

Asparagus, fresh or frozen; low sodium, canned, cooked	½ cup
Beets, fresh, sliced, cooked	½ cup
Broccoli, fresh or frozen, cooked	½ cup
Brussels sprouts, fresh or frozen	½ cup
Carrots, fresh, cooked	½ cup
Cauliflower, frozen, cooked	½ cup
Chard, Swiss, cooked	½ cup
Collards, fresh, cooked	½ cup
Corn, frozen, cooked	½ cup
Dandelion greens, fresh, cooked	½ cup
French-fried potatoes	5 pieces
Kohlrabi, fresh, raw or cooked	½ cup
Mustard greens, fresh, cooked	½ cup
Peppers, green, fresh, cooked	½ cup
Potato, boiled without skin, diced	½ cup
Radishes, sliced	½ cup
Squash, winter, frozen, cooked	½ cup
Sweet potato, canned	½ cup
Tomato, canned, low sodium	½ cup
Tomato, fresh, 2" diameter	1 slice
Vegetables, mixed, frozen	½ cup

Continued.

Table 11-3 Exchange lists for renal diets—cont'd

	Calorie Supplements	

Each of the foods listed in the amounts indicated yields approximately 100 calories

GROUP A
Carbohydrates
Average Analysis

Protein	0.1 g	Phosphorus	4.0 mg
Sodium	9.0 mg	Calcium	4.0 mg
Potassium	9.0 mg	Calories	100

Bright 'N' Early	8 oz	Jelly	2 tbsp
Cranberry juice	8 oz	Jelly beans	1 oz.
Cranberry sauce	¼ cup	Low-protein bread	1 slice
Fruit ice	½ cup	Low-protein noodles:	
Ginger ale	10 oz	anellini, cooked	½ cup
Grape soda	8 oz	rigatoni, cooked	½ cup
Hard candy	1 oz	tagliatelle, cooked	½ cup

Hi-C	8 oz
Honey	1½ tsp
Jam	3 tbsp
Low-protein porridge	¾ cup
Marshmallows	4 large
Mints	37
Orange soda	8 oz.
Root beer	8 oz.
Table syrup	2 tbsp

GROUP B

Maltodextrin supplements (3 tbsp)
Average Analysis

Protein	0.0 g
Sodium	19.0 mg
Potassium	trace
Phosphorus	trace
Calcium	trace
Calories	93

Cal-Plus
Controlyte
Hy-Cal
Moducal liquid
Moducal powder
Polycose liquid
Polycose powder
Sumacal

Continued.

Table 11-3   Exchange lists for renal diets—cont'd

	Calorie Supplements—cont'd		

GROUP C
Dairy substitute
Average Analysis

Protein	0.3 g	Phosphorus	24.0 mg
Sodium	24.0 mg	Calcium	17.0 mg
Potassium	23.0 mg	Calories	100

Dessert topping, pressurized can	¾ cup	Powdered dessert topping	1 cup
Frozen dessert topping	½ cup	Rich's liquid	3 tbsp

GROUP D
Fat—salt-free (1 tbsp)
Average Analysis

Protein	trace	Phosphorus	trace
Sodium	trace	Calcium	trace
Potassium	trace	Calories	115

Unsalted butter
Unsalted margarine

Vegetable oils
Vegetable shortenings

GROUP E
Alcoholic beverages

Average Analysis

Protein	trace	
Sodium	5.0 mg	
Potassium	1.0 mg	
Phosphorus	0.0 mg	
Calcium	0.0 mg	
Calories	100	

Cordials and liqueurs	1 oz	
Gin, rum, vodka, whiskey	1½ oz	

GROUP F
Wines (3½ oz)

Average Analysis

Protein	1.5 g	
Sodium	8.0 mg	
Potassium	1.0 mg	
Phosphorus	13.0 mg	
Calcium	0.0 mg	
Calories	78	

White wine (chablis)	3½ oz	
Burgundy	3½ oz	

Modified from Walser M and others: *Nutritional management,* Philadelphia, 1984, WB Saunders.

Table 11-4   Sample diet patterns for protein-restricted diets

Exchange List	Grams of Protein/Day			
	25	40	70	100
Meat	2	3	6	9
Milk	1	2	3	3
Bread A or B	2	5	6	9
Vegetable A or B	2	2	2	3
Fruit A or B	2	3	3	4
Fat	10	9	8	10
Calorie supplements				
A	7	6	5	—
B	3	3	—	—
C	—	1	—	—
D	*	*	*	*
E or F	—	1	—	1

NOTE: If essential amino acid supplements are given, the diet can include less meat and milk and more breads, vegetables, and fruits.
*As needed for kcal.

monohydrate used in the dialysate provides 3.4 kcal/g. Thus the client receives:

$$42.5 \text{ g/L} \times 70\% \times 3.4 \text{ kcal/g} = 101 \text{ kcal/L of } 4.25\% \text{ dialysate}$$

or

$$15 \text{ g/L} \times 70\% \times 3.4 \text{ kcal/g} = 36 \text{ kcal/L of } 1.5\% \text{ dialysate}$$

Approximately 55% to 60% of total kcal should come from carbohydrate. Thus if the dialysate is providing 25% to 30% of kcal, the diet is calculated so that 30% to 35% of its kcal comes from carbohydrate.

Minerals

Calcium. A calcium intake of 1000 mg/day is needed to prevent or delay the progression of renal osteodystrophy, or demineralization of the bones, resulting from chronic acidosis and altered vitamin D metabolism. Because milk intake is usually restricted to about 1 cup/day to reduce phosphorus and protein intake, a supplement (most commonly calcium carbonate) is needed. Calcium supplements should not be given if serum phosphate is not under control because of the danger of precipitation of calcium phosphate in the kidney.

Phosphorus. Progression of renal insufficiency has been shown to be delayed with diets containing less than 600 mg of phosphorus per day. By reducing milk intake to no more than 1 cup/day, omitting soft drinks and beer, and reducing the intake of meats, poultry, fish, eggs, cereals, and breads (especially whole grains) sufficiently to comply with protein restrictions, it is usually possible to achieve this level of intake.

Aluminum hydroxide antacids are given orally when necessary to bind dietary phosphorus and prevent its absorption. They can be added to cookie dough to increase acceptability. Current trends, however, are to reduce dietary phosphorus rather than to rely routinely on phosphorus binders. Chronic use of aluminum hydroxide has resulted in aluminum toxicity, with ataxia, dementia, and exacerbation of renal osteodystrophy.

Vitamin-mineral supplementation
Water-soluble vitamins and minerals. The renal diet may be low in water-soluble vitamins, iron, and zinc. Supplements providing the RDA of these are often prescribed. Additional supplements of vitamin B_6 (5 to 10 mg/day), vitamin C (70 to 100 mg/day), and folic acid (1 mg following dialysis) are needed by dialyzed clients.

Fat-soluble vitamins. Supplements of fat-soluble vitamins (vitamins A, E, D, and K), including multivitamin preparations containing these vitamins, are not usually appropriate in the renal diet. Both parenterally and enterally fed patients have experienced toxicity of these vitamins. Products containing only water-soluble vitamins are available commercially. Some examples are Iberet (Abbott) and Beminal (Ayerst) for oral use and Berocca-C (Roche) for parenteral use.

The kidney is responsible for producing 1,25-dihydroxyvitamin D_3, the active form of vitamin D, which stimulates calcium and phosphorus absorption from the intestine. To prevent renal osteodystrophy, dialyzed clients with CRF may need calcitriol, a synthetic form of 1,25-dihydroxyvitamin D_3. Clients must consume 800 to 1200 mg of calcium per day from food or supplements for calcitriol to be effective.

Emotional support

Renal failure and subsequent dependence on dialysis creates severe emotional demands on the individual. Furthermore, the diet includes many restrictions to which the individual must adjust. Health care professionals must provide reinforcement and encouragement.

Client teaching

Dietary restrictions and their rationale

Exchange lists for diets restricted in protein, sodium, and potassium (Table 11-3) can be used in teaching dietary options to the client and family. Although sample diet patterns are provided in Table 11-4, it is essential to individualize the diet as much as possible rather than forcing the client to adhere to standardized patterns. This improves the client's quality of life and compliance with the diet.

Protein. Clients and their families need to be able to recognize sources of high biologic value (HBV) and low biologic value (LBV) protein. The following foods provide approximately 7 g of HBV protein: 1 oz of meat, fish, or poultry; 1 egg; 7 fluid oz of whole, low-fat, or skim milk. Cereals, breads, vegetables, and legumes are the primary sources of LBV protein. An individual who is allotted 34 g of HBV protein and 11 g LBV protein daily can consume the equivalent of 5 oz of meat, 3 slices of bread (2 g of protein per slice), 3 vegetables (1 g of protein per serving), and 2 fruits (0.5 g of protein per serving).

To provide a source of calories with minimal protein, low-protein pasta and bread products are sold commercially.

Kilocalories. Fats, such as unsalted butter or margarine and cooking oils, and simple carbohydrates, such as sugar, jam, syrup, hard candy, gumdrops, jelly beans, and popsicles, are widely used as calorie sources because they contribute little or no sodium, potassium, and protein. However, hyperlipidemia is common among individuals with renal failure. Individuals with hypercholesterolemia should use oils and margarine containing primarily liquid safflower, sunflower, corn, soybean, or cottonseed oil; lean meats, fish, or skinned poultry; and skim milk products. Individuals with hypertriglyceridemia should reduce their intake of simple carbohydrates. Their fat intake may need to be as high as 35% of their total kcal (as opposed to the recommended 30% for healthy individuals), since high carbohydrate intakes exacerbate hypertriglyceridemia. If hyperlipidemia does not respond to these changes, more extensive dietary modifications to control heart disease are needed (see Chapter 13).

Sodium. High-sodium foods are listed in the box on pp. 261-262. Some clients receiving dialysis have no need to avoid these, but individuals with fluid retention, edema, and hypertension do need to avoid them. Salt substitutes are not usually used because of their high potassium content.

Many over-the-counter drugs, including antacids (except magaldrate), aspirin, cough medicines, and laxatives, are high in sodium. Clients should avoid these products.

Potassium. The richest sources of potassium are meats, milk products, fruits, and vegetables. Potassium intake can be reduced by choosing canned, drained fruits or vegetables (processed without salt) rather than their fresh or frozen counterparts. Potassium content of fresh vegetables and fruits can be decreased by cutting them into small pieces and soaking or cooking them in a large amount of water, then discarding the water.

Fluid. The client or family members must learn to measure body weight and check daily for edema, especially in the lower extremities and around the eyes.

Foods that are liquids at room temperature should be counted in the fluid allowance. Gelatins can be considered to be 100% water, and ice cream is 33%, fruit ices and sherbet 50%, and custard 75% water.

Prevention of constipation

Constipation often occurs with regular use of phosphate binders. High-fiber foods (see Appendix C) and regular exercise help prevent constipation.

Nephrotic Syndrome

Pathophysiology

Nephrotic syndrome results in massive proteinuria (greater than or equal to 3.5 g/day), hypoalbuminemia, edema, and hyperlipidemia. It may result from conditions such as glomerulonephritis, diabetes mellitus, collagen vascular diseases, or sickle cell anemia.

Treatment

Drug therapy includes corticosteroids, which help lessen protein-uria, and diuretics. If massive edema is present, salt-poor albumin is given to draw fluid into the intravascular space so that it can be excreted. If hypercholesterolemia or hypertriglyceridemia are severe, drugs may be used to control them. These include bile acid-binding resins, nicotinic acid, HMGCoA reductase inhibitors (lovastatin), and fibric acids.

Nutritional Care

Goals of nutritional care are to replace protein losses, improve serum albumin levels, and reduce edema.

Assessment

Assessment is summarized in Table 11-1.

Intervention

Plan a high-protein, low-sodium diet to replace losses and decrease fluid retention

Protein intake should be greater than or equal to 1.5 g/kg/day. Children need 2 to 3 g/kg/day. Emphasis should be placed on HBV protein.

Adequate kcal should be provided to prevent use of protein for energy (35 to 50 kcal/kg/day in adults, 75 to 100 kcal/kg/day for children).

Sodium. Sodium should be limited, usually to 1000 to 2000 mg (40 to 90 mEq)/day, to help control edema. See the box on pp. 261-262.

Control of hyperlipidemia

A diet that is low in saturated fat and cholesterol (see Chapter 13) will help to reduce serum cholesterol. Because diets very low in fat could worsen hypertriglyceridemia, a moderate intake (30% to 35% of kcal) is recommended. In addition, weight reduction if the client is overweight will help reduce serum cholesterol.

Prevention of hyperglycemia

Steroid administration is commonly associated with a decrease in glucose tolerance. To control this problem, intake of simple carbohydrates such as desserts, soft drinks, and pastries should be reduced, and instead, complex carbohydrates such as breads, cereals, legumes, and starchy vegetables should be emphasized.

Supplementation
Supplementation is rarely necessary since the diet can be planned to be adequate in all nutrients.

Client teaching

Principles of high-protein, low-sodium diet; rationale for diet
The client should be encouraged to consume 2 to 3 servings of meat, fish, poultry, or legumes (2 to 3 oz per serving for children, 4 to 5 oz for adolescents and adults), and 3 to 4 servings of milk, cheese, or yogurt daily. To reduce cholesterol and saturated fat intake, lean meat, fish, and skinned poultry should be used, and dairy products should be made with skim milk. Fresh, uncured meat products and unsalted cheeses are preferable to reduce the sodium content of the diet. The box on pp. 261-262 list specific foods that should be avoided on a low-sodium diet. The client may be encouraged to know that the desire for salty foods decreases after about 3 months of following a sodium-restricted diet.

Monitoring of fluid retention
The client should be taught to check his or her weight daily, as well as to check for edema, particularly in the feet and pretibial areas and around the eyes.

Renal Calculi

Pathophysiology
Calculi, or stones, can precipitate in any part of the urinary tract. Most stones contain calcium compounds.

Treatment
Medical management includes removal of the calculi, if they are not passed spontaneously, analgesics to relieve the pain associated with calculi, and treatment of any underlying causative factors such as urinary tract infection, obstruction, or gout (excessive uric acid production).

Nutritional Care

The goals of intervention and teaching are to produce a dilute urine in which calculi are unlikely to precipitate, to limit dietary substrates that contribute to calculi formation, and to encourage mobility, which reduces release of calcium from the bones.

Assessment

Assessment is summarized in Table 11-5.

Intervention and client teaching

Increase fluid intake

Fluid intake should be at least 50 ml/kg/day to produce dilute urine, which reduces the risk of precipitation of calculi. The use of water should be encouraged, but juices, tea, coffee, and soft drinks can also provide some of the liquid. Unconscious individuals may need to receive extra fluid via a feeding tube or intravenous infusions.

Reduce dietary substrates contributing to calculi formation

Calcium. If stones are calcium-containing, restriction of calcium to approximately 400 mg/day may be of benefit. Consumption of milk, yogurt, buttermilk, or cheese must be restricted to about one serving (1 cup of milk or yogurt or 1 oz of cheese)/day.

Oxalic acid. If the stones consist of calcium oxalate, the client should avoid "megadoses" (greater than or equal to 1 g/day) of

Table 11-5 Assessment for renal calculi

Area of Concern	Significant Findings
Inadequate Fluid Intake	*History*
	Failure to consume at least 50 ml/kg of water, juice, or other fluids/day; history of previous calculi

vitamin C, since this vitamin yields oxalate when it is metabolized and could potentially contribute to calculi formation, and restrict or omit oxalate-containing foods such as cocoa, chocolate, coffee, plums, berries (except cranberries), celery, beans (dried, baked, green, and wax), peanuts, deep green, leafy vegetables (spinach, kale, and collards), rhubarb, and artichokes.

Acid ash. Foods are metabolized in the body to yield acid or alkaline "ash," or end products. The original pH of the food has no relationship to the acidity or alkalinity of its end products. Acid ash diets are sometimes used to help acidify the urine and prevent precipitation of calcium stones.

Foods to Include	Foods to Avoid
Cereals and yeast-leavened breads	Fruits and vegetables, except those specifically allowed
Meat, poultry, fish, eggs	Baking powder, baking soda
Cranberries, plums, prunes	Salt, salt substitute
Corn	Chocolate
Peanuts	

Encourage mobility

Whenever possible, individuals should have daily weight-bearing exercise. The stress of this type of exercise helps prevent hypercalciuria caused by the release of calcium from the bone. It is especially important that caregivers in long-term care and rehabilitation facilities be aware of this problem and make every attempt to assist clients to obtain exercise.

Supplementation

Individuals with a calcium-restricted diet need a daily riboflavin supplement. Those consuming an acid ash diet need a supplement providing the RDA of vitamins C and A and folic acid.

Table 11-6 Meal plan of man with CRF

Menu	Pro (g)	Na (mg)	K (mg)	Kcal
Breakfast				
Shredded wheat, ½ cup	2	1	38	70
Frozen strawberries, ½ cup	0.5	1.5	115	80
Sugar, 1 tsp	—	—	—	16
Half and half, ½ cup	4	60	170	160
Cinnamon toast:				
Low-protein bread, 1 slice	0.1	9	9	100
Margarine, 2 tsp	—	100	2	90
Sugar, 2 tsp	—	—	—	32
Snack				
Jelly beans, 1 oz	0.1	9	9	100
Lunch				
Shrimp salad:				
Shrimp, 2 oz	13.8	60	190	150
Mayonnaise, 3 tsp	—	150	3	135
Lettuce, ¼ cup shredded	0.5	4.5	57	13
Matzo, 1 piece	2	1	38	70
Margarine, 2 tsp	—	100	2	95
Cranberry juice, 1 cup	0.1	9	9	100
with Polycose powder, 1 tbsp	—	6	—	31
Tangerine, 1 medium	0.5	1.5	115	40
Snack				
Hard candy, 1 oz	0.1	9	9	100
Dinner				
Grilled chicken, 2 oz	13.8	60	190	75
Rigatoni, low protein, ½ cup	0.1	9	9	100
with margarine, 2 tsp	—	100	2	90
Stirfry:				
mushrooms, ½ cup	1	9	113	25
zucchini, ½ cup	1	9	113	25
oil, 3 tsp	—	—	—	115
Hi-C, 1 cup	0.1	9	9	100
with Polycose powder, 1 tbsp	—	6	—	31

Pro, Protein; *Na,* sodium; *K,* potassium.

Table 11-6   Meal plan of man with CRF—cont'd

Menu	Pro (g)	Na (mg)	K (mg)	Kcal
Peaches, ½ cup, canned, drained	0.7	3.5	215	75
Sugar mints, 37	0.1	9	9	100
Snack				
Low-protein toast, 2 slices	0.2	18	18	200
Margarine, 3 tsp	—	150	3	135
Honey, 1 tbsp	0.1	9	9	100
Milk, whole, ½ cup	4	9	9	100
with Polycose powder, 1 tbsp	—	6	—	31
TOTALS	44.8	979	1626	2664
HBV protein = 35.6 g Fluid = 720 ml				

CASE STUDY

Mr. J., a 75 kg man with CRF, is not receiving dialysis. His diet order is for 45 g protein (34 g HBV), 1000 mg sodium, 1650 mg potassium, 2650 + kcal, and 720 ml of fluid per day. The meal plan in Table 11-6 illustrates his usual intake.

Bibliography

Alvestrand A: Protein metabolism and nutrition in hemodialysis patients, *Contrib Nephrol* 78:102, 1990.

Gahl GM, Hain H: Nutrition and metabolism in continuous ambulatory peritoneal dialysis, *Contrib Nephrol* 84:36, 1990.

Grodstein GP and others: Glucose absorption during continuous ambulatory peritoneal dialysis, *Kidney Int* 19:564, 1981.

Grundy SM, Vega GL: Rationale and management of hyperlipidemia of the nephrotic syndrome, *Am J Med* 87(5N):3N, 1989.

Guarnieri G and others: The assessment of nutritional status in chronically uremic patients, *Contrib Nephrol* 72:73, 1989.

Hellerstein S and others: Nutritional management of children with chronic renal failure: Summary of the task force on nutritional management of children with chronic renal failure, *Pediatr Nephrol* 1:195, 1987.

Ihle BU and others: The effect of protein restriction on the progression of renal insufficiency, *N Engl J Med* 321:1773, 1989.

Mitch WS, Klahr S: *Nutrition and the kidney,* Boston, 1988, Little, Brown & Co.

Diabetes Mellitus 12

Diabetes mellitus (DM) is a disorder characterized by impaired carbohydrate, fat, and protein metabolism. Hyperglycemia and glucosuria commonly occur.

Pathophysiology

There are two types of DM:

Type I, or insulin-dependent DM (IDDM), which results from insulin deficiency caused by destruction of the beta cells of the pancreas. Most individuals with IDDM are normal weight or underweight. Classic symptoms of untreated IDDM include polyuria, polydipsia (increased fluid intake), polyphagia (increased food intake), and weight loss.

Type II, or non-insulin-dependent DM (NIDDM), is characterized by impaired pancreatic β-cell function and insulin resistance or by decreased tissue uptake of glucose in response to insulin. Insulin levels may be normal, decreased, or increased, but secretion of insulin is impaired in relation to the degree of hyperglycemia. It is usually diagnosed after age 30, and 75% of individuals with type II are obese or have a history of obesity.

DM is associated with many complications. The major chronic ones are accelerated macrovascular disease (coronary heart disease, peripheral vascular disease, and cerebrovascular disease), retinopathy, nephropathy, and neuropathy. Acute complications of type I include diabetic ketoacidosis (DKA) and hypoglycemia, and those of type II include hyperglycemic hyperosmolar nonketotic coma (HHNC), hypoglycemia, and infections such as pneumonia, cellulitis, bacteriuria, and vulvovaginitis. DKA results from insulin deficiency—too small a dosage, omission of a dose or doses, increased need for insulin, or elevation of the insulin-antagonizing counterregulatory hormones (glucagon, catecholamines, cortisol, and growth hormone), such as occurs during infection or trauma. Metabolic hallmarks of DKA include hyperglycemia, osmotic diuresis and dehydration, hyperlipidemia caused by increased lipolysis, and acidosis resulting from increased production of ketones from fatty acids (Fig. 12-1). HHNC, on the other hand, is almost always precipitated by some stressor that increases glycemia (surgery; trauma; burns; chronic disease; infection; drugs, such as corticosteroids or diuretics; dialysis). It results in marked hyperglycemia (often greater than 1000 mg/dl), absence of or only mild ketosis, elevation of serum osmolality, and dehydration.

Treatment

Treatment of diabetes hinges on a controlled diet and medications, if necessary. Many clinicians feel that near-perfect control, or maintaining the blood glucose within the normal range almost all of the time, will delay the onset, reduce the incidence, or lessen the severity of long-term complications.

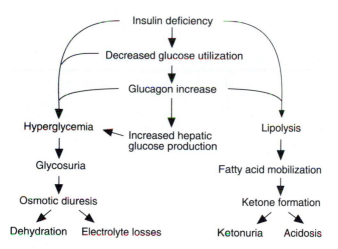

Fig. 12-1
Pathophysiology of diabetic ketoacidosis. (From *Crit Care Nurs Q,* Vol 13, No 3, p. 53, 1990, with permission of Aspen Publishers, Inc.,)

Diet

Diet is essential in management of both types of DM. Food intake must be evenly distributed throughout the day, and it must be consistent from day to day. It is especially important that clients receiving insulin coordinate their food intake with insulin activity. Furthermore, people with type II DM tend to be overweight, which is associated with insulin resistance and hyperglycemia. Glucose tolerance often improves with weight reduction.

Medications

Some individuals with DM are treated either with insulin or oral hypoglycemic agents.

Insulin

Insulin is available in three forms: short-acting, intermediate-acting, or long-acting (Table 12-1). Most insulin-dependent individuals need at least two daily doses, usually given before breakfast and before the evening meal and often providing both short- and intermediate-acting insulin. Other schedules are: (1) three injections per day — short- and intermediate-acting in the morning, short-acting before the evening meal, and intermediate-acting at bedtime, (2) multidose — injections of short-acting before each

Table 12-1   Insulin activity*

| Insulin | (Approximate Number of Hours After Injection) | | |
	Onset	Peak	Duration
Short Acting			
Regular	0.5-1	2-5	6-8
Intermediate Acting			
NPH	1.5-5	4-12	14-24
Lente	2.5-5	4-12	18-24
Long Acting			
Ultralente	6-10	10-30	24-36

*The times of onset, peak activity, and duration may vary widely from individual to individual and at different times in the same individual. Therefore these times are guidelines only. In general, human insulins have a more rapid onset, earlier peak, and shorter duration than animal (beef and pork) insulins.

meal, combined with 1 or 2 daily injections of long- or intermediate-acting, and (3) continuous subcutaneous insulin infusion
(CSII), or insulin pump therapy, which delivers short-acting insulin continuously to provide basal levels and allows the patient
to administer boluses with meals or snacks. The last two methods
are the most intensive, designed to maintain near-euglycemia.
They require the most client/family commitment for accurate
blood glucose monitoring and delivery of insulin, and they carry
the greatest risk of hypoglycemia and development of obesity.

Oral hypoglycemic agents

Oral hypoglycemic agents are used only in treatment of some
individuals with type II DM. They stimulate either insulin release
from the β-cells of the pancreas or uptake of glucose by the peripheral tissues. The duration of action and frequency of administration of oral hypoglycemic agents is shown in Table 12-2.

Monitoring of blood glucose

Self-monitoring of blood glucose (SMBG), using glucose reagent
strips, has become an important part of care and is preferred over
urine glucose measurements. Urine glucose measurements are
not useful in detecting hypoglycemia, nor are they reliable, because they are only positive when the renal threshold for glucose
is exceeded, and this can vary greatly from individual to individual. Careful teaching and continual reassessment is essential to
ensure that SMBG is accurate enough to guide treatment deci-
sions. To evaluate the need for changes in diet or insulin dosage,
monitoring should be done at least twice a day. In stable clients,
SMBG done four times a day, 3 days a week is often sufficient.
When more intensive insulin therapy is used with near-normal-

Table 12-2 Activity of oral hypoglycemic agents

Agent	Duration (hr)	Usual Doses/Day
Chlorpropamide (Diabinese)	60	1
Glipizide (Glucotrol)	12-24	1-2
Glyburide (Diaβeta, Micro-nase)	16-24	1-2
Tolazamide (Tolinase)	14-16	1-2
Tolbutamide (Orinase)	6-12	1-3

Table 12-3   Assessment of nutritional care

Area of Concern	Significant Findings
Overweight	*History*
	Type II DM; sedentary life-style; excessive insulin or kcal intake
	Physical examination
	Wt > 120% of desirable or BMI > 27.3 (women) or 27.8 (men); triceps skinfold > 95th percentile
Underweight	*History*
	Type I DM
	Physical examination
	Wt < 90% of desirable or BMI < 19.1 (women) or 20.7 (men); triceps skinfold < 5th percentile; failure of children to follow established growth patterns (see Appendix F)
	Laboratory analysis
	Urine contains > 0.5% glucose
Glucose Tolerance	
Hyperglycemia	*History*
	Type I and II DM with inadequate treatment (too low a drug dosage or too great a kcal allowance), noncompliance to the treatment regimen, or stress such as infection or surgery
	Physical examination
	Flushed skin, thirst, polyuria, poor skin turgor; drowsiness, dizziness, weakness; pain in abdomen; nausea, vomiting
	Laboratory analysis
	↑ Blood glucose; urine positive for glucose; urine positive for ketones (in ketoacidosis); ↑ serum osmolality (in nonketotic hyperosmolar coma); Hb A_{1c} > 6% (hyperglycemia over a period of several weeks)

Table 12-3   Assessment of nutritional care—cont'd

Area of Concern	Significant Findings
Glucose Tolerance—cont'd	
Hypoglycemia	*History*
	Excessive intake of insulin; unusual exertion without increased food intake; omission of scheduled meal or snack; gastroenteritis or other illness with vomiting; excessive alcohol use; use of drugs that reduce blood glucose (e.g., salicylates, chloramphenicol)
	Physical examination
	Hunger, headache; trembling, excessive perspiration, faintness, double vision
	Laboratory analysis
	↓ Blood glucose
Adequacy of Mineral Nutriture	
Zinc (Zn)	*History*
	↑ Excretion
	Physical examination
	Anorexia; hypogeusia; poor wound healing; diarrhea; dermatitis
	Laboratory analysis
	↓ Serum Zn

ization of blood glucose being the goal, SMBG must be done four to eight times daily. In all clients, more frequent monitoring is needed during times of acute illness or changes in schedules.

Nutritional Care

Assessment

Assessment is summarized in Table 12-3.

Intervention and client teaching

The goals of intervention and teaching are to control blood glucose, minimize complications, and maximize self-care abilities. The client can be aided in achieving these goals through:

Planning the diet and using the exchange lists

The primary concerns in planning and following the diet are achieving an optimum kcal intake, with intake distributed throughout the day; coordination of food intake with insulin; use of the Exchange Lists for Meal Planning; use of optimum types and amounts of carbohydrates and fat in the diet; use of alcohol and diabetic foods; and regular exercise.

Exchange Lists for Meal Planning, available from the American Diabetes Association or the American Dietetic Association, are tools for diet planning and client education. Foods are assigned to the various lists depending on their protein, carbohydrate, or fat content (Table 12-4).

In using the exchange lists to plan the diet, these steps are used:

1. Calculate the daily kcal requirement (Table 12-5).
2. Divide the kcal allowance among protein, carbohydrate, and fat; protein usually provides 12% to 20% (0.8 g/kg body weight), carbohydrates 50% to 60%, and fat 30% of kcal.
3. Determine the number of exchanges from each list that will provide the desired amount of carbohydrates, protein, and fat.

Table 12-4 Composition of food exchange groups (per exchange)

Group	Carbohydrate (g)	Protein (g)	Fat (g)	Kcal
Starch/bread	15	3	trace	80
Meat				
Lean	0	7	3	55
Medium fat	0	7	5	75
High fat	0	7	8	100
Vegetable	5	2	0	25
Fruit	15	0	0	60
Milk				
Skim	12	8	trace	80
Low fat	12	8	5	120
Whole	12	8	8	150
Fat	0	0	5	45

Table 12-5   Estimating daily kcal needs

Age	Kcal Needed/kg Desired Body Wt*
15-20 yr	
Female	29-33
Male	33-40
Adults	
Active	31-35
Moderately active	26-31
Sedentary	22-26
Sedentary >55 yr, or obese	22
Pregnancy and Lactation	
First trimester	26-35
Second and third trimester (may be reduced if woman is obese, has excessive gain, or is very sedentary)	29-37
Lactation	33-37

For children: Total needs = 1000 kcal for 1st yr + 100 kcal/yr over age 1

For 12- to 15-year-old: Female = 1500 to 2000 kcal + 100 kcal/yr over age 12. Male = 2000 to 2500 kcal + 200 kcal/yr over age 12

These are only guidelines; kcal allowances must be adjusted as necessary to compensate for growth and changes in activity or weight.

Used with permission from *Physician's guide to insulin-dependent (type 1) diabetes: diagnosis and treatment*, 1988, the American Diabetes Association.

*For an adult, consult Appendix E for the table of desirable weight or use the following rule: Ideal wt for female (kg) = (100 lb + 5 lb for every inch in ht over 5 ft) ÷ 2.2; ideal wt for male (kg) = (106 lb + 6 lb for every inch in ht over 5 ft) ÷ 2.2. For a child, use the current weight if appropriate for height and age. If the child is unusually over- or underweight, the weight for the 50th percentile for age (see the growth charts in Appendix F) can be used.

4. Assign the exchanges to meals and snacks distributed throughout the day. The client must consume the same number of exchanges each day at the same times. Each feeding should contain carbohydrates with protein or fat to slow the rate of digestion and absorption. If insulin is used, meals and snacks must be coordinated with onset of action, peak activity, and duration of activity (Table 12-1). Carbohydrates must be available during insulin activity to prevent hypoglycemia. For example, if the client takes a dose of NPH insulin at 6 AM, the client should eat breakfast by 7 or 8 AM. The client needs a midday meal and also an afternoon snack, since the peak activity will occur between noon and late afternoon. A snack before bedtime is also required because the insulin activity can last up to 24 hours. Even if the client does not receive insulin, kcal should be spread as evenly as possible among the meals, and meals should be far enough apart (4 to 5 hours) to allow blood glucose to return to basal levels before each one.

Once the diet is planned, the exchange lists are used to educate the client. The diet plan provides an individualized pattern showing how many exchanges from each list are to be eaten at each meal or snack. It is important to work with the client until he or she is skilled in determining which foods belong to each list and in planning meals utilizing the exchange lists and the individualized diet plan. The Case Study on p. 245 illustrates the use of the exchange lists in planning meals. The educator should emphasize the variety made possible by the use of the diverse foods in each list. Self-care skills are crucial for individuals with DM because of the necessity of lifelong modifications in their diets and life-styles. The exchange lists are an aid to achieving self-care, since they increase the flexibility of the diet and make meal planning easier.

Carbohydrates. Complex carbohydrates (fibers and starches) should be emphasized. A fiber intake of 35 to 40 g/day is recommended. Soluble fibers, including pectins, gums, and hemicelluloses, have a glucose- and cholesterol-lowering effect. Good sources are fruits, legumes, tubers, oats, and oat bran (see Appendix C). Insoluble fibers, which include cellulose, lignin, and some hemicelluloses, are found in bran, whole grains, and some vegetables. They have a beneficial effect on bowel function but do not improve control of blood glucose or cholesterol. The "glycemic index," which is the change in the blood glucose after consumption of a particular food in comparison with the change in blood glucose after eating white bread, is largely determined by the carbohydrate composition of the food. For individuals with DM, foods with a lower glycemic index (those which raise the blood glucose little) are preferred over those with higher indexes. Some foods with low glycemic indexes are pasta, barley, legumes, pumpernickel bread, and All Bran; foods with higher glycemic indexes include potatoes, white or whole-wheat bread, cornflakes, Müeslix, puffed rice, and shredded wheat.

Fat. Because of the prevalence of coronary heart disease in DM, saturated fats should be limited to one third or less of the fat calories, and polyunsaturated fats should provide one third of the fat calories. Cholesterol intake should be limited to 300 mg/day. Chapter 13 provides more information about modifying diets to decrease the risk of heart disease.

Alcohol. Alcohol has many disadvantages for the person with DM: it provides 7 kcal/g, which can contribute to overweight; it may exacerbate hypertriglyceridemia; and it may precipitate hypoglycemia, especially if meals are also skipped. However, if the individual desires, and the physician agrees, alcohol can be consumed. Preferably, no more than 2 oz are taken at a time, and the frequency is no more than 1 to 2 times a week. Food should be taken with alcohol or at bedtime, if alcohol is consumed late in the evening. Drinks containing sweetened mixers, liqueurs, and after-dinner drinks are not recommended because of their carbohydrate content. It is best if obese individuals omit alcohol altogether.

Sodium. It is recommended that individuals with DM consume no more than 3 g of sodium daily because of their propensity for hypertension. The box on pp. 261-262 provides guidelines for this level of sodium restriction.

Sweeteners and diabetic foods. Nutritive, or kcal-containing, and nonnutritive, or kcal-free, sweeteners can be used in moderation by individuals with DM.

Nutritive sweeteners. Nutritive sweeteners include sucrose (table sugar), fructose, and sorbitol, a sugar alcohol. Small amounts of these can be used when the diet is planned to incorporate them. Fructose and sorbitol are frequently used in "sugar-free" or "diabetic" commercial products, but these products can be as high in kcal as similar sugar-containing products and thus cannot be used freely. Also, excessive amounts of sorbitol can cause abdominal cramping and diarrhea.

Nonnutritive sweeteners. Nonnutritive sweeteners on the market are aspartame and saccharin. Powdered aspartame and saccharin are packaged with dextrose or dextrin and provide approximately 4 kcal/packet. This must be considered if these products are used often. Individuals with phenylketonuria should not use aspartame (NutraSweet).

Exercise

Although it is not without risks (e.g., hypoglycemia), regular exercise (continuous activity lasting at least 20 to 30 minutes and performed at least 3 to 4 days a week) improves insulin sensitivity and sometimes glucose tolerance in individuals with both type I and II DM. In addition, exercise promotes weight loss in overweight individuals. The guidelines in Chapter 5, for becoming and remaining physically fit, are appropriate for individuals with DM, but these individuals should undertake an exercise program only under a physician's supervision.

It is best if individuals with type I monitor their blood glucose before, during, and after exercise to determine whether insulin or food intake need to be adjusted. Moderate exercise lasting 30 to 45 minutes or less rarely requires adjustment in insulin, but often a small snack is needed just before exercise, especially if blood glucose is less than or equal to 80 mg/dl. For longer periods of exercise, snacks are usually needed every 30 to 60 minutes. Either 15 to 20 g of rapidly-absorbed carbohydrate, such as fruit or juice, or a combination of protein with complex carbohydrate, such as half a meat or milk exchange with half a bread exchange, works well. Some individuals become hypoglycemic several hours after exercise ends, and they need a snack or meal after exercise. During sustained, intensive activities such as backpacking or cross-country skiing, a decrease in insulin dosage is usually needed. Individuals with DM must take care to consume enough fluid before, during, and after exercise to prevent dehydration.

Coping with acute illness

All individuals will have occasional bouts of illness with vomiting, which can have serious consequences for individuals with type I DM. These individuals should be instructed to con-

Foods and Fluids for Sick Days*

Foods	Replacement Fluids
⅓ cup regular gelatin dessert	¾ cup regular ginger ale
½ cup vanilla ice cream	½ cup regular cola or lemon-lime soda
¼ cup sherbet or sorbet	½ cup orange juice
3 squares graham crackers	1 frozen fruit juice bar
7 saltine crackers	
1 cup cream soup (prepared with milk)	
½ cup custard	

*Each serving provides approximately 15 g carbohydrate.

tinue taking insulin when acute illnesses occur; the physician usually provides guidelines as to the amount. Blood glucose and urine ketones need to be monitored as often as every 2 to 3 hours. Although the client may not be able to adhere to the usual meal pattern, he or she needs to consume 10 to 20 g carbohydrate every 1 to 2 hours. When vomiting occurs, small amounts of kcal-containing liquids taken every 15 to 20 minutes will help to prevent dehydration and replace sodium, potassium, and kcal. Some suitable foods are listed in the accompanying box. If it is impossible to take and retain carbohydrate-containing foods and fluids for 4 hours or more, or if blood glucose is difficult to control or ketonuria is present, the client should notify the physician.

Pregnancy

Hormonal changes during pregnancy, including elevations of cortisol and production of human placental lactogen by the placenta, contribute to glucose intolerance, insulin resistance, and lipolysis. The incidence of major congenital malformations may be as high as 20% to 25% among women with poor control during the first trimester. Thus intensive therapy to maintain near-normal blood glucose levels is preferred during pregnancy; it is best if intensive therapy begins before conception, since most organogenesis occurs very early in pregnancy. Normal-weight women need approximately 30 to 35 kcal/kg/day, while obese women are often prescribed approximately 25 kcal/kg/day. The kcal are usually divided as follows: 10% at breakfast, 30% at lunch, 30% at the evening meal, and 30% in snacks. Even moderate periods of fasting (such as sleeping through the night) are associated with accelerated production of ketones in pregnancy. Therefore a bedtime snack is usually advisable.

Minimizing the occurrence and complications of hypoglycemia or hyperglycemia

Hypoglycemia. Hypoglycemia occurs in both types of DM. Instruction should be planned to help the client:

1. Be aware of and avoid precipitating factors: failing to eat scheduled meals and snacks, eating meals or snacks late, vomiting or poor food intake during acute illness, prolonged or intense physical activity without a compensatory increase in carbohydrate intake or decrease in insulin dosage, impaired hepatic gluconeogenesis with alcohol intake, and impaired mentation and self-care skills, resulting from alcohol intoxication or illicit drug use.
2. Recognize signs and symptoms of hypoglycemia: hunger, irritability, headache, shakiness, sweating and altered neurologic status ranging from drowsiness to unconsciousness and convulsions.
3. Correct hypoglycemia if it occurs; the client should have a carbohydrate source, such as glucose tablets, granulated sugar, or hard candy, always available for use if symptoms occur; it is a good idea for individuals with DM to wear a "Medic-Alert" bracelet so that treatment can be given if the client becomes confused or unconscious.

Diabetic ketoacidosis. Instruction should help the client:

1. Be aware of precipitating factors, such as acute infectious illnesses or failure to take the prescribed dosage of insulin or oral hypoglycemic agents
2. Recognize signs and symptoms: thirst, warm dry skin, nausea and vomiting, "fruity" smelling breath, pain in abdomen, drowsiness, and polyuria
3. Check blood glucose if the symptoms occur, and obtain medical treatment if blood glucose is excessively elevated

Hyperglycemic hyperosmolar nonketotic coma. Instruction should make the client aware of precipitating factors, such as infections or other stress. In addition, the client and family should be able to recognize the symptoms: excessive thirst, polyuria, dehydration, shallow respirations, and altered sensorium. If SMBG is practiced, blood glucose should be checked if these symptoms occur; medical attention should be obtained if blood glucose is high or if the symptoms occur in a client who does not use SMBG.

Follow-up instruction

The individual with DM should meet with a dietitian every 6 months for adjustment of the diet and meal pattern to accommodate growth and changes in weight and life-style. The dietitian can also reinforce the diet instruction, assist in handling special circumstances (eating out or eating fast foods, ethnic foods, or convenience foods), and suggest resources such as cookbooks.

CASE STUDY

Tables 12-6 and 12-7 illustrate the meal plan and 1 day's food intake for a moderately active young man with type II DM. His weight, which is close to the desirable weight for his height, is 81 kg.

Table 12-6   Diet for a man with type II DM

Group	No. Exchanges	Carbohydrate (g)	Protein (g)	Fat (g)	Kcal
Starch/bread	15	225	45	15*	1200
Meat, medium fat	5	0	35	25	375
Vegetable	6	30	12	0	150
Fruit	4	60	0	0	240
Milk, low fat	2	24	16	10	240
Fat	5	0	0	25	225
TOTALS		339 (56%)	108 (18%)	75 (28%)	2430

*Because of the large number of servings, the starch/bread group contributes to the fat intake. For further information regarding calculation of the diet, see Powers MA: *Nutrition guide for professionals: diabetes education and meal planning,* Alexandria, Va, and Chicago, 1988, The American Diabetes Association, Inc, and The American Dietetic Association.

Table 12-7 Sample daily intake

Meal	No. Exchanges
Breakfast	
1 cup bran flakes	2 starch
¾ cup blueberries	1 fruit
1 whole-grain bagel	2 starch
1 tbsp cream cheese	1 fat
1 cup 2% milk	1 low-fat milk
Lunch	
1 cup bean soup	1 starch + 1 meat + 1 vegetable
Tuna-stuffed tomato	
¼ cup water-packed tuna	1 meat
1 large tomato	1 vegetable
1 tsp mayonnaise	1 fat
1 cup cucumbers and onions marinated in vinegar	1 vegetable
8 rye crackers	2 starch
1 small pear	1 fruit
Afternoon Snack	
1 cup low-fat yogurt	1 low-fat milk
1 sliced nectarine	1 fruit
1 bran muffin	1 starch + 1 fat
Dinner	
½ cup vegetable juice	1 vegetable
2 oz roast pork loin	2 meat
1 cup sweet potato	3 starch
2 tsp margarine	2 fat
1 cup broccoli, stir-fried in nonstick spray	2 vegetable
½ cup baked beans	2 starch
Bedtime Snack	
2 slices whole-wheat bread	2 starch
1 tbsp peanut butter	1 meat
1 tbsp sugar-free jelly	Free
2 tangerines	1 fruit

Bibliography

Beebe CA and others: Nutrition management for individuals with non-insulin-dependent diabetes in the 1990s: a review by the Diabetes Care and Education dietetic practice group, *J Am Diet Assoc* 91:196, 1991.

Brink SJ: Pediatric, adolescent, and young-adult nutrition issues in IDDM, *Diabetes Care* 11:192, 1988.

Diabetes mellitus and exercise, *Diabetes Care* 14(suppl 2):36, 1991.

Nutritional recommendations and principles for individuals with diabetes mellitus, *Diabetes Care* 14(suppl 2):20, 1991.

Exchange lists for meal planning, Alexandria, Va, and Chicago, 1989, American Diabetes Association, Inc, and American Dietetic Association.

Graves L III: Diabetic ketoacidosis and hyperosmolar hyperglycemic nonketotic coma, *Crit Care Nurs Q* 13(3):50, 1990.

Jenkins DJA, Wolever TMS, Jenkins AL: Starchy foods and glycemic index, *Diabetes Care* 11:149, 1988.

O'Connell KA and others: Symptom beliefs and actual blood glucose in type II diabetes, *Res Nurs Health* 13:145, 1990.

Physician's guide to insulin-dependent (type I) diabetes: diagnosis and treatment, Alexandria, Va, 1988, American Diabetes Association.

Physician's guide to non-insulin-dependent (type II) diabetes: diagnosis and treatment, ed 2, Alexandria, Va, 1988, American Diabetes Association.

Heart Disease

13

Heart disease, the leading cause of death in the United States, encompasses a variety of conditions, including atherosclerosis, hypertension, and congestive heart failure.

Coronary Heart Disease

Pathophysiology

Coronary heart disease (CHD) occurs when plaques containing lipoproteins, cholesterol, tissue debris, and calcium form on the intima, or interior surface of blood vessels. The plaques roughen the intima, and platelets are attracted to the roughened areas, forming clots. When the plaques enlarge sufficiently to occlude the blood flow, tissues are deprived of oxygen and nutrients, creating an area of infarct. CHD is manifested when a myocardial infarction (MI) occurs or when there is myocardial ischemia such as angina pectoris.

Serum cholesterol is carried by several lipoproteins classified by their density. In order of increasing density, the lipoproteins are: chylomicrons, very low-density lipoproteins (VLDLs), low-density lipoproteins (LDLs), and high-density lipoproteins (HDLs). LDLs carry the most cholesterol and are the most atherogenic. HDLs reduce the risk from CHD by transporting cholesterol from the tissues to the liver, where it is metabolized and excreted. Adults can be classified as at risk for CHD on the basis of total and LDL-cholesterol levels (Table 13-1).

Risk factors for coronary heart disease: In addition to LDL-cholesterol, risk of CHD is increased by other factors: male sex, CHD before age 55 in a parent or sibling, smoking more than 10 cigarettes per day, hypertension, HDL-cholesterol concentration below 35 mg/dl, diabetes mellitus, history of cerebrovascular or

Table 13-1   Classification of serum cholesterol levels

Classification	Serum Cholesterol (mg/dl)
Total Cholesterol	
Desirable	<200
Borderline-high	200-239
High	≥240
LDL-Cholesterol*	
Desirable	<130
Borderline-high risk	130-159
High risk	≥160

From the National Cholesterol Education Program: report of the expert panel on detection, evaluation, and treatment of high blood cholesterol in adults, NIH Pub No
89-2925, Washington, DC, 1989, US Department of Health and Human Services.
*Routinely measured only in individuals with high total cholesterol levels and indi-
viduals with borderline-high total cholesterol plus definite CHD *or* two other risk
factors for CHD (p. 248). From the lipoprotein analysis, LDL-cholesterol can be
calculated by using the following equation:
LDL-cholesterol = total cholesterol − HDL-cholesterol − (triglycerides/5)

peripheral vascular disease, and being more than 30% overweight.

Treatment

Dietary modifications are a part of treatment for all individuals
with CHD, since reduction of saturated fat and cholesterol intake
helps reduce serum cholesterol. In severe cases, drug therapy
may be needed. Commonly used drugs are the bile acid seques-
trants cholestyramine and colestipol; nicotinic acid, which lowers
total and LDL-cholesterol, as well as triglycerides; inhibitors of
cholesterol synthesis, such as lovastatin; fibric acid derivatives
such as gemfibrozil and clofibrate, which reduce triglycerides and
raise HDL-cholesterol; and prubocol, which reduces LDL-cholesterol and also HDL-cholesterol.

Nutritional Care

Goals of nutritional care are to reduce the risk of CHD in adults
with elevated LDL-cholesterol levels by:
  1. Reducing LDL-cholesterol levels below 130 mg/dl in indi-

Table 13-2   Assessment in heart disease

Areas of Concern	Significant Findings
Overweight	*History* Excessive kcal intake; sedentary life-style *Physical examination* Wt > 120% of ideal or BMI >27.8 (men) or >27.3 (women); triceps skinfold >95th percentile for age and sex
Underweight (seen primarily in congestive heart failure)	*History* Poor intake because of dyspnea or fatigue; impaired absorption because of inadequate bowel perfusion; increased kcal needs if dyspneic or suffering from concomitant infection *Physical examination* Wt <90% of ideal or BMI <19.1 (women) or <20.7 (men) or ht or wt <5th percentile for age (children); triceps skinfold <5th percentile for age and sex
Elevated serum lipid levels	*History* Daily use of foods high in saturated fat and cholesterol; sedentary life-style; family history of hyperlipidemia; cultural food pattern that emphasizes foods high in fat or cholesterol (e.g., Southern diet with regular use of corn bread, biscuits, fried meats and vegetables, and bacon drippings or salt pork as seasonings) *Physical examination* Xanthomas, or yellowish plaques deposited on the skin (not found in the majority of the individuals) *Laboratory analysis* ↑ Total serum cholesterol; HDL <35 mg/dl; LDL-cholesterol >130 mg/dl

Table 13-2   Assessment in heart disease—cont'd

Areas of Concern	Significant Findings
Elevated blood pressure	*History*
	Daily use of high-sodium foods and salt at the table; psychosocial stress; family history of hypertension; cultural food patterns emphasizing foods high in sodium (e.g., kosher diet)
	Physical examination
	Edema; elevated blood pressure

viduals with definite CHD or two CHD risk factors (p. 248) other than high-risk levels of LDL-cholesterol

2. Reducing LDL-cholesterol levels below 160 mg/dl in individuals with neither definite CHD nor two risk factors other than high levels of LDL-cholesterol

Reduction of saturated fat and cholesterol intake, along with weight reduction if the individual is overweight, are the means used to achieve these goals. Although control of cholesterol levels is also desirable in children, specific goals for them have not yet been published.

Assessment

Assessment is summarized in Table 13-2.

Intervention and client teaching

Through the following measures, clients can achieve the nutritional goals safely.

Recognize the need to make permanent diet and life-style changes to reduce risk

Permanent diet and life-style changes include achieving weight control, decreasing dietary fat and cholesterol, not smoking, and developing constructive ways of coping with stress. These changes may be better accepted and less overwhelming if clients are counseled to make changes gradually. For instance, they can be guided in selecting one or two habits, such as smoking cigarettes or eating 8 or more ounces of red meat daily, and making a plan to alter those. Once these initial changes are made, the client can select a few more habits to work on.

Reduce fat and cholesterol in the diet

The National Cholesterol Education Program has advocated that individuals with LDL-cholesterol greater than or equal to 160 mg/dl and those with borderline-high-risk LDL-cholesterol who also have definite CHD or two other risk factors (p. 248) should receive intensive dietary therapy. A two-step diet program to reduce saturated fat and cholesterol intake has been established (Table 13-3). Total fat intake is limited, as well, to aid in weight reduction. Initially, the client receives counseling regarding Step-One, which reduces the most common and obvious sources of saturated fatty acids and cholesterol in the diet and can be implemented without drastic diet or life-style changes for most clients. If, after adhering to the diet for 3 months, the client does not succeed in lowering LDL-cholesterol to the desirable level, he or she may progress to the Step-Two Diet. While the physician and nurse can often provide education regarding the Step-One Diet, referral to a dietitian is valuable for clients who have difficulty adhering to the diet or who have a disappointing response to the diet. The dietitian's help is particularly needed by clients who progress to the Step-Two Diet.

Diet teaching should emphasize the fact that the changes do not have to result in a restrictive or unpalatable diet. Tasty, attractive dishes can be readily prepared within the guidelines. Table 13-4 outlines the Step-One Diet modifications used to lower blood cholesterol. Additional information useful in teaching is provided below. The American Heart Association has published a detailed manual for clients who need more specific guidelines regarding both the Step-One and Step-Two Diets.[1]

Specific information about each food grouping

1. *Meats:* No more than 6 oz of lean meat, chicken, turkey, and fish daily. A 3 oz serving of meat is approximately the size of a deck of cards. Lean cuts of meat should be used: extra-lean ground beef, sirloin tip, round steak, rump roast, arm roast or center-cut ham, loin chops, and tenderloin. Trim away all visible fat before cooking, and pour off fat after browning beef. The skin and underlying fat should be removed from poultry before cooking. The organ meats, including brains, liver, heart, kidney, and

Table 13-3 Dietary therapy of high blood cholesterol

Nutrient	Recommended Intake	
	Step-One Diet	Step-Two Diet
Total fat	Less than 30% of Total Calories	
Saturated fatty acids	Less than 10% of total calories	Less than 7% of total calories
Polyunsaturated fatty acids	Up to 10% of total calories	
Monounsaturated fatty acids	10 to 15% of total calories	
Carbohydrates	50 to 60% of total calories	
Protein	10 to 20% of total calories	
Cholesterol	Less than 300 mg/day	Less than 200 mg/day
Total calories	To achieve and maintain desirable weight	

From the National Cholesterol Education Program: Report of the expert panel on detection, evaluation, and treatment of high blood cholesterol in adults, NIH Pub No 89-2925, Washington, DC, 1989, U.S. Department of Health and Human Services.

Table 13-4   Recommended diet modifications to lower blood cholesterol: the Step-One Diet

Food Group	Choose	Decrease
Fish, chicken, turkey, and lean meats	Fish, poultry without skin, lean cuts of beef, lamb, pork or veal, shellfish	Fatty cuts of beef, lamb, pork; spare ribs, organ meats, regular cold cuts, sausage, hot dogs, bacon, sardines, roe
Skim and low-fat milk, cheese, yogurt, and dairy substitutes	Skim or 1% fat milk (liquid, powdered, evaporated)	Whole milk (4% fat): regular, evaporated, condensed; cream, half-and-half, 2% milk, imitation milk products, most nondairy creamers, whipped toppings
	Buttermilk	
	Nonfat (0% fat) or low-fat yogurt	Whole-milk yogurt
	Low-fat cottage cheese (1% or 2% fat)	Whole-milk cottage cheese (4% fat)
	Low-fat cheeses, farmer, or pot cheeses (all of these should be labeled no more than 2-6 g fat/oz)	All natural cheeses (e.g., blue, roquefort, camembert, cheddar, swiss)
		Low-fat or "light" cream cheese, low-fat or "light" sour cream
		Cream cheeses, sour cream
	Sherbet	Ice cream
	Sorbet	
Eggs	Egg whites (2 whites = 1 whole egg in recipes), cholesterol-free egg substitutes	Egg yolks

	Choose	Decrease
Fruits and vegetables	Fresh, frozen, canned, or dried fruits and vegetables	Vegetables prepared in butter, cream, or other sauces
Breads and cereals	Homemade baked goods using unsaturated oils sparingly, angel food cake, low-fat crackers, low-fat cookies	Commercial baked goods: pies, cakes, doughnuts, croissants, pastries, muffins, biscuits, high-fat crackers, high-fat cookies
	Rice, pasta	Egg noodles
	Whole-grain breads and cereals (oatmeal, whole wheat, rye, bran, multigrain, etc.)	Breads in which eggs are major ingredient
Fats and oils	Baking cocoa	Chocolate
	Unsaturated vegetable oils: corn, olive, rapeseed (canola oil), safflower, sesame, soybean, sunflower	Butter, coconut oil, palm oil, palm kernel oil, lard, bacon fat
	Margarine or shortening made from one of the unsaturated oils listed above	
	Diet margarine	
	Mayonnaise, salad dressings made with unsaturated oils listed above	Dressings made with egg yolk
	Low-fat dressings	
	Seeds and nuts	Coconut

From the National Cholesterol Education Program: Report of the expert panel on detection, evaluation, and treatment of high blood cholesterol in adults, NIH Pub No 89-2925, Washington, DC, 1989, U.S. Department of Health and Human Services.

sweetbreads, are especially high in cholesterol and should be used rarely. Processed meats, such as regular hot dogs (even if made from turkey), cold cuts, bacon, and sausage are high in fat and should be avoided. Shrimp are relatively high in cholesterol but low in fat and can be used occasionally.

Some fish (e.g., salmon, mackerel, herring, tuna, and swordfish) are good sources of "omega-3" fatty acids. These fatty acids have been reported to reduce serum triglycerides and to inhibit platelet aggregation and inflammation, which contributes to CHD, although they have no effect on LDL-cholesterol. There is no evidence that fish oil supplements are of value in reducing the risk of CHD. However, in epidemiologic studies, frequent consumption of fish, whether it is a type that is rich in omega-3 fatty acids or not, is associated with reduced risk of CHD.

To avoid having servings seem scanty and to emphasize the importance of shifting away from planning the meal around meat, combine small amounts of meat with larger amounts of rice, pasta, or vegetables to make more filling entrees. Dried beans and peas and tofu are low-fat, high-protein, and cholesterol-free and can be used to replace meats.

2. *Dairy products:* At least two servings of skim milk or the equivalent daily. Milk fat is largely saturated, and therefore milk products made with skim milk should be emphasized. Natural and processed cheeses are generally rich in fat. Low-fat or nonfat cottage cheese made with skim milk, and synthetic cheeses made with vegetable oils are good choices. Low-fat cottage cheese or yogurt can be substituted for sour cream in dips and salad dressings or on potatoes.

3. *Eggs:* Limit yolks to three per week on the Step-One Diet and one per week for the Step-Two Diet. Egg yolks are rich in fat and cholesterol. Egg whites are free of fat and cholesterol and can be used frequently. Cholesterol-free egg substitutes are also acceptable.

4. *Fruits and vegetables:* Use liberally. Fruits and vegetables provide color, texture, vitamins, minerals, and fiber and should be a part of every meal. Plant products do not contain cholesterol, and almost all fruits and vegetables are

low in fat. Exceptions are avocados and olives, which are discussed below under fats and oils. Frying or adding butter, cream, or cheese sauces increases the fat content of fruits and vegetables to undesirable levels.

5. *Breads and cereals:* Increase intake to replace meats in the diet. Breads and cereals are good sources of vitamins and minerals, and whole grains provide fiber, as well. However, commercial bakery items and even some cereals (e.g., granola) are often high in fat. In addition, quick breads (muffins, banana and other fruit or nut breads, corn bread, pancakes, and waffles) contain significant amounts of egg. Homemade products made with egg whites or egg substitutes and the fats and oils allowed are acceptable.

6. *Fats and oils:* Limit to 6 to 8 tsp/day. Fats and oils high in saturated fat and/or cholesterol should be avoided as much as possible. Butter, lard, and other animal fats are high in both saturated fat and cholesterol. Vegetable fats are cholesterol-free, but coconut, palm, and palm kernel oil are high in saturated fat. These are commonly used in bakery products, processed foods, popcorn oils, and nondairy creamers.

"Unsaturated" fats are those containing one (monounsaturated) or more than one (polyunsaturated) double bond. They do not raise blood cholesterol, but they are high in kcal and low in most other nutrients. Margarine made from unsaturated oils (Table 13-4) is preferable to butter. However, both margarine and shortening are partially hydrogenated and thus contain *trans* fatty acids, which are not naturally occurring and should not be taken in excess. (On the Step-Two Diet, shortening should be avoided altogether.)

Most nuts and seeds contain unsaturated fats, but their high fat content makes them high in kcal. Thus 1 tbsp of nuts or 2 tsp of peanut butter is equivalent to 1 tsp of fat. Other foods equivalent to 1 tsp of fat are: regular salad dressings, 1 tbsp; mayonnaise or diet margarine, 2 tsp; olives, 5 large or 10 small; and avocado, one-eighth medium.

Preparation methods

Cooking methods that add little or no fat are preferred. Steaming, baking, broiling, microwaving, frying in a nonstick pan, or stir-frying in a small amount of fat are all acceptable. Soups, stews, and broths should be prepared in advance so that they can be chilled after cooking and the fat layer that forms on top can be skimmed off.

Snacks and desserts. Fruits and fruit ices make good desserts and snacks. Chips and high-fat crackers should be avoided. Appropriate substitutes include melba toast, Ry Krisp, graham crackers, bagels, English muffins, and vegetables. Sherbet, angel food cake, fruit-flavored gelatin, low-fat cookies such as gingersnaps and Newton cookies, and occasionally low-fat frozen yogurt or ice milk are also acceptable. Cakes, pies, and cookies made with egg whites, egg substitutes, skim milk, and unsaturated oils can be used occasionally.

Eating out. Avoid fried foods; in fast-food restaurants, choose from the salad bar or from grilled items. Order foods without sauces, butter, and sour cream. Use margarine rather than butter, and use only small amounts. Ask that salad dressings be served on the side, and use limited amounts. Avoid high-fat toppings such as bacon, chopped eggs, and cheese; eat only small amounts of sunflower seeds and olives.

Convenience foods. Many convenience foods are high in saturated fats or cholesterol. One approach to this problem is to prepare casseroles, breads, and desserts with low-fat, low-cholesterol ingredients in advance and to freeze them for occasions when preparation time is short. Also, several manufacturers now make low-fat, low-kcal frozen entrees and meals.

Increase intake of dietary fibers

"Soluble" fibers, including pectin, gums, and some hemicelluloses are hypocholesterolemic. They are found in oat bran, barley, legumes, and many fruits and vegetables. "Insoluble" fibers such as cellulose, found in wheat bran, have no such effect. A dietary fiber intake of 25 to 30 g/day is desirable. Appendix C provides a listing of dietary fiber content of common foods.

Take steps to reduce hypertriglyceridemia (if applicable)

Hypertriglyceridemia can be defined as fasting plasma triglyceride levels greater than 500 mg/dl. "Borderline hypertriglyceridemia" includes levels between 250 and 500 mg/dl. Although hypertriglyceridemia has been found to be positively associated with CHD, it is not as highly predictive of CHD as the other risk factors (p. 248). Nevertheless, very high triglyceride levels are associated with abdominal pain and pancreatitis, with significant morbidity and even mortality.

Weight reduction and increased physical activity will help to correct borderline hypertriglyceridemia. The Step-One Diet can be used to reduce fat intake to approximately 30% of kcal, which will aid in weight reduction. Limiting alcohol intake also helps reduce serum triglycerides.

For individuals with higher triglyceride levels, especially if greater than 1000 mg/dl, a very low-fat diet (10% to 20% of total kcal) will help reduce the risk of pancreatitis. In clients with diabetes, good control of glycemia usually reduces hypertriglyceridemia. Elimination of alcohol intake is also beneficial.

Achieve or maintain ideal weight
Chapter 19 provides information about weight control. Weight loss often increases HDL and decreases triglyceride levels.

Perform regular aerobic exercise
Chapter 5 gives guidelines for developing physical fitness. HDL levels often increase with regular exercise, and exercise is a useful adjunct to weight loss programs. Individuals with a history of CHD and those over age 40 need a physician's evaluation before beginning an exercise program.

Facilitate cardiac rest in the client with an acute myocardial infarction
If the CHD client experiences an acute myocardial infarction (MI), efforts are made to avoid stressing the heart as much as possible during the early recovery period. Generally, a low-kcal (1200 to 1500) diet with small meals is used to avoid the metabolic demands caused by larger intakes. The diet should be low in saturated fat and cholesterol, and it is generally moderately low in sodium to control any tendency for edema and congestive heart failure to develop. Foods at temperature extremes are generally avoided. Recent research indicates that most clients tolerate cold fluids (ice water) well, but a subset of clients has electrocardiographic changes after drinking ice water.

Hypertension

Hypertension is usually defined as a blood pressure of 160/95 or greater. Normotension is a blood pressure less than 140/90. Measurements between these two values reflect borderline hypertension.

Pathophysiology

Increases in blood volume, heart rate, or peripheral vascular resistance lead to hypertension. Ninety percent of cases are "essential" hypertension—that is, no cause is known. Hypertension is a risk factor for cerebral vascular accident (CVA), myocardial infarction, and renal failure.

Treatment

Drugs used in treatment of hypertension include diuretics, β-adrenergic blocking agents such as propanolol, α-adrenergic blocking agents such as phentolamine, and antihypertensive agents such as methyldopa. Diet and life-style changes are also important in treatment of hypertension.

Nutritional Care

The goal of nutritional care is to establish and maintain normotension.

Assessment

Assessment is summarized in Table 13-2.

Intervention and client teaching

Intervention and teaching include the following measures.

Recognition of the need to make diet and life-style changes

The client should participate in assessing personal diet, exercise pattern, and weight and in planning strategies for permanent change. Gradual changes may be more successful than sweeping ones.

Reduction of sodium intake

Sodium restriction helps lower blood pressure in many individuals with hypertension. The physician usually determines the level of restriction by the severity of hypertension. The box below demonstrates levels of restriction. Clients may be encouraged to know that the taste preference for salt decreases after about 3 months on a sodium-restricted diet.

Low-sodium seasonings. Herbs and spices (except high-sodium ones such as celery seeds; parsley flakes; and garlic, onion, or celery salts) and flavorings such as lemon juice can be used to replace salt. Some examples include:

Foods	Suggested Seasonings
Beef	Horseradish, mustard, cloves, pepper, bay, garlic
Poultry	Curry, sage, coriander, ginger, tarragon
Stews	Bay, garlic, basil, oregano, thyme
Vegetables	Mace, nutmeg, dill, rosemary, savory

Foods to be Avoided on Sodium-Restricted Diets*

Mild Restriction (2-3 g/day)

Do not use:

Salt at the table (use salt lightly in cooking; 1 tsp salt ≈ 2300 mg sodium)

Smoked, cured, or salt-preserved foods such as salted fish, ham, bacon, sausage, cold cuts, corned beef, kosher meats, sauerkraut, olives

Salted snack foods such as chips, pretzels, popcorn, nuts, crackers

Seasonings such as onion, garlic, and celery salt and monosodium glutamate, bouillon, and meat tenderizers; condiments such as catsup, prepared mustard, relishes, soy sauce, Worcestershire sauce, and pickles

Cheese, peanut butter

Moderate Restriction (1 g/day)

Do not use:

Salt in cooking or at the table
Any food prohibited under "Mild Restriction"

---

*Low-sodium versions of many of the products are available. These may be included in the diet.

Continued.

Foods to be Avoided on Sodium-Restricted Diets*— cont'd

Moderate Restriction (1g/day)— cont'd

Do not use:

Canned meat or fish, vegetables, and vegetable juice (except low-sodium)

Frozen fish fillets, peas, limas, mixed vegetables, or any frozen vegetables to which salt has been added

More than one serving of any of these in a day: artichoke, beet greens, beets, carrots, celery, dandelion greens, kale, mustard greens, spinach, Swiss chard, turnips

Buttermilk

Regular bread, rolls, crackers

Dry cereals (except puffed wheat), puffed rice, and shredded wheat

Instant oatmeal and grits

Shellfish (except oysters)

Salted butter or margarine, commercial salad dressings and mayonnaise

Regular baking powder, baking soda, or any products containing them (e.g., biscuits, corn bread, muffins, cookies, cakes); self-rising flour

Prepared mixes such as breads, muffins, pancakes, entrees, cake, pudding

Frozen waffles and French toast

Water treated with a water softener

Bottled water (mineral, sparkling, spring, or other waters), unless information obtained from the bottler indicates it is low in sodium

Regular or diet soft drinks, unless information obtained from the bottler indicates them to be low in sodium

Strict Restriction (0.5 g/day)

Do not use:

Any food listed under Mild or Moderate Restrictions

More than 2 cups milk/day

Commercial foods made with milk, such as ice milk, ice cream, shakes

Artichokes, beet greens, beets, carrots, celery, dandelion greens, kale, mustard greens, spinach, Swiss chard, turnips

Commercial candy, except hard candies, gumdrops, or jelly beans (limit to 10 pieces daily)

The American Heart Association can provide low-sodium recipes, including one for a spice mixture that serves as a salt substitute. Commercial salt substitutes contain potassium chloride, rather than sodium chloride. The physician may allow their use if the client has no renal impairment.

Kosher diets. Koshered meats contain 2 to 3 times as much sodium as nonkoshered. Soaking meats in tap water for 1 hour, then discarding the water and cooking the food is effective in reducing the sodium content, while still adhering to the Jewish food laws.

Medications. Some drugs, including antibiotics (especially the penicillins), sulfonamides, and barbiturates, are high in sodium. Their sodium content should be considered for the individual who is following a sodium-restricted diet. The pharmacist can provide information about the sodium content of these drugs. Clients should be cautioned about using over-the-counter medications without physician approval. Antacids (except those containing magaldrate), aspirins, cough medicines, and laxatives are often high in sodium.

Limitation of alcohol intake

Hypertensive individuals should limit their alcohol to 1 oz/day, which is equivalent to 2 oz of 100-proof whiskey, 8 oz of wine, or 24 oz of beer. Excessive alcohol intake contributes to hypertension.

Increase in potassium intake

A high potassium intake (4.5 to 7 g or 120 to 175 mEq/day) may have a mild blood pressure-lowering effect. It also helps replace potassium lost as a result of diuretic use. Fresh fruits and vegetables are generally low in sodium and rich in potassium. Potassium content of some common foods is:

Apple, raw, 1 medium, 159 mg
Spinach, cooked, ½ cup, 291 mg
Milk, skim, 1 cup, 406 mg
Hamburger patty, lean, cooked, 480 mg

Orange, 1 medium, 250 mg
Tomato, raw, 1 medium, 366 mg
Banana, 1 medium, 451 mg
Potato, baked, 1 medium, 503 mg

Increase in calcium intake

Adequate calcium may be important in preventing or treating hypertension. Two to three cups of milk or yogurt per day, or 4 oz of low-sodium cheese, will provide the needed calcium. Obese individuals who lose weight often lower their blood pressure even if they do not achieve their ideal body weight. Loss of 1 kg (2.2 lb) reduces diastolic and systolic blood pressure by an average of 1 mm Hg. See Chapter 19 for weight control information.

Development of effective ways of reacting to stress

The client can be aided in evaluating present coping mechanisms and planning better ones, if necessary.

Congestive Heart Failure

Pathophysiology

Congestive heart failure (CHF), which results from decreased myocardial efficiency, can be caused by myocardial infarction, disease of the heart valves, hypertension, thiamin deficiency, and many other conditions. Renal blood flow may decrease, with impaired excretion of sodium and water. Peripheral edema, pulmonary edema, and ascites often result.

Treatment

Diuretics are used to reduce total body water, and inotropic agents such as digitalis are often given to improve cardiac contractility. Morphine sulfate may be given to relieve anxiety and induce venous dilation.

Nutritional Care

The goals of nutritional care are to reduce total body water sodium and water to reduce the work load of the heart. Children with CHF frequently have impaired growth and poor weight gain. This may be due to a combination of factors (See Table 13-2 for a listing). For these children, improvement of growth is a goal.

Assessment

Assessment is summarized in Table 13-2.

Intervention and client teaching

The following measures are designed to alleviate the effects of CHF.

Reduction of dietary sodium to decrease fluid retention

The amount of sodium allowed ranges from 45 to 70 mg/kg/ day in infants to 2 g/day in adults. The box on pp. 261 and 262 provides guidelines for achieving sodium restriction. Usually these will be needed for a prolonged period, so the client and family will need instruction about sodium restriction.

Reduction of fluid intake to help reduce circulatory volume

Fluid allowance ranges from 80 to 160 ml/kg/day in infants to 1.5 to 2 L/day in adults. This includes dietary sources, as well as fluids given with medications. Some foods that are solid at room temperature are liquids at body temperature. Gelatins can be considered to be 100% water, ice cream 33%, fruit ices and sherbet 50%, and custard 75%. Nutrients must be provided in as small a volume as possible. If the client is tube fed, a formula providing 2 or more kcal/ml (Magnacal [Biosearch], Isocal HCN [Mead Johnson], TwoCal HN [Ross], Nutrisource [Sandoz]) should be used. If parenteral nutrition is necessary, 20% fat emulsions (2 kcal/ml) can be used as a kcal source.

Increase potassium intake to 4.5 to 7 g/day unless renal impairment is present

Diuretics increase potassium losses, and hypokalemia predisposes to digitalis toxicity. See p. 263 for potassium sources.

Divide daily food intake into several small meals

Five to six small meals are often better tolerated by the dyspneic individual than three large meals a day.

Achieve optimum body weight in adults and growth in children

The overweight individual with CHF has an increased burden on the myocardium. Weight reduction is essential. (See Chapter 19.) Malnourished clients, especially children, have shown improved growth without a worsening of CHF when given continuous tube feedings. Modular ingredients (Table 6-2) can be used to increase the kcal-density of standard infant formulas to allow provision of adequate kcal within the fluid volume tolerated.

Table 13-5 Dietary changes to reduce risk of heart disease

Previous Intake	Revised Intake
Breakfast	Breakfast
Doughnut	Shredded wheat (Fi, F)*
Orange juice	Sliced strawberries (Fi)
Coffee	Coffee
Nondairy creamer	Skim milk (F, C)
Lunch	Lunch
Quarter-pound hamburger	Salad of lettuce, spinach, green pepper, and garbanzo beans with low-kcal dressing (F, C, Fi, Na)
French fries, salted	Unsalted whole wheat crackers (Fi, F, Na)
Soft drink	Diet soft drink
Fried fruit pie	Fresh pears (F, Fi, Na)
Dinner	Dinner
Prime rib	Curried chicken, without salt (F, Na)
Baked potato with sour cream	Brown rice (F, C)
Green beans cooked with salt	Green beans cooked with thyme (Na)
Lettuce wedge with Thousand Island dressing	Lettuce wedge with low-kcal dressing (F)
Whole milk	Skim milk (F, C)
Chocolate cake with icing	Blueberry-oatmeal crisp (F, Fi)

*Abbreviations refer to reduction in cholesterol (C), fat (F), sodium (Na) and increase in fiber (Fi) intake.

CASE STUDY

On a routine physical examination, Mr. F., 42 years old, was noted to have a serum cholesterol level of 242 mg/dl. He was 5 kg (11 pounds) overweight, and his blood pressure on two occasions was in the range for "borderline hypertension." After recording his food intake for 3 days, Mr. F. consulted the dietitian, and together they planned dietary changes. Table 13-5 demonstrates a typical day's intake with his previous and revised food habits.

Reference

1. *Dietary treatment of hypercholesterolemia,* Dallas, 1988, American Heart Association.

Bibliography

Boegehold MA, Kotchem TA: Importance of dietary chloride for salt sensitivity of blood pressure, *Hypertension* 17(1 suppl):1158, 1991.

Burns ER, Neubort S: Sodium content of koshered meat, *JAMA* 252:2960, 1984.

Connor WE, Connor SL: Diet, atherosclerosis, and fish oil, *Adv Intern Med* 35:139, 1990.

Cutler JA and others: An overview of randomized trials of sodium reduction and blood pressure, *Hypertension* 17(1 suppl):127, 1991.

Fletcher GF and others: Exercise standards: a statement for health professionals from the American Heart Association, *Circulation* 82:2286, 1990.

Kirchhoff KT and others: Electrocardiographic response to ice water ingestion, *Heart Lung* 19:41, 1990.

Korch GC: Sodium content of potable water: dietary significance, *J Am Diet Assoc* 86:80, 1986.

Lampe JW and others: Serum lipid and fecal bile acid changes with cereal, vegetable, and sugar beet fiber feeding, *Am J Clin Nutr* 53:1235, 1991.

National Cholesterol Education Program: Report of the Expert Panel on Detection, Evaluation, and Treatment of High Blood Cholesterol in Adults. NIH Pub No 89-2925, Washington, DC, 1989, US Department of Health and Human Services.

National Education Programs Working Group report on the management of patients with hypertension and high blood cholesterol, *Ann Intern Med* 114:224, 1991.

Schwartz SM and others: Enteral nutrition in infants with congenital heart disease and growth failure, *Pediatrics* 86:368, 1990.

Pulmonary Disease

14

Chronic Obstructive Pulmonary Disease

Chronic obstructive pulmonary disease (COPD) is a group of diseases that includes asthma, bronchitis, emphysema, and bronchiectasis. These diseases are estimated to affect 15% of older adults.

Pathophysiology

The common feature in COPD is chronic obstruction of airflow. Airflow obstruction can result from bronchospasm (asthma), overproduction of mucus in the respiratory system (bronchitis), destruction of elastin, the elastic lung tissue, with air trapping and poor gas exchange (emphysema), or bronchial obstruction caused by a tumor, foreign body, or infection (bronchiectasis).

Treatment

Bronchodilators such as theophylline and aminophylline are often used in treatment of COPD. Antibiotics are prescribed when secondary infections (e.g., pneumonia) occur. Chest percussion and postural drainage may be used in individuals producing large amounts of sputum.

Nutritional Care

Malnutrition is common among clients with COPD, especially those with emphysema. As many as 70% have weight loss, are underweight, or show signs of muscle or fat wasting. Poor intake of vitamin A has been found in 61%. Deficiency of vitamin A reduces the replication of epithelial cells and causes degeneration of mucus-secreting cells in the respiratory tract, thus making the client more susceptible to infection. Vitamin C intakes have been found to be low in approximately 25% of clients, which further predisposes them to infection.

Interventions are designed to promote comfort and maintain adequate, although not excessive, nutrient intake. Optimal nutritional status will help the client avoid infection and maintain as much functional ability as possible.

Assessment

Assessment is summarized in Table 14-1.

Intervention

Prevention or correction of underweight

Some studies have shown nutritional depletion to correlate with increased airflow obstruction in COPD clients. Furthermore, mortality is higher in clients who have lost weight than in those who have not. It is not known whether nutritional repletion of clients who have lost weight lowers the risk of death. However, prevention or correction of weight loss may help maintain strength and a feeling of well-being.

Specific interventions include:

1. Increase kcal intake through use of kcal-dense foods or supplements; the box on p. 161 provides a list of suggestions; clients with moderate to severe dyspnea may prefer liquid supplements (shakes, instant breakfast, or commercial nutrient drinks; see Tables 6-1 and 6-2).

2. Offer underweight COPD clients feedings between meals, or save items such as fruit, sherbet, ice cream, or sandwiches for the client's later consumption if not eaten at mealtimes; weight gain is usually greater when small, frequent feedings are consumed than when the individual tries to eat 3 large meals a day; small feedings minimize the restriction of diaphragmatic movement caused by a full stomach.

3. Ensure that clients have sufficient resources to secure an adequate diet; many individuals with COPD are elderly or retired, they may have a limited income, or they may have a poor diet because of loneliness, apathy about food, or few food preparation skills (especially elderly men); these clients may need assistance in enrolling in the food stamp program, encouragement to utilize the congregate feeding

Table 14-1 Assessment in pulmonary disease

Areas of Concern	Significant Findings
Protein Calorie Malnutrition (PCM)	*History* COPD: Poor intake of protein and kcal resulting from breathing difficulty caused by pressure of a full stomach on the diaphragm, unpleasant taste in the mouth from chronic sputum production, gastric irritation from bronchodilator therapy, inadequate income, loneliness, apathy, inadequate food preparation skills; increased needs because of increased work of breathing, frequent infections Respiratory failure: inadequate intake of protein and kcal caused by upper airway intubation, altered state of consciousness, dyspnea; increase in protein and kcal requirements because of increased work of breathing or acute pulmonary infections *Physical examination* Evidence of wt loss (muscle wasting, lack of fat); wt for ht < 90% of standard or ideal or BMI < 19.1 (women) or 20.7 (men); triceps skinfold or AMC < 5th percentile (see Appendix G) *Laboratory analysis* ↓ Serum albumin, transferrin, or prealbumin; ↓ lymphocyte count; nonreactive skin tests; ↓ creatinine-height index (see Table 1-4) — Uncommon in COPD
Overweight	*History* COPD: Decreased kcal needs resulting from decreased basal metabolic rate with aging, decreased activity to compensate for impaired respiratory function *Physical examination* Wt for ht > 120% of desirable or ideal or BMI > 27.3 (women) or 27.8 (men); triceps skinfold >95th percentile (see Appendix G)

Table 14-1   Assessment in pulmonary disease—cont'd

Areas of Concern	Significant Findings
Vitamin Deficiencies	
A	*History*
	Failure to consume at least 1 serving of a food rich in vitamin A or its precursor, carotene, at least every other day (see Appendix B for such foods)
	Physical examination
	Follicular hyperkeratosis; poor light-dark visual adaptation; dryness of the skin or cornea
	Laboratory analysis
	↓ Serum retinol
C	*History*
	Failure to consume at least one serving of vitamin C-rich foods (see Appendix B)/ day
	Physical examination
	Petechiae, ecchymoses; gingivitis
	Laboratory analysis
	↓ Serum or leukocyte ascorbic acid
Phosphate (P) Deficiency	*History*
	Refeeding of client with malnutrition; use of carbohydrate to provide most of kcal
	Physical examination
	Muscle weakness; acute respiratory failure
	Laboratory analysis
	↓ Serum P
Elevated Respiratory Quotient (RQ)	*History*
	Use of glucose or other carbohydrate to provide 70% or more of nonprotein kcal; administration of excess kcal
	Physical examination
	Tachypnea (> 20 breaths/min in a nonmechanically ventilated adult); shortness of breath
	Laboratory analysis
	$RQ \geq 1$ (see Intervention, p. 275, for explanation of RQ; RQ measurements are not available in many institutions); ↑ partial pressure of CO_2 (P_{CO_2})

Continued.

Table 14-1 Assessment in pulmonary disease—cont'd

Areas of Concern	Significant Findings
Fluid Excess	*History*
	Administration of more than 35-50 ml fluid /kg/day in an adult, include fluids in IVs, IV medications, tube feedings, TPN, and oral intake; ventilator dependency, which causes ↑ release of antidiuretic hormone (ADH)
	Physical examination
	Bounding pulse; sacral or peripheral edema; shortness of breath; pulmonary rales
	Laboratory analysis
	↓ Serum Na
Excess IV Lipid	*History*
	Rapid administration (over 10 to 12 hours or less) of IV lipid emulsions, especially if > 2 g lipid/kg/day are administered
	Laboratory analysis
	↑ Serum triglycerides; ↓ Po_2, ↑ Pco_2

program for the elderly, or, if they are homebound, referral to the Meals on Wheels program.

Promotion of comfort

Nutrient intake will be improved if attention is paid to client comfort:

1. Provide mouth care often, especially before meals, to clear the palate of the taste of sputum and improve the appetite.
2. Schedule treatments and exercise so that the client has a chance to rest before meals.

Client teaching

Maintenance of ideal body weight

Underweight individuals have increased morbidity as a result of weakness and susceptibility to infection. On the other hand, excess weight increases the work of breathing.

Underweight clients

Nutrient intake can often be improved by helping the client learn to cope with frequently encountered symptoms that impair food intake. Problems reported by individuals with COPD, along with strategies for dealing with them, are listed below.

Early satiety: Eat high-kcal foods first, then foods of low kcal-density (beverages, raw vegetables) at the end of the meal or between meals. Experiment to see if foods served cold cause fewer problems.

Bloating: Eat small, frequent meals and avoid hurrying through meals, to reduce air swallowing.

Anorexia: Eat high-kcal foods first and save lower kcal ones to eat at the end of the meal; have favorite foods available; use fat-containing foods, which have higher caloric density (p. 161).

Dyspnea: Rest before meals; take bronchodilators before meals; eat slowly; use pursed lip breathing between bites. Avoid excessive protein, which increases ventilatory drive; consume a moderate (up to 50% of kcal) carbohydrate diet, since excess increases CO_2 production.

Fatigue: Rest before meals; eat larger meals when less tired; have easy-to-prepare foods readily available for times when fatigued.

Overweight/Obese clients

1. Increase activity within physical limitations; walking is an example of a good exercise for individuals with COPD; it is important that they start with brief periods of light exercise and gradually increase the duration and intensity
2. Decrease kcal intake by following the guidelines in Chapter 19

Acute Respiratory Failure

Respiratory failure is one of the leading reasons for admission to intensive care units (ICUs). ICU clients are at increased risk of malnutrition, with more than 40% being malnourished at the time of admission.

Pathophysiology

Respiratory failure is not a disease but instead is a ventilatory disorder caused by a variety of different conditions. It can result from increased pulmonary capillary pressure or permeability (e.g., pulmonary edema, pneumonia, near drowning), inadequate excretion of carbon dioxide (e.g., chronic bronchitis, emphysema), and depression of the respiratory center or failure of neuromuscular transmission (e.g., drug overdose, spinal cord injury, multiple sclerosis).

Malnutrition adversely affects respiratory function by causing: (1) wasting of the diaphragm and intercostal muscles, making respiratory efforts so weak that it is difficult to wean clients from the ventilator, (2) decreased ventilatory response to hypoxia, (3) decreased surfactant production, (4) decreased replication of respiratory epithelium with predisposition to infection, (5) decreased cell-mediated immunity with increased susceptibility to infection, and (6) decreased colloid osmotic pressure with increased likelihood of pulmonary edema.

Treatment

Treatment of respiratory failure includes administration of oxygen or use of mechanical ventilation to maintain near-normal partial pressures of oxygen and carbon dioxide in the blood, use of antibiotics if infection is present, and, in some cases, use of corticosteroids to decrease pulmonary edema and stabilize pulmonary membranes.

Nutritional Care

Nutritional care is aimed at the prevention or correction of nutritional deficiencies or excesses that may worsen respiratory function and predispose the individual to secondary infections.

Assessment

Assessment is summarized in Table 14-1.

Intervention

Prevention or correction of PCM

Because these clients tend to have multiple medical problems requiring simultaneous attention, it is easy to neglect nutrition. Clients with acute respiratory failure should be started on nutrition support within the first 3 or 4 days of hospitalization to prevent progression of nutritional deficits. Clients given nutrition support are more readily weaned from ventilators than those given only intravenous (IV) glucose solutions.

Clients able to eat should be given a diet of nutrient-dense foods. Those unable to eat but having functioning gastrointestinal (GI) tracts should be given nasogastric (NG) or nasoduodenal/nasojejunal feedings. Those who are unable to be fully fed by the GI tract should be given TPN. Excessive amino acid administration should be avoided, since it stimulates the ventilatory drive and may increase minute ventilation, fatigue respiratory muscles, and contribute to respiratory arrest.

Prevention of elevated respiratory quotient (RQ), or carbohydrate excess

Glucose is usually the primary kcal source in TPN. Unfortunately, carbon dioxide (CO_2) is a major product of carbohydrate metabolism. This is reflected in an increased RQ—the amount of CO_2 produced in metabolism ÷ the amount of oxygen consumed. The amount and type of kcal delivered have a major impact on RQ.

RQ when carbohydrates alone are used as fuel = 1.0

RQ when fat (lipid) alone is used as fuel = 0.7

RQ when a mixture of carbohydrates and lipid is used = 0.87

RQ when overfeeding results in accumulation of body fat > 1.0

RQ is measured by indirect calorimetry, a technique that is not available in many institutions. However, some of the effects of rising RQ can be assessed clinically.

When most of the kcal are provided as glucose or other carbohydrates, the resulting increase in CO_2 production forces the client to increase minute ventilation to rid himself or herself of CO_2. Increased Pco_2 (partial pressure of CO_2 in the blood) may be noted. These factors make it difficult to wean some clients from the ventilator. Non-ventilator-dependent clients with respiratory compromise can become tachypneic and complain of shortness of breath when given excess carbohydrate.

For hypercapnic clients, whether they are freely breathing or ventilator-dependent, administering a portion of the kcal as fat may help to reduce CO_2 production. Pulmocare (Ross) is a high-fat enteral formula designed for clients with respiratory compromise. Overfeeding is especially to be avoided in clients with respiratory insufficiency.

Avoidance of fluid excess

The fluid required for delivery of tube feedings or TPN, along with medications, to pulmonary clients puts them at risk for over-hydration. To provide concentrated kcal in minimal fluid:

1. Emphasize foods containing fat, which is a concentrated kcal source, for clients who can eat. The box on p. 161 provides suggestions. Lipomul (Upjohn), an oral fat supplement containing 6 kcal/ml, can also be used.

2. Use concentrated formulas for clients receiving tube feedings. These include Magnacal (Biosearch), Isocal HCN (Mead Johnson), and Pulmocare (Ross), which provide 1.5 to 2 kcal/ml, and Nutrisource (Sandoz), which can be reconstituted to provide more than 2 kcal/ml.

3. Use 20% lipid emulsions daily as a kcal source for clients receiving TPN. These supply 2 kcal/ml, while 10% emulsions provide only 1.1 kcal/ml.

Prevention of lipid excess

Rapid infusion of intravenous lipid emulsions may interfere with pulmonary diffusion capacity in clients with impaired respiratory function. Neonates are at increased risk. If the individual has elevated triglycerides or turbid serum, the volume of lipid emulsion should be decreased, or the emulsion should be stopped temporarily until the individual's serum is clear of triglycerides. Infusion of the lipid over at least 12 to 24 hours each day is associated with the least likelihood of diffusion defects.

CASE STUDY

Mr. S., a 42-year-old man with adult respiratory distress syndrome, is to receive TPN. The accompanying box demonstrates a TPN solution designed to provide him with an adequate protein and kcal intake, with little potential for elevation of the RQ, in a limited fluid volume.

Sample TPN Regimen for a Client in Acute Respiratory Failure

Estimated nonprotein kcal need = 2400 kcal
Estimated protein need = 90 g
Nutrient solutions:

Glucose-amino acid solution, each liter containing:

	Nonprotein kcal/L	Protein (g/L)
400 ml 70% glucose	952	0
600 ml 85% amino acids	0	51
Minerals, electrolytes and vitamins as needed		
20% lipid emulsion	2000	0

Nutritional prescription:

Infuse 1.8 L glucose-amino acid solution (1714 nonprotein kcal and 92 g amino acids) and 0.25 L lipid emulsion (500 kcal) per day.

Bibliography

Benotti PN, Bistrian B: Metabolic and nutritional aspects of weaning from mechanical ventilation, *Crit Care Med* 17:181, 1989.

Donahoe M, Rogers RM: Nutritional assessment and support in chronic obstructive pulmonary disease, *Clin Chest Med* 11:487, 1990.

Greene HL, Hazlett D, Demaree R: Relationship between Intralipid-induced hyperlipidemia and pulmonary function, *Am J Clin Nutr* 29:127, 1976.

Keim NL and others: Dietary evaluation of outpatients with chronic obstructive pulmonary disease, *J Am Diet Assoc* 86:902, 1986.

Rothcopf MM and others: Nutritional support in respiratory failure, *Nutr Clin Prac* 4:166, 1989.

Neurologic and Mental Disorders

15

Nutritional care is rarely, if ever, the primary therapy in neurologic and mental disorders. However, most of these disorders are long term in nature. Thus nutritional care is an important supportive measure that can assist in maintaining optimal functioning and well-being.

Seizure Disorders

Pathophysiology

Seizure disorders, or epilepsy, are characterized by brain dysfunction with alteration of consciousness. Generalized seizures are observed in grand mal epilepsy. Petit mal epilepsy, on the other hand, is associated with brief alteration of consciousness and twitching of the mouth or eyelids.

Treatment

Anticonvulsant medications are the primary means of treatment. Anticonvulsants used include carbamazepine, hydantoins (phenytoin and ethotoin), ethosuximide, valproic acid, and phenobarbital.

Nutritional Care

Goals are to maintain optimal nutrition and, in some instances, to induce ketosis in an effort to control seizures.

Assessment

Nutritional assessment is summarized in Table 15-1.

Table 15-1   Assessment in neurologic disorders

Area of Concern	Significant Findings
Protein Calorie Malnutrition (PCM)	*History* Restricted protein intake (e.g., ketogenic diet in seizure disorder, low-fat diet in multiple sclerosis); unpalatable diet (e.g., ketogenic diet); feeding/swallowing difficulties such as dribbling of food and beverages from the mouth, dysphagia, weakness of muscles required for chewing, incoordination or spasticity interfering with chewing and swallowing; dementia or memory loss (refusing or forgetting to eat); use of corticosteroids *Physical examination* Muscle wasting; triceps skinfold or AMC <5th percentile (see Appendix G); weight <90% of standard or BMI <19.1 (women) or 20.7 (men) or weight-for-height or weight-for-age <5th percentile (children); edema, ascites *Laboratory analysis* ↓ Serum albumin, transferrin, or prealbumin; ↓ lymphocyte count; nonreactive skin tests
Overweight/Obesity	*History* ↓ kcal needs resulting from inactivity; reliance on soft or pureed foods, which are often more dense in kcal than higher fiber foods *Physical examination* Triceps skinfold >95th percentile (see Appendix G); weight >120% of standard or BMI >27.3 (women) or 27.8 (men) or weight-for-height or weight-for-age >95th percentile (children)

Continued.

Table 15-1   Assessment in neurologic disorders—cont'd

Area of Concern	Significant Findings
Vitamin and Mineral Deficiencies	
Folate	*History*
	Phenytoin use
	Physical examination
	Pallor; glossitis
	Laboratory analysis
	↓ Hct, ↑ MCV; ↓ blood folate
D	*History*
	Use of phenobarbital, primidone, or phenytoin, especially when combined with ketogenic diet; lack of sun exposure (e.g., institutionalization)
	Physical examination
	Rickets; osteomalacia
	Laboratory analysis
	↓ Serum 1,25-dihydroxyvitamin D; ↓ serum Ca (uncommon); ↑ alkaline phosphatase
Iron (Fe)	*History*
	Inadequate intake (ketogenic diet used in seizure disorders, low-fat diet used in MS, difficulty chewing meats)
	Physical examination
	Pallor, blue sclerae; koilonychia
	Laboratory analysis
	↓ Hct, Hgb, MCV, MCH, MCHC; ↓ serum Fe; ↑ serum transferrin or TIBC
Zinc (Zn)	*History*
	Inadequate intake (ketogenic diet, low-fat diet, difficulty chewing meats)
	Physical examination
	Diarrhea; dermatitis; hypogeusia, dysgeusia
	Laboratory analysis
	↓ Serum Zn

Table 15-1 Assessment in neurologic disorders—cont'd

Area of Concern	Significant Findings
Vitamin and Mineral Deficiencies—cont'd	
Calcium (Ca)	*History*
	Phenytoin use (↓ Ca absorption) or corticosteroid use with increased losses; inadequate intake (ketogenic diet, low-fat diet used in MS, lactose intolerance);
	Physical examination
	Rickets; osteomalacia
	Laboratory analysis
	↓ Serum Ca (uncommon); ↑ serum alkaline phosphatase
Fluid Deficiencies	*History*
	Poor intake caused by difficulty swallowing fluids (as in CP or ALS) or inability to express thirst
	Physical examination
	Poor skin turgor; ↓ urinary output; dry, sticky mucous membranes
	Laboratory analysis
	↑ Serum Na, serum osmolality, BUN, Hct, urine specific gravity

Intervention and client teaching

For most individuals, no special diet is needed. In a few cases, especially when anticonvulsants are not effective in controlling seizures, a "ketogenic" diet is used in conjunction with medication. High levels of ketones in the blood appear to decrease seizure activity.

Ketogenic diet

A ketogenic diet relies primarily on fat for kcal. The diet prescription usually specifies the ratio of dietary fat to the combined carbohydrate and protein, with ratios of 3:1 to 4:1 (by weight) being the most common. Other concerns in planning the diet and instructing parents:

1. The diet usually includes 1 g of protein per kg per day.

2. Kcal are limited to approximately 75 kcal/kg/day for children ages 1 to 3, 68 kcal/kg/day for children ages 4 to 6, and 60 kcal/kg/day for children ages 7 to 10.

3. Fluids are restricted to approximately 80 to 100 ml/day, with no more than 120 ml taken in a 2-hour period, to prevent expansion of plasma volume with dilution of the ketones. Urine specific gravity must be maintained between 1.020 and 1.025. Beverages can contain no aspartame or caffeine, which inhibit ketosis. Diet soft drinks should provide no more than 1 kcal/day.

4. Exchange lists[1] are available to assist in planning daily food intake.

The diet is usually initiated in the hospital to ensure that severe hypoglycemia does not occur, ketosis is established, and the parents or other caregivers are fully instructed.

Limitations of the diet. The diet is effective only if adherence is rigid, since a small excess of carbohydrate will inhibit ketosis. Adherence becomes much more difficult as children age, unless they are severely retarded. The high fat intake is unpalatable to many clients, and the strict diet is onerous. Hyperlipidemia is common, but it apparently resolves once the diet is discontinued. Parents should be encouraged to choose margarine and polyunsaturated oils (see Chapter 13) more often than butter and cream to avoid increasing serum lipid levels unnecessarily.

Some physicians prefer the use of medium-chain triglycerides (MCT) to long-chain triglycerides (see Chapter 6). MCT appear to be more ketogenic than the long-chain triglycerides commonly found in foods, and this allows the combined carbohydrate and protein content of the diet to be increased to 20% to 40% of the kcal and the kcal and fluid allowances to be more liberal. However, results are still better if moderate kcal and fluid restrictions are practiced. The MCT diet has the same limitations as the traditional ketogenic diet. In addition, MCT are not available in supermarkets, as dietary fats are, and they are expensive. Furthermore, excessive intakes of MCT can result in abdominal cramping and diarrhea. One of the most successful ways of administering MCT is to blend them in skim milk and serve small amounts throughout the day.

Supplementation

Because of the restrictions of the diet, a daily supplement of vitamins C, A, and B complex, iron, zinc, and calcium is advisable.

Cerebral Palsy

Pathophysiology

Cerebral palsy (CP) is usually the result of hypoxia during the perinatal period. Motor centers of the brain are affected, with resulting incoordination; physical disabilities; and sometimes impairments of speech, sight, and hearing. There are several types of CP: spastic paralysis, with hyperactivity of the extensor muscles; choreoathetosis, with involuntary muscle movements; ataxia, or incoordination; and flaccidity, or decreased muscle tone.

Treatment

Physical therapy and judicious use of devices, such as computers, which make communication by nonverbal individuals possible, can help clients with CP achieve their maximum potential. Orthopedic surgery is sometimes used to correct deformities.

Nutritional Care

Goals of care are to maintain adequate intake of nutrients and to prevent obesity, which further impairs mobility in individuals with CP.

Assessment

Assessment is summarized in Table 15-1.

Intervention and client teaching

Coping with chewing and swallowing problems

Provision of adequate nutrients may be difficult because of neuromuscular impairments and persistence of primitive reflexes. To minimize these problems:

1. Foods offered should be tailored to the needs of the individuals. Beverages often leak out of the mouth. Leakage can be decreased by thickening fluids with infant cereals or yogurt, or liquids can be offered in the form of gelatin, fruit ices, ice cream, or sherbet.

2. Children with CP should be placed in good anatomic position for feeding. Those with spastic CP are especially likely to hyperextend their necks, which makes swallowing difficult. Positioning them with back straight and hips and knees flexed reduces hyperextension. Separating the legs promotes stability.

3. Underweight is a common problem, largely because of difficulty ingesting food. Parents of some children with CP have been found to spend between 3 and 7 hours daily feeding the children. Because of the prolonged mealtimes, provision of snacks is often not effective in increasing intake. Thus increasing the kcal content of foods eaten at mealtimes is the best alternative. Skim milk powder, margarine, oils, or modular ingredients (see Table 6-2) can be added to foods to increase kcal density. Tube feedings may also be used.

Promotion of self-feeding

To facilitate self-feeding:

1. Utilize plates with rims to allow food to be scooped up by pushing it against the rim.
2. Insert spoon or fork handle into a rolled washcloth to make it easier to grip.
3. Prevent scooting of plates or bowls by putting suction cups, such as those used for soap holders, under them.

Constipation

Inactivity promotes constipation. Bran (2 tbsp), whole grains, legumes, or fruits and vegetables should be served daily.

Amyotrophic Lateral Sclerosis

Pathophysiology

Amyotrophic lateral sclerosis (ALS) is a progressive degenerative neurologic disease that results in atrophy of the muscles. Eventually it affects most of the body, including the muscles involved in chewing and swallowing.

Treatment

There is no specific therapy and no cure for ALS. Physical therapy can help maintain as much muscle mass as possible.

Nutritional Care

Goals of care are to prevent nutritional deficits and maintain feeding safety.

Assessment

Assessment is summarized in Table 15-1.

Intervention and client teaching

Prevention of nutritional deficits

A. Weight loss is inevitable because of muscle wasting. Nutritional deficits, however, accelerate loss. Where loss in 6 months is greater than 10% of usual weight, kcal deficits should be suspected. Chair or bed scales are often necessary to obtain weight measurements. To minimize weight loss, encourage small, frequent feedings to maintain optimal intake. The box on p. 161 offers suggestions for increasing kcal intake. Supplements in the form of puddings or thick liquids may be the easiest to consume.

B. Protein foods may be difficult to chew, especially if dry. Encourage use of:
   1. Tender, chopped meats and poultry. Gravies and sauces make chewing and swallowing easier. Moist casseroles made with meat, fish, or poultry are good protein sources.
   2. Cheese and cottage cheese.
   3. Poached, soft-cooked, or scrambled eggs.

   Commercial supplements (high-protein puddings and beverages or protein powders to be added to other foods, see Tables 6-1 and 6-2) are available, but home-prepared products are often tastier.

C. Vitamins and minerals may be lacking because of impaired intake. A daily multivitamin-multimineral supplement can be recommended if assessment indicates a need.

D. Fluids are among the most difficult foods to swallow. Plain water is especially likely to cause choking. Semi-solid sources of fluid (e.g., sherbet, sorbet, fruit ices, and gelatin) can be used to promote adequate intake. Fluids can also be thickened with baby cereal to make swallowing easier.

Reducing dysphagia and potential for pulmonary aspiration

Suggestions that may be beneficial are:

1. To reduce choking, serve soft, moist foods, for example, casseroles, meats and vegetables with gravies and sauces, applesauce, mashed potatoes, cooked cereals.
2. Do not rush the individual while eating. Serving foods in insulated dishes or on a warming tray can help maintain their temperature during prolonged mealtimes.
3. Suggest that the client try turning the head to the side while swallowing or swallowing twice after each bite. Also, speech or physical therapists may help the individual in dealing with dysphagia.
4. If excessive mucus is a problem, reduce intake of milk, which is thought to increase mucus production. Calcium can be obtained from cheese or calcium carbonate supplements.
5. Keep suction equipment available.

Gastrostomy feedings are sometimes instituted where dysphagia is severe and the risk of aspiration is high. Blended foods or commercial formulas may be used. Fluoroscopic examination while the individual is swallowing foods and liquids containing small amounts of barium has been used to evaluate the likelihood of aspiration and to determine when gastrostomy is necessary.

Prevent constipation

Inactivity and muscle weakness contribute to decreased bowel motility and constipation. Increase fiber intake with daily servings of bran, cooked legumes, whole grains, fruits, and vegetables. If tube feedings are used, choose a blended formula made of regular foods or a commercial formula containing added fiber (see Chapter 6). A fluid intake of 50 ml/kg/day also helps produce larger, softer stools.

Compensate for weakness and tiring during feedings

Feedings should be small and frequent to avoid exhausting the individual. Utensils with loops to fit over the hands help prevent dropping of utensils and improve grip.

Multiple Sclerosis

Pathophysiology

Multiple sclerosis (MS), a disease of the central nervous system, affects the myelinated nerve fibers and the muscles they innervate. Patches of the myelin surrounding the nerves degenerate, and the myelin is replaced by scars. The cause of MS is unknown, but the most promising theories are that it is a slow response to viral infection or a viral-induced immune disease. The disease tends to follow a pattern of exacerbations and remissions.

Treatment

Although there is no cure for MS, steroids are sometimes used as palliative therapy. Avoidance of physical and psychologic stress appears to help prevent relapses.

Nutritional Care

Assessment

Assessment is summarized in Table 15-1.

Intervention and client teaching

There is no proof that a special diet is effective in alleviating the effects of MS. However, long-term use of a low-fat diet, especially one low in saturated fat, is postulated to reduce the number of acute exacerbations and slow the progress of the disease. Although firm evidence for the efficacy of this diet is lacking, it should not be harmful if clients are carefully instructed so that the diet is nutritionally adequate.

Low-fat diet

The low-fat diet should consist of protein, 60 to 70 g/day; total fat, 50 to 60 g/day; and carbohydrates sufficient to provide the balance of needed kcal. Saturated fat is restricted to 10 g/day. This necessitates reducing meat, fish, and poultry to about 2 oz/day and using dairy products that are prepared from skim milk. The balance of the fat should be primarily polyunsaturated. Cod liver oil, 1 tsp/day (equivalent to 4.5 g fat), is recommended. Other sources of polyunsaturated fat include safflower, sunflower, corn, soybean, and cottonseed oils.

Supplementation

Intake of calcium, iron, and zinc should be investigated. Supplements are usually needed because of the restriction of animal products.

Constipation

Constipation is reported by more than 40% of clients. Generalized muscle weakness, immobility, and constipating medications probably are etiologic factors. Increased intake of fiber-containing foods (see Appendix C) and consumption of 35 to 50 ml of fluid per kg per day will help to alleviate the problem.

Parkinsonism, or Parkinson's Disease

Pathophysiology

Parkinsonism is a progressive neuromuscular disorder characterized by low content of dopamine in the basal ganglia of the central nervous system. This results in tremor, rigidity, a characteristic "pill rolling" movement of the fingers, and hypoactivity.

Treatment

Levodopa, a precursor of dopamine, or a combination of levodopa and carbidopa is used to treat parkinsonism.

Nutritional Care

Assessment

Assessment is summarized in Table 15-1.

Intervention and client teaching

Optimization of drug therapy

Vitamin B_6 (pyridoxine) is an antagonist of dopamine. The individual should not take vitamin supplements containing more than the RDA of vitamin B_6. Alcohol can antagonize levodopa, therefore it is best if alcohol is omitted from the diet.

After several years of levodopa therapy, clients may become less responsive to the drug. Restricting protein intake during the day to less than or equal to 7 g improves responsiveness of some clients. Clients can be taught to consume only fruits; green, leafy vegetables; juices; candies; and small amounts of bread and cereal during the day. They can eat meats and dairy products at dinner, since control of Parkinson symptoms is less important during the night.

Prevention of constipation

Hypoactivity promotes constipation. Bran, whole grains, legumes, fresh fruits, and fresh vegetables, along with a large fluid intake, help alleviate the problem.

Coping with feeding difficulties

Fluids may be especially difficult to swallow. Semisolids such as gelatin, sherbet, ice cream, or fruit ices may be easier to handle than liquids.

Eating is apt to be slow, so insulated dishes or a warming tray can be used to keep foods warm and palatable. Any distraction can cause the elderly client with Parkinsonism to lose focus on the task at hand. If interrupted during eating, clients may have difficulty starting again. Thus it is best to plan care to avoid interruptions such as medication administration during mealtimes.

Since coordination of hand movements is poor, plate guards or special eating utensils may be needed to help clients scoop up food and convey it to their mouths. Chewing and biting movements also tend to be relatively ineffective. Especially tough, hard, or chewy foods should be avoided. It may be necessary to provide soft-textured foods for these individuals.

Cerebrovascular Accident, or Stroke

Pathophysiology

Cerebrovascular accident (CVA) results from decreased blood supply to the brain and is manifested by persistent neurologic signs and symptoms. The cause can be embolism, thrombosis, or intracerebral and subarachnoid hemorrhages. Symptoms vary, depending on the extent and location of the CVA. Some clients experience hemiplegia, or paralysis of one side of the body; visual field defects (e.g., hemianopia, or failure to see half of the visual field); apraxia (inability to perform a known task in response to verbal instructions); and dysphagia.

Treatment

Pharmacologic therapy is aimed at decreasing or preventing extension of the damage. Anticoagulants are used in selected clients, especially those with emboli arising from the heart, to reduce the formation of a clot. Steroids or osmotic agents such as mannitol may be used to reduce cerebral edema. Antifibrinolytic agents such as aminocaproic acid are used to prevent recurrence of bleeding in some clients with stroke resulting from a ruptured aneurysm. Surgery (thrombectomy or embolectomy) is sometimes required to reestablish cerebral perfusion.

Nutritional Care

The extent and location of the CVA will determine the severity and exact type of problems experienced by the client. Thorough assessment to provide the basis for an individualized plan of care is thus essential.

Assessment

Assessment is summarized in Table 15-1.

Intervention and client teaching

Coping with feeding difficulties

1. *Hemiplegia:* The client may need assistance in opening packages of utensils or condiments, cutting or buttering foods, or feeding himself or herself if the dominant hand is affected. Some clients experience "pocketing" of food in the cheek on the affected side during meals, since they cannot sense that the food is there. The nurse should check for the presence of food and provide good mouth care after meals. The family or other caregivers will need to be taught to do this before discharge.

2. *Visual field defects:* The client may fail to eat half the food on the tray because he or she does not see it. The client can be taught to compensate by scanning, or routinely turning the head and moving the eyes toward the affected side.

3. *Dysphagia:* Muscle weakness or incoordination, impaired gag or swallowing reflexes, and impaired cough contribute to dysphagia and increased likelihood of pulmonary aspiration. The client should be positioned upright, if possible, during and for at least 30 minutes after a meal. Thick liquids such as shakes, or liquids thickened with infant cereals, cornstarch, instant potatoes, or mashed potatoes may be easier to swallow than thin liquids such as water or tea.

Slick foods (e.g., gelatin, pasta salad) are likely to cause difficulty. Foods served at temperature extremes, either chilled or hot, and foods with interesting textures may stimulate the swallowing reflex. The client with dysphagia should not be left alone during meals, and suction should be available. Enteral tube feedings may be necessary if the problem is severe.

Correction of constipation

Immobility and altered muscle function frequently lead to constipation. Dietary measures to correct constipation include increased fiber intake (see Appendix C), consumption of prunes or prune juice, and ensuring that fluid intake is 35 to 50 ml/kg/day.

Alzheimer's Disease and Dementia

Pathophysiology

Alzheimer's disease is the most common cause of dementia, or progressive loss of mental function because of an organic cause. The cause is unknown, but the most common findings in the brains of individuals with Alzheimer's disease are cerebral atrophy, senile plaques and neurofibrillary tangles. Clients experience memory loss, shortening of the attention span, expressive and receptive language disorders, apraxia (inability to perform a task in response to verbal commands), loss of reasoning skills, and intolerance of frustration.

Treatment

There is no definitive therapy at present, and therefore most therapy is directed toward management of specific symptoms and supportive care.

Nutritional Care

Progressive loss of self-care skills affects food intake and nutritional status. Longitudinal studies of clients in extended care facilities have shown that weight loss in clients with Alzheimer's disease is greater than in clients without the disease.

Assessment

Assessment is summarized in Table 15-1.

Intervention

Nutrition interventions are designed to encourage an adequate intake so that weight and strength will be maintained, morbidity (e.g., decubitus ulcers and pneumonia) will be lessened, and client comfort will be optimized.

Encourage adequate intake

The following list summarizes management of problems commonly experienced by the client with Alzheimer's disease.

1. *Memory loss:* Provide verbal and nonverbal cues that it is mealtime (e.g., announce the meal to the client; put utensils in the client's hand). Eating in a group setting may improve intake because the client observes models of eating behavior.

2. *Poor swallowing:* Food consistency may have to be altered to cope with swallowing difficulties (see Interventions for cerebrovascular accident). Positioning the client upright, with chin slightly downward to reduce the possibility of aspiration, will help to reduce dribbling of food from the mouth, coughing, and choking.

3. *Poor intake:* Provide adequate time for the client to eat, and avoid distractions during mealtimes. Feed client if necessary. Many clients experience "sundowning," or restlessness and agitation in the evening, and food intake is poor at this time. For these individuals, maximize intake at the noon and morning meals when cognitive abilities are better. Many clients with Alzheimer's disease seem to prefer sweet items to other types of foods. Alternating bites of sweetened with unsweetened foods can improve their intake. If the client is combative or resistive when being fed, diversions (singing, cheerful conversation, touching, holding hands) are sometimes effective in redirecting behavior.

Alcoholism

Pathophysiology

Heavy alcohol use has adverse effects on nutrition both because it displaces other, more nutritious, foods in the diet and because chronic use impairs absorption and metabolism of nutrients. Chronic alcohol abuse results in low hepatic stores of folate, niacin, and vitamins B_6 and B_{12}, as well as impaired utilization of folate and vitamins B_1 and B_6. In addition, zinc and magnesium levels may be low as a result of increased urinary excretion of these minerals during heavy drinking.

Wernicke-Korsakoff syndrome is a serious disorder of the central nervous system, occurring in alcoholism. Symptoms are mental confusion, memory loss, confabulation, ataxia, abnormal ocular motility (ophthalmoplegia and nystagmus), and peripheral neuropathy. The cause appears to be multifactorial, but both genetics and vitamin B_1 deficiency play a role.

Treatment

Effective therapy of alcoholism comes only after the individual has acknowledged the illness. Comprehensive therapy includes individual or group counseling and a nutritious diet. Diazepam (Valium) may be used to reduce anxiety during alcohol withdrawal. Disulfiram (Antabuse) is sometimes used to help the individual resist the compulsion to drink.

Nutritional Care

Goals are to support the individual in avoiding alcohol and to correct nutritional deficits.

Assessment

Assessment is summarized in Table 15-2.

Intervention

Provision of a nutritious diet to promote hepatic regeneration and correct nutritional deficits
The diet should be tailored to the individual's needs:

Problem	Diet
Alcoholic hepatitis	≥100 g protein, high carbohydrate
Hepatic encephalopathy	15 to 20 g protein/day; ↑ as tolerated; see Chapter 9, p. 143
Steatorrhea	≤50 g fat/day
Ascites	Sodium restriction (usually 1 g/day); see box on pp. 261-262
Esophageal varices	Bland foods, soft in texture

All alcoholics should abstain from alcohol.

Table 15-2   Assessment in alcoholism and disruptions of mental health

Area of Concern	Significant Findings
Protein Calorie Malnutrition (PCM)	*History* Chronic alcohol or other drug abuse (inadequate intake of nutritious foods or impaired absorption of nutrients); paranoia, delusions (e.g., fear that food is poisoned); confusion, disorientation, inability to care for self (e.g., schizophrenia, Alzheimer's disease) *Physical examination* Hepatomegaly (can be from both malnutrition and toxic effects of alcohol); ascites, edema; muscle wasting; triceps skinfold or AMC <5th percentile (see Appendix G); weight <90% of standard or BMI <19.1 (women) or 20.7 (men) (↓ body weight may be masked by presence of ascites and edema) *Laboratory analysis* ↓ Serum albumin, transferrin, or prealbumin; (↓ levels may indicate liver failure instead of or in addition to malnutrition); ↓ lymphocyte count; nonreactive skin tests
Overweight/ Obesity	*History* Excessive intake of kcal (sometimes occurs in depression or alcoholism) *Physical examination* Weight >120% of standard or BMI >27.3 (women) or 27.8 (men); triceps skinfold >95th percentile (see Appendix G)

Table 15-2   Assessment in alcoholism and disruptions
of mental health—cont'd

Area of Concern	Significant Findings
Vitamin Deficiencies	
B Complex especially B_1, B_6, folate	*History* Alcohol abuse; severely restricted diet (e.g., canned soups, soft drinks, candy, snack foods) *Physical examination* Peripheral neuropathy; dermatitis; glossitis; cheilosis; edema, congestive heart failure; confusion, memory loss *Laboratory analysis* ↓ Hct, ↑ MCV; ↑ activity coefficients for thiamin pyrophosphate and erythrocyte glutamic oxaloacetic transaminase (for vitamins B_1 and B_6, respectively); NOTE: assessment of activity coefficients is rarely done; these vitamins have low toxicity; large doses are given and response is evaluated clinically
Mineral Deficiencies	
Zinc (Zn)	*History* Alcohol abuse, with poor intake and ↑ excretion of Zn *Physical examination* Hypogeusia, dysgeusia; diarrhea; dermatitis *Laboratory analysis* ↓ Serum Zn
Magnesium (Mg)	*History* Alcohol abuse, with poor intake and ↑ excretion of Mg *Physical examination* Tremor, ataxia; mental disorientation *Laboratory analysis* ↓ Serum Mg

Supplementation

Supplements usually used include folate and vitamins B_1 and B_6. In Wernicke-Korsakoff syndrome, the dose of vitamin B_1 is about 100 times the RDA. The other vitamins are given in amounts equal to two or three or more times the RDA. If serum levels are low, zinc and magnesium supplements are used. Careful observation should be made of response to supplements. Ocular changes of Wernicke-Korsakoff syndrome respond quickly to vitamin B_1, but ataxia and confusion respond slowly and may never resolve.

Client teaching

Adequate diet

The recovering alcoholic will need instruction in consuming an appropriate nutritious diet. See Intervention, p. 293.

Reinforcement of the need to abstain from alcohol

Recovered alcoholics need continued help, particularly advice for coping with social events and holidays when alcohol is usually served. Role playing before these occasions can be helpful.

Disorders of Mental Health

Pathophysiology

Mental illnesses have a variety of diverse etiologies too extensive to describe here. It is important to note that the vast majority of mental illnesses have no nutritional cause. "Orthomolecular psychiatry," a treatment approach utilizing vitamin supplements containing 10 to 500 times the RDA, is not supported by scientific evidence or recognized as acceptable therapy by the American Psychiatric Association. There is also no reason to believe, as some individuals do, that many cases of mental illness arise from allergies or hypersensitivity to common foods. In most cases, nutritional care is primarily a supportive measure during the treatment of mental health disorders.

Treatment

A variety of treatment modalities may be used in mental disorders, including psychoanalysis, behavioral therapy, and family therapy. Some of the medications used are major and minor tranquilizers and lithium. Chapter 18 lists effects of these drugs on appetite and nutrient needs.

Nutritional Care

The goal of care is for the client to be able to cope with nutrition-related symptoms often seen in disruptions of mental health.

Assessment

Table 15-2 describes assessment in mental disorders.

Intervention

A variety of nutrition-related symptoms are found among individuals with disruptions of mental health. Most of these are corrected when the individual receives adequate treatment for the underlying disorder. However, Table 15-3 summarizes approaches that can be used until the client has responded to treatment.

Table 15-3 Intervention in mental disorders

Symptoms	Example of Mental Disorder	Suggested Interventions
Anorexia/apathy about food	Depression	Provide small, frequent feedings of foods high in kcal; determine likes and dislikes, and try to accommodate these; serve foods in an attractive manner; use nutritional supplements (Tables 6-1 and 6-2) as needed
Constipation	Depression	Encourage high-fiber foods and large fluid intake
Overeating	Depression	Make low-kcal foods available, but avoid emphasizing weight control until mental condition stabilizes

Continued.

Table 15-3   Intervention in mental disorders—cont'd

Symptoms	Example of Mental Disorder	Suggested Interventions
Confusion/ disorientation	Schizophrenia, organic brain syndrome, Alzheimer's disease (AD, or senile dementia)	Remind client to eat, if necessary; may need to direct client to take each bite; feed the client in an unhurried manner if he is unable to feed himself
Excessive activity with "no time to eat"	Manic behavior	Provide high-kcal foods that can be carried with the person who is too active to sit for a meal: sandwiches; muffins; sliced cheese; fruit, custard, or pudding served in unbreakable containers; liquid nutritional supplements (see Table 6-1) in plastic glasses
Delusions (e.g., fear that food is poisoned, or, conversely, belief that certain foods have magical powers)	Schizophrenia	Allow client to choose foods and beverages until delusions have responded to treatment; try to avoid tube feeding of clients with paranoia since this may increase the feeling of persecution

CASE STUDY

Mr. J., a 52-year-old man with amyotrophic lateral sclerosis, began having symptoms of choking on water and other fluids and difficulty in chewing and swallowing meats. He was also noted to have tachypnea. A chest radiograph revealed a right upper lobe infiltrate consistent with aspiration pneumonia. Mr. J. underwent placement of a percutaneous gastrostomy tube (one inserted without a surgical incision). His wife was instructed in the preparation and administration of a formula prepared from pureed meat and vegetables, milk powder, orange juice, and oil. Mr. J. tolerated the feedings well and experienced no further episodes of aspiration.

Reference

1. Walser M and others: *Nutritional management: the Johns Hopkins handbook,* Philadelphia, 1984, WB Saunders.

Bibliography

Athlin E and others: Aberrant eating behavior in elderly Parkinsonian patients with and without dementia: analysis of video-recorded meals, *Res Nurs Health* 12:41, 1989.

Biery JR, Williford JH Jr, McMullen EA: Alcohol craving in rehabilitation: assessment of nutrition therapy, *J Am Diet Assoc* 91:463, 1991.

Buelow JM, Jamieson D: Potential for altered nutritional status in the stroke patient, *Rehab Nurs* 15:260, 1990.

Evers, S., and others: Nutritional rehabilitation of developmentally disabled residents in a long-term care facility, *J Am Diet Assoc* 91:471, 1991.

Gasch AT: Use of the traditional ketogenic diet for treatment of intractable epilepsy, *J Am Diet Assoc* 90:1433, 1990.

Gray GE, Gray LK: Nutritional aspects of psychiatric disorders, *J Am Dietet Assoc* 89:1492, 1989.

Hinds JP, Eidelman BH, Wald A: Prevalence of bowel dysfunction in multiple sclerosis, *Gastroenterology* 98:1538, 1990.

Norberg AI, Athlin E: Eating problems in severely demented patients: issues and ethical dilemmas, *Nurs Clin North Am* 24:781, 1989.

Pincus JH, Barry K: Influence of dietary protein on motor fluctuations in Parkinson's disease, *Arch Neurol* 44:270, 1987.

Sanders KD and others: Growth response to enteral feeding by children with cerebral palsy, *J Parenter Enteral Nutr* 14:23, 1990.

Sushi NS, and Nielsen CC: Factors affecting food intake of women with Alzheimer's type dementia in long-term care, *J Am Diet Assoc* 89:1770, 1989.

Inborn Errors of Metabolism

16

Inborn errors of metabolism are congenital traits causing impaired metabolism of some nutrient(s), resulting from absence or reduced activity of an enzyme or cofactor. Many of these result in mental retardation or other severe clinical manifestations.

In many instances, dietary therapy can "bypass" the affected enzyme or cofactor, thus ameliorating the disorder. A multitude of inborn errors exist, but only a few of the more common ones with well-established nutritional therapies can be discussed here.

As the child on a severely restricted diet becomes older, peer influences and advertising are increasingly important, and the child becomes aware of a variety of foods never offered by his or her parents. The child may sample these surreptitiously or beg the parent for them. Parent-child struggles over the diet will be reduced if the child is taught gradually, from an early age, to take responsibility for adhering to the diet. The parents may feel guilty that they have produced a child with a defect. They need someone to listen to their concerns and provide emotional support.

Galactosemia

Pathophysiology

Galactosemia results from an inability to metabolize galactose to glucose as a result of the lack of one of two enzymes, galactokinase or galactose-1-phosphate uridyltransferase. Cataracts are the major problem in individuals with galactokinase deficiency, and these can be effectively prevented with a galactose-free diet. Deficiency of the transferase enzyme is associated with more symptoms: vomiting, failure to thrive, hepatomegaly, jaundice, cataracts, and susceptibility to *Escherichia coli* sepsis. Learning disorders, delayed growth, and ovarian dysfunction are reported to be common even in those children who receive treatment. Severe retardation occurs in untreated individuals. Most states require screening of all infants for elevated blood galactose within 7 days of birth.

Nutritional Care

The goal of nutritional care is to avoid galactose intake and to prevent any deficiencies that might result from avoiding galactose-containing foods.

Assessment

Assessment is summarized in Table 16-1.

Table 16-1 Assessment in inborn errors of metabolism

Area of Concern	Significant Findings
Protein Deficiency	*History*
	Excessive restriction of amino acids needed for protein synthesis (e.g., failure to add sufficient phenylalanine-containing foods to the diet of a child with PKU)
	Physical examination
	Edema; changes in hair pigmentation and texture; hepatomegaly; diarrhea; dermatitis
	Laboratory analysis
	↓ Serum albumin, transferrin, or prealbumin
Vitamin Deficiencies	
A	*History*
	Restriction of fruit and vegetable intake (e.g., in glycogen storage disease [GSD])
	Physical examination
	Dry skin or cornea; follicular hyperkeratosis; delayed growth; poor appetite
	Laboratory analysis
	↓ Serum retinol

Continued.

Table 16-1 Assessment in inborn errors of metabolism—cont'd

Area of Concern	Significant Findings
Vitamin Deficiencies—cont'd	
C	*History*
	Restriction of fruit and vegetable intake (e.g., in GSD)
	Physical examination
	Gingivitis; petechiae, ecchymoses; swollen joints; rickets
	Laboratory analysis
	↓ Serum or lymphocyte vitamin C
B$_2$	*History*
	Restriction of milk products in galactosemia, GSD, or PKU
	Physical examination
	Cheilosis; seborrheic dermatitis; corneal vascularization
	Laboratory analysis
	↑ Activity coefficient for erythrocyte glutathione reductase (rarely done)
Folate	*History*
	Restriction of fruits and vegetables (e.g., in GSD)
	Physical examination
	Pallor; glossitis
	Laboratory analysis
	↓ Hct, ↑ MCV; ↓ RBC folate

Intervention

Eliminate galactose intake

Eliminate galactose (and lactose, which is composed of galactose and glucose) from the diet throughout life.

1. All dairy products are to be avoided. Human milk is excluded, as well. Soy infant formulas (Prosobee [Mead Johnson], Nursoy [Wyeth], or Isomil [Ross]) are appropriate for infants. Soy milk can be used by older children and adults.

Table 16-1   Assessment in inborn errors of metabolism—cont'd

Area of Concern	Significant Findings
Mineral Deficiencies	
Calcium (Ca)	*History*
	Restriction of dairy products in galactosemia, GSD, or PKU
	Physical examination
	Rickets; osteomalacia; bone pain
	Laboratory analysis
	↑ Alkaline phosphatase; ↓ serum Ca (uncommon)
Iron (Fe)	*History*
	Restriction of animal protein products in GSD or PKU
	Physical examination
	Pallor, blue sclerae; koilonychia
	Laboratory analysis
	↓ Hct, Hgb, MCV, MCH, MCHC; ↓ serum Fe; ↑ serum transferrin
Zinc (Zn)	*History*
	Restriction of animal protein intake in GSD or PKU
	Physical examination
	Hypogeusia, dysgeusia; diarrhea; dermatitis
	Laboratory analysis
	↓ Serum Zn

2. Galactoside-containing products (soy and organ meats such as kidneys, liver, and brains) were previously restricted, but recent evidence indicates that this is unnecessary.

3. Many medications in tablet form contain lactose as fillers or coating ingredients. Composition of all medications should be ascertained before use by galactosemics.

Supplementation

Fortified soy formula or soy milk or supplements providing the RDA for calcium and vitamin B_2 should be used daily.

Client teaching

Sources of galactose/lactose

Dairy products are the most obvious source of lactose. However, the family should be informed that lactose is added to many commercial products (e.g., frankfurters, margarine, dry cereals, instant mashed potatoes, and some commercial fried potatoes). Any products containing lactose, milk sugar, and milk solids should be avoided. Some casein and whey proteins (milk proteins often added in food processing) contain small amounts of lactose. These should be avoided unless they are known to be lactose-free. Parents (and later the affected child) should learn to read all food labels.

Diet for subsequent pregnancies

The mother of a galactosemic child is often advised to follow a galactose-restricted diet during subsequent pregnancies, although following such a diet has not been documented to improve long-term outcome.

Glycogen Storage Diseases

Pathophysiology

At least 12 types of glycogen storage disease (GSD), each involving a defect in some step of glycogen synthesis or degradation, are known. Glucose-6-phosphatase, or G-6-P, deficiency (GSD I) is the most common GSD. It results in marked hypoglycemia after a fast of only 2 to 4 hours, elevated serum lactate, hyperlipidemia, hyperuricemia (gout), platelet dysfunction, and impaired growth. Diagnosis is made by performing a liver biopsy and finding low levels of G-6-P in the tissue.

Nutritional Care in GSD I

The goals of care are to prevent fasting, provide a constant source of glucose, and avoid overweight. Through prevention of hypoglycemia, it is possible to prevent the metabolic complications and growth failure associated with GSD I.

Assessment

Assessment is summarized in Table 16-1.

Intervention

Proportions of macronutrients in the diet

Plan the diet to include about 10% to 15% protein, 60% to 70% carbohydrates, and 20% to 30% fat. Fat is restricted because it makes little immediate contribution to the blood glucose and may lead to obesity.

Avoid hypoglycemia through elimination of fasting

1. During the day, give small feedings of complex carbohydrates (pasta; unsweetened cereals or rice; *uncooked* cornstarch suspended in water, served in artificially sweetened drink mixes, or mixed with water, lemon juice or other flavorings, and artificial sweetener to form a "pudding"; or breads) approximately every 3 to 4 hours.

2. Give one third of the daily calories as a continuous tube feeding during the night. The formula must contain minimal fat and no carbohydrates except glucose or glucose oligosaccharides, which provide energy readily usable by all cells. One such formula is Vivonex (Norwich Eaton). These feedings are used every night until the individual is able to maintain the blood glucose through an 8-hour fast. This point varies with the individual, but has occurred at about 18 to 22 years of age in some individuals studied.

   Recent data indicate that it is possible to replace continuous nightly tube feedings with intermittent feedings of uncooked cornstarch, as long as they are given at least every 5 hours. Further study of long-term effects of such treatment is needed, but it offers a promising alternative to tube feedings, which can be burdensome for the child and family.

3. Use published exchange lists for planning GSD diets[1] to provide variety and simplify client teaching.

Limit carbohydrate sources other than glucose or starch

Galactose, lactose, fructose, and sucrose tend to replace glucose and starch in the diet and are not directly utilized by the cell for energy. Intake of candy, sweetened bakery items, honey, sugar, and sugar-coated cereals should be avoided. Limited amounts of fruits, juices, and milk are usually allowed.

Supplementation

A nutritionally complete tube feeding formula is used, but the volume given is unlikely to meet vitamin and mineral needs. A multivitamin-mineral supplement should be given to provide the RDA for vitamin C, vitamin A, and folate and at least one half the RDA for iron, zinc, and calcium.

Explore emotional and financial concerns

Use of nocturnal feedings is expensive, since it requires a costly elemental formula and an enteral feeding pump, along with other tube feeding supplies, for 18 to 20 years. The family may have insurance that will cover the majority of costs, or they may need referral to the appropriate social service agencies. In addition, emotional support of the family is vital, since the diet and nocturnal feedings require much commitment. Because of the severe sequelae (e.g., mental deficits, potentially malignant liver tumors), which appear to be preventable by dietary control, every effort should be made to ensure that families have adequate resources to maintain the diet.

Client teaching

Dietary modifications (see Interventions)

The family should be taught foods to limit, foods to emphasize (those with readily available glucose or starch), and the need for an unvarying feeding schedule with no more than 3 to 4 hours between daytime feedings.

Nocturnal tube feedings

Teaching needs include: (1) preparation of the formula, (2) operation of the enteral feeding pump (gravity drip administration is too irregular to maintain a stable blood glucose), and (3) maintenance of the feeding route. Maintenance of the feeding route entails insertion of a nasogastric (NG) tube, if applicable; care of the insertion site, if a gastrostomy or jejunostomy is used; and irrigation of the tube. These procedures are discussed in Chapter 6.

Avoidance of fasting

Once receiving nutritional therapy, the child tolerates fasting poorly. If pump failure occurs, the parents must wake the child every 3 hours during the night to consume cornstarch or a meal similar to those given during the day, and they should secure a replacement pump the next day.

If severe gastroenteritis prevents the child from retaining foods or fluids, the physician must be notified so that intravenous therapy can be started.

Phenylketonuria

Pathophysiology

Because of a defect in the enzyme phenylalanine hydroxylase, individuals with phenylketonuria (PKU) do not convert phenylalanine to tyrosine. Blood phenylalanine levels are high (16 to 20 mg/dl, compared with less than 4 mg/dl in normal individuals), and mental retardation occurs if treatment is not instituted within the first few weeks of life. All states require screening of infants for PKU.

Nutritional Care

The goals of care are to prevent retardation by controlling blood phenylalanine levels.

Assessment

Assessment in summarized in Table 16-1.

Intervention

Restrict dietary phenylalanine to maintain blood phenylalanine between 2 to 10 mg/dl

1. Infants less than 6 months of age use a low-phenylalanine formula (Lofenalac [Mead Johnson] or PKU 1 [Milupa]). Because this formula is so low in phenylalanine that it may not be adequate for growth, the physician will prescribe small amounts of milk to be added to the formula. Blood phenylalanine levels are measured regularly (often weekly or biweekly) to evaluate the success of therapy. With careful monitoring, it is possible for the infant to be breastfed if the mother so desires.

2. Individuals over 6 months of age normally use a phenylalanine-free milk replacement (Phenyl-free [Mead Johnson] or PKU 2 [Milupa]). Foods with a low phenylalanine content, including fruits, vegetables, cereals, low-protein bread and pasta products, fats and oils, are added to the diet to supply phenylalanine and to normalize the diet as much as possible.

3. Exchange lists are used to simplify diet teaching and assist in planning diets for individuals with PKU.[2] The approximate requirement for phenylalanine is 47 mg/kg/day for infants and 200 to 500 mg/day for children. The total number of exchanges allowed should be planned with this in mind.

4. The diet is often discontinued by 8 to 10 years of age or even before, since brain development is considered to be largely complete by that time, but considerable evidence has accumulated that outcome is improved if control is maintained through age 12 and possibly into adulthood.

5. Women with PKU should achieve good control of phenylalanine levels before becoming pregnant and stay in control throughout pregnancy. Infants of mothers with elevated phenylalanine levels during pregnancy have an increased likelihood of microcephaly, reduced birth weight, and congenital defects, especially cardiac defects. Controlling the mother's diet only after conception seems to provide much less benefit than pre- and postconceptual control.

Client teaching

Dietary restrictions (see Intervention)

Although sweets such as sugars, most candies, syrups, jams, and jellies are low in phenylalanine, parents should be discouraged from allowing children unlimited amounts of these. Some parents feel guilty about their children's illness and allow large amounts of sweets to compensate.

It is difficult for the woman who has not been on a controlled diet to return to it during pregnancy, and much support is needed, both from her family and health professionals, for her to adhere to the diet.

Table 16-2   Diet for a 4-year-old with GSD I*

Time	Feeding
7:30 AM	Oatmeal, ½ cup; whole milk, ½ cup; fresh orange, ½
10:00 AM	Cornstarch, 16 g
12:00 PM	Water-packed tuna, 1½ ounce; whole wheat bread, 1½ slice; mayonnaise, 1 tsp; carrot sticks, ½ cup
3:00 PM	Boiled potatoes, 2 small
5:30 PM	Baked chicken, 1 oz (skinned); spaghetti, ¾ cup; tomato juice, ½ cup (over spaghetti)
8:00 PM	Cheddar cheese, ½ oz; macaroni, cooked, plain, ¾ cup
9:00 PM-8:00 AM	Elemental formula (1 kcal/ml), 42 ml/hr

*Weight = 16.5 kg. kcal needs = wt × RDA = 16.5 kg × 85 kcal/kg ≈ 1400 kcal. Tube feedings should supply one third of kcal (≈ 462 kcal). The remainder of kcal are allocated to protein, fat, and carbohydrates as described in the text.

CASE STUDY

Table 16-2 shows a sample diet for a 4-year-old child with GSD I.

References

1. Folk CC, Greene HL: Dietary management of Type I glycogen storage disease, J Am Diet Assoc 84:293, 1984.
2. Acosta P, Elsas L: *Dietary management of inherited metabolic disease: phenylketonuria, galactosemia, tyrosinemia, maple syrup urine disease,* Atlanta, 1976, ACELMU Publishers.

Bibliography

Azen CG and others: Intellectual development in 12-year-old children with phenylketonuria, *Am J Dis Child* 145:35, 1991.
Committee on Nutrition, American Academy of Pediatrics: Special diets for infants with inborn errors of metabolism, *Pediatrics* 57:783, 1976.
Holton JB: Galactose disorders: an overview, *J Inherited Metab Dis* 13:476, 1990.

McCabe L and others: The management of breast feeding among infants with phenylketonuria, *J Inherited Metab Dis* 12:467, 1989.

Schmidt K: A primer to the inborn errors of metabolism for perinatal and neonatal nurses, *J Perinat Neonatal Nurs* 2(4):60, 1989.

Smith I, Glossop J, Beasley M: Fetal damage due to maternal phenylketonuria: effects of dietary treatment and maternal phenylalanine concentrations around the time of conception, *J Inherited Metab Dis* 13:651, 1990.

Wolfsdorf JI and others: Continuous glucose for treatment of patients with type I glycogen storage disease: comparison of the effects of dextrose and uncooked cornstarch on biochemical variables, *Am J Clin Nutr* 52:1043, 1990.

Low Birth Weight Infants

17

Low birth weight (LBW) infants are those with birth weights less than 2500 g. They are premature and/or small-for-gestational age (SGA). Very low birth weight (VLBW) infants have birth weights less than 1500 g, and extremely low birth weight (ELBW) infants weigh less than 1000 g at birth. Premature or preterm infants are those born before 37 weeks of gestation.

Pathophysiology

The smaller and the more premature the infant is, the greater the nutritional risk. Some of the factors contributing to nutritional problems are:

1. Decreased nutrient stores. Most fat, glycogen, and minerals, such as iron, calcium, phosphorus, and zinc, are deposited during the last 8 weeks of pregnancy. Thus preterm infants have increased potential for hypoglycemia, rickets, and anemia.

2. Increased kcal needs for growth. The LBW infant requires approximately 120 kcal/kg/day, compared with the term neonate's 108 kcal/kg/day.

3. Immature mechanical function of the gastrointestinal (GI) tract. A coordinated suck and swallow, with closure of the epiglottis to prevent pulmonary aspiration, does not develop until 32 to 34 weeks of gestation. Delayed gastric emptying and poor intestinal motility are common in preterm infants.

4. Reduced digestive capability. Preterm infants have a smaller pool of bile salts, which are required for fat digestion and absorption, than term infants. Production of pancreatic amylase and lipase, enzymes involved in carbohy-

drate and fat digestion, is also reduced. Lactase (the enzyme required for milk sugar digestion) levels are low until about 34 weeks of gestation.

5. Immature lungs with increased work of breathing and increased kcal needs. Respiratory problems also interfere with enteral feedings. A tachypneic infant, with a respiratory rate greater than 60/min, cannot be safely nipple fed, nor can an infant requiring mechanical ventilation. Furthermore, enteral feedings are not usually given while umbilical artery catheters (UACs), used for monitoring blood gases, are in place. Feedings during UAC use increase the risk of necrotizing enterocolitis (NEC), a serious disease that can result in GI perforation and even death.

6. Potential for heat loss due to large body surface area in relation to body weight, as well as little subcutaneous fat to provide insulation. Loss of heat increases kcal needs.

Treatment

Immaturity of the lungs (particularly inadequate surfactant production, resulting in respiratory distress syndrome or RDS) is the primary problem for many preterm infants. Oxygen therapy and mechanical ventilation are often needed until respiratory function improves. Surfactant replacement therapy is increasingly being utilized in preterm infants.

Nutritional Care

Assessment

Assessment is summarized in Table 17-1.

Intervention

Commonly used feeding methods

Total parenteral nutrition

Total parenteral nutrition (TPN) is needed in severe RDS, congenital bowel anomalies, NEC, or intolerance of enteral feedings, where enteral intake is expected to be delayed for 5 to 7 days or more. Lipid emulsions (2 to 4 g/kg/day) are often given to provide part of the needed kcal. Lipids are not usually started until the indirect bilirubin is low enough that phototherapy is not needed, since free fatty acids can displace bilirubin from its bind-

Table 17-1   Assessment in low birth weight infants

Area of Concern	Significant Findings
Protein Calorie Malnutrition	*History*
	Increased kcal needs for growth and physiologic stress—cold, infection, respiratory disease; poor kcal reserves; poor enteral feeding tolerance caused by immature GI function; impaired digestive ability; limited fluid tolerance, which limits the amount of nutrients delivered (excess fluid contributes to patent ductus arteriosus, which worsens cardiorespiratory function)
	Physical examination
	Poor weight gain (gain should average 20-30 g/day once LBW infants are stable)
	Laboratory analysis
	Serum albumin <3.0 g/dl or prealbumin <11 mg/dl
Vitamin Deficiencies	
A	*History*
	Poor stores; oxygen therapy, with ↑ need for antioxidants such as vitamin A
	Physical examination
	Poor growth
	Laboratory analysis
	Serum retinol <20 μg/dl
E	*History*
	Poor stores; use of oxygen and IV lipid emulsions, with ↑ need for antioxidants such as vitamin E
	Physical examination
	Pallor, tachycardia, mild generalized edema
	Laboratory analysis
	↓ Serum tocopherol, Hct, Hgb (hemolytic anemia)

Continued.

Table 17-1 Assessment in low birth weight infants—cont'd

Area of Concern	Significant Findings
Electrolyte/Mineral Deficiencies	
Sodium (Na)	*History*
	Poor renal conservation caused by immaturity; increased Na needs for growth; use of diuretics in infants with cardiorespiratory disease
	Laboratory analysis
	↓ Serum Na
Iron (Fe)	*History*
	Poor stores; iatrogenic blood loss—frequent laboratory testing
	Physical examination
	Pallor; tachycardia
	Laboratory analysis
	↓ Hct, Hgb, MCV, MCH, MCHC
Calcium (Ca)	*History*
	Decreased reserves with great needs for bone mineralization; limited amount of Ca soluble in formulas or IV fluids
	Laboratory analysis
	↓ Serum Ca; ↑ alkaline phosphatase; radiographic evidence of poor mineralization or fractures
Phosphorus (P)	*History*
	Decreased reserves with great needs for bone mineralization; limited amount of P soluble in formulas or IV fluids
	Laboratory analysis
	↓ Serum P; ↑ alkaline phosphatase; radiographic evidence of poor mineralization
Zinc (Zn)	*History*
	Poor stores; great needs for tissue anabolism during rapid growth; use of Fe supplements, which compete with Zn for absorption
	Physical examination
	Delayed growth; diarrhea; seborrheic dermatitis
	Laboratory analysis
	↓ Serum Zn

ing sites on serum albumin. Also, it may be necessary to avoid lipids, or to use low doses, in septic infants, since they experience impaired metabolism of lipids. Moreover, excessive doses may decrease the partial pressure of oxygen in the blood (PO_2).

TPN may be delivered by a catheter inserted via the subclavian vein, as in adults (Chapter 6), or by a long catheter inserted percutaneously through the basilic or cephalic vein.

Enteral tube feedings

Tube feedings can be used when there is GI motility (active bowel sounds) and absence of UACs.

Types of tube feedings include:

Intermittent oral-gastric (gavage) feedings. These are usually given at frequent (1 to 3 hour) intervals.

Indications: Method of choice for routine feedings.

Shortcomings: Not tolerated well by infants with delayed gastric emptying and in some infants recovering from severe RDS, who have decreased arterial oxygen tension and lung volumes with bolus feedings. Potential for pulmonary aspiration.

NOTE: Several studies have shown that allowing the infant to suck a pacifier during gavage feedings accelerates growth.

Continuous oral-gastric feedings.

Indications: Infants recovering from severe RDS or those with diminished absorptive capacity (such as short-bowel syndrome).

Shortcomings: Potential for pulmonary aspiration.

Continuous transpyloric (nasoduodenal) feedings.

Indications: Delayed gastric emptying, severe gastroesophageal reflux and aspiration, use of CPAP (continuous positive airway pressure) where the stomach may be distended with air.

Shortcomings: May result in bacterial overgrowth of the upper intestine, impaired absorption of potassium and fat, potential for dumping syndrome (influx of plasma fluid into the small bowel, resulting from the hyperosmolar state caused by rapid hydrolysis of nutrients delivered into the duodenum) and diarrhea, potential for intestinal perforation if tube is advanced past the second portion of the duodenum or if polyvinyl chloride or polyethylene tube is used. No advantage over oral-gastric feedings in promotion of kcal intake or weight gain.

Nipple feedings

Nipple feedings are used for infants with a coordinated suck or swallow and a normal respiratory rate. Preterm infants often have difficulty forming a seal around the nipple and sucking in a functional manner. The nurse or parent can assist the infant, e.g., by placing one finger under the chin to provide gentle pressure, stimulating complete closure of the mouth.

Although it has been common practice to allow infants to breastfeed only after they take bottle feedings well, recent research demonstrates that even infants as small as 1300 g tolerate breastfeeding as well as or better than nipple feeding. Breastfeeding does not compromise their respiratory status or temperature stability. If there is concern about the adequacy of the small infant's intake, the infant can be weighed on an electronic scale before and after breastfeeding. The number of grams gained is approximately equal to the milliliters of milk consumed. Mechanical scales are not sufficiently accurate to measure the small weight change resulting from feeding.

Milk and formulas

Human milk. Milk from mothers of preterm infants (preterm milk) has higher levels of minerals and protein than milk of mothers delivering at term (term milk). Nevertheless, levels of calcium, phosphorus, calories, zinc, and sodium in preterm milk are probably too low for rapidly growing premature infants. Levels of these nutrients decline rapidly and reach term levels after 2 to 4 weeks of lactation.

Fortifiers containing protein, carbohydrates, lipid, minerals, and vitamins (e.g., Similac Natural Care [Ross] or Enfamil Human Milk Fortifier [Mead Johnson]) are available for addition to human milk. These fortifiers make it possible to achieve optimum growth while feeding LBW infants their own mothers' milk.

Formulas. Specially prepared formulas with greater protein, mineral, vitamin, and kcal content than formulas for term infants are available for preterm infants. Composition of some of these is shown in Table 17-2. They are usually used until the infant's weight is about 1800 g (approximately 4 lb). Modifications of

Table 17-2 Selected formulas for low birth weight infants (nutrient content per 100 kcal)

Nutrient	Advisable Intakes for Birth Weight*		Similac Special Care 24 kcal (Ross)	Enfamil Premature 24 kcal (Mead Johnson)
	1 kg	1.5 kg		
Protein (g)	3.1	2.7	2.7	2.5
Minerals and Vitamins				
Sodium (mEq)	2.7	2.3	2.2	1.7
Calcium (mg)	160	140	180	100
Phosphorus (mg)	108	95	90	50
Zinc (mg)	0.5	0.5	1.5	0.9
Vitamin E (IU)	0.7†	0.7†	4	1.8

Both formulas above provide 0.8 kcal/ml. Both are low in iron; iron should be supplied by other sources.
*From Committee on Nutrition: Nutritional needs of low birth weight infants, *Pediatrics* 75:976, 1985.
†There is some evidence that this should be higher.

these to make them appropriate for preterm infants include:

1. Using corn syrup solids or glucose oligosaccharides in addition to lactose as a calorie source, to take advantage of more mature enzyme systems.
2. Using medium-chain triglycerides (MCTs) in addition to long-chain triglycerides. MCTs require fewer bile salts for absorption.
3. Concentrating calories into a smaller volume (24 kcal/oz rather than 20 kcal/oz).
4. Increasing levels of minerals and vitamins to promote more adequate growth.

Safe delivery of nutrition support

LBW infants are especially vulnerable to mechanical and infectious complications of nutrient delivery. To prevent these, nutrition support must be carefully administered and monitored (see Chapter 6). In addition to the guidelines in Chapter 6:

During TPN. Check blood glucose at least every 8 hours until stable. LBW infants often have poor glucose tolerance and a low renal glucose threshold. Thus they can experience hyperglycemia and glucosuria, with loss of kcal and excessive fluid in the urine, on relatively low doses of glucose.

During enteral feedings. Evaluate the color of the gastric residual before each intermittent feeding or every 2 to 3 hours during continuous feedings. Bile-stained (green or yellow) fluid usually indicates reduced GI motility and should be reported to the physician. Feedings may need to be decreased or stopped until the problem resolves.

Supplementation

Some physicians prescribe 5 to 25 IU of vitamin E and 400 IU of vitamin D per day for LBW infants. Once the LBW infant receiving human milk reaches 2000 g (4 lb 6½ oz) or goes home from the hospital, the infant needs 2 to 3 mg/kg/day of elemental iron as ferrous sulfate drops. Iron-fortified formula usually provides enough iron to meet needs.

CASE STUDY

Betty J. was born at 30 weeks of gestation, weighing 1400 g (3 lb 1 oz). She received TPN and lipid emulsions during her first 7 days of life. Once her respiratory disease resolved, she was begun on oral-gastric tube feedings of her mother's milk, diluted to half strength. She tolerated feedings well, without vomiting, bile-stained residual, or abdominal distention. Volume and concentration of the milk were increased daily. From the sixth day of feedings until she reached 1800 g, a commercial fortifier was added to the milk. By 34 weeks postconceptual age, she was taking half of her feedings by nipple, and gradually she made the transition to breastfeeding. She was discharged 6 weeks after her birth, weighing 2050 g.

Bibliography

Antonowicz I, Lebenthal E: Developmental pattern of small intestinal enterokinase and disaccharidase activities in the human fetus, *Gastroenterology* 72:1299, 1977.

Bauer K and others: Body composition, nutrition, and fluid balance during the first two weeks of life in preterm neonates weighing less than 1500 grams, *J Pediatr* 118:615, 1991.

Committee on Nutrition, American Academy of Pediatrics: Nutritional needs of low-birth-weight infants, *Pediatrics* 75:976, 1985.

Field T and others: Nonnutritive sucking during tube feedings: effects on preterm neonates in an intensive care unit, *Pediatrics* 70:381, 1982.

Heird WC: Advances in infant nutrition over the past quarter century, *J Am Coll Nutr* 8:228, 1989.

Leick-Rude MK: Use of percutaneous silastic intravascular catheters in high-risk neonates, *Neonatal Netw* 9(1):17, 1990.

Meier P: Bottle- and breast-feeding: effects on transcutaneous oxygen pressure and temperature in preterm infants, *Nurs Res* 37:36, 1988.

Meier PP and others: The accuracy of test weighing for preterm infants, *J Pediatr Gastroenterol Nutr* 10:62, 1990.

Peidboeuf B and others: Total parenteral nutrition in the newborn infant: energy substrates and respiratory gas exchange, *J Pediatr* 118:97, 1991.

Saunders RB, Friedman CB, Stramoski PR: Feeding preterm infants: schedule or demand, *JOGNN* 20(3):212, 1991.

Shaker CS: Nipple feeding premature infants: a different perspective, *Neonatal Netw* 8(5):9, 1990.

Drug-Nutrient Interactions 18

Drug therapy is part of the treatment of most diseases. Drugs can affect a person's nutritional status by altering his or her food intake or absorption, metabolism, and excretion of nutrients. On the other hand, food intake can alter the absorption, metabolism, and excretion of certain drugs. Awareness of these potential interactions can help prevent nutrient deficiencies and impairment or exaggeration of the drug's effects.

Pathophysiology

Several types of individuals are at particular risk for drug-nutrient interactions. These are individuals with inadequate or marginal nutrient intake (e.g., alcoholics); those with increased nutritional demands resulting from catabolic illnesses (e.g., cancer), recent surgery, or infection; those with impaired ability to absorb, metabolize, or excrete drugs and nutrients (e.g., individuals with chronic renal or gastrointestinal diseases; the elderly); and individuals requiring long-term drug therapy (e.g., individuals with organ transplants, hypertension, or rheumatoid arthritis).

Some of the specific effects of drugs on nutritional status are:
1. Alteration of food intake caused by appetite changes (see the accompanying box), changes in the senses of taste and smell (see the box on p. 322), or nausea and vomiting.
2. Alteration of nutrient absorption caused by changes in gastrointestinal (GI) pH or motility, reduction of bile acid activity, formation of drug-nutrient complexes, inactivation of the nutrient transport mechanisms in the bowel, or GI mucosal damage.
3. GI irritation with blood loss.

Drugs Affecting Appetite

Appetite Depressants

Amphetamines and related compounds
Benzphetamine (Didrex)
Fenfluramine (Pondimin)
Phenmetrazine (Preludin)
Phenylpropanolamine (Dexatrim, Dimetapp, Triaminic)
Antibiotics
Amphotericin B (Fungizone)
Gentamicin (Garamycin)
Metronidazole (Flagyl)
Zidovudine (AZT)
Carbonic anhydrase inhibitors
Acetazolamide (Diamox)
Dichlorphenamide (Daranide)
Digitalis preparations
Methylphenidate (Ritalin)

Appetite Stimulants

Antidepressants
Amitriptyline (Elavil)
Antihistamines
Astemizole (Hismanal)
Cyproheptadine (Periactin)
Tranquilizers
Lithium carbonate (Lithane)
Benzodiazipines: all, including
Prazepam (Centrax)
Diazepam (Valium)
Phenothiazines: all, including
Chlorpromazine (Thorazine)
Promethazine (Phenergan)
Steroids
Anabolic steroids
Oxandrolone (Anavar)
Glucocorticoids
Dexamethasone (Decadron)
Methylprednisolone (Medrol)
Tetrahydrocannabinol (marijuana)

From Levitsky DA: Drugs, appetite, and body weight. In Roe DA, Campbell TC, editors: Drugs and nutrients: the interactive effects, *New York, 1984, Marcel Dekker; Drug Evaluations Annual 1991, Milwaukee, 1990, American Medical Association.*

Some Drugs That Affect Taste Sensitivity*

Amphetamines ($\downarrow$ sweet, $\uparrow$ bitter)
Ampicillin
Amphotericin B
Aspirin
Captopril
Chlorpheniramine maleate†
Clindamycin (bitter aftertaste)
Clofibrate ($\downarrow$ sensitivity, aftertaste)
Diazoxide
Dinitrophenol
Ethacrynic acid
Griseofulvin
Insulin
Lincomycin
Lithium carbonate (strange, unpleasant taste)
Meprobamate
Methicillin (aftertaste)
Metronidazole
Oxyfedrine
Penicillamine
Phenindione
Phenytoin
Propantheline
Sodium lauryl sulfate‡
Streptomycin
Tetracyclines
Zidovudine

Modified from Carson JAS, Gormican A: Disease-medication relationships in altered taste sensitivity, J Am Diet Assoc 68:550, 1976; Roe DA: Interactions between drugs and nutrients, Med Clin North Am 63:985, 1979.
*Sensitivity decreased unless otherwise noted.
†Antihistamine found in many over-the-counter cold/allergy products.
‡Toothpaste ingredient.

4. Alteration of nutrient metabolism and excretion.

Nutritional effects of commonly used drugs are described in Table 18-1. Nutrients (or nutrient deficiencies) alter drug therapy in the following ways:

1. Alteration of absorption of enterally administered drugs by affecting GI transit time and motility, GI pH, ionization of the drug, stability of the drug, solubility of the drug, or formation of a complex between the drug and food components. The box on p. 327 lists drugs whose absorption is affected by food intake.
2. Acceleration or delay of the drug's metabolism or excretion.
3. Antagonism of the drug's effect by a food component.

Table 18-1   Nutritional effects of selected drugs

Drug	Effect on Nutrition
Alcohol	$\uparrow$ excretion of mg, K^+, Zn; impaired folate utilization
Antacids	
All	$\downarrow$ Fe absorption caused by $\uparrow$ gastric pH
Aluminum hydroxide	$\downarrow$ Phosphate absorption
Antibiotics/Antifungals/ Antitubercular Agents	
Amphotericin B	Hypokalemia; $\uparrow$ urinary excretion of Mg
Cephalosporins	False positive urine glucose by Clinitest (enzyme-based tests such as Tes-Tape or Clinistix not affected)
Chloramphenicol	$\downarrow$ Hgb synthesis (interferes with response to Fe, folate, or vitamin B_{12} therapy)
Cycloserine	$\downarrow$ Serum levels of vitamins B_{12}, B_6, folate
Gentamicin	$\uparrow$ Urinary excretion of Mg, K^+, Ca (>10 g cumulative dose)
Isoniazid	Depletion of vitamin B_6, supplement should be given
Neomycin	Diarrhea and mucosal injury; $\downarrow$ absorption of fat, lactose, protein, vitamins A, D, K, B_{12}, Ca, Fe, K^+
Para-amino-salicylic acid	$\downarrow$ Absorption of fat, folacin, vitamin B_{12}
Anticonvulsants	
Phenytoin	$\downarrow$ Absorption of Ca
Phenobarbital	$\downarrow$ Absorption of Ca
Primidone	$\downarrow$ Absorption of Ca

Roe DA: Drug and nutrient interactions. In Schneider HA, Anderson CE, Coursin DB, editors: *Nutritional support of medical practice,* Philadelphia, 1983, Harper & Row; Drug Evaluations Annual 1991, Milwaukee, 1990, American Medical Association; *Physicians' Desk Reference,* ed 45, Oradell, NJ, 1991, Medical Economics.

Continued.

Table 18-1   Nutritional effects of selected drugs—cont'd

Drug	Effect on Nutrition
Antidiarrheal Agent	
Sulfasalazine	↓ Absorption of folate; megaloblastic anemia
Antihypertensive Agents	
Diazoxide	Hyperglycemia
Hydralazine	↑ Excretion of vitamin B_6
Nitroprusside	↓ Serum vitamin B_{12}
Antiinflammatory Agents	
Aspirin	↑ Urinary loss of vitamin C; Fe deficiency caused by GI blood loss
Colchicine	↓ Absorption of vitamin B_{12}, fat, carotene, lactose, protein, Na, K^+
Indomethacin	↑ Urinary loss of vitamin C; Fe deficiency caused by GI blood loss
Antineoplastic drugs	See Chapter 8
Carbonic Anhydrase Inhibitors	
All	Hyperglycemia; ↑ excretion of K^+
Cardiac Drugs	
Digitalis, digoxin, digitoxin, etc.	Diarrhea, malabsorption of all nutrients
Chelating Agents	
Penicillamine	↓ Absorption of Cu, Zn, Fe
Corticosteroids	
All	↑ Protein catabolism; ↓ protein synthesis; hyperglycemia; ↑ serum triglycerides and cholesterol; ↓ absorption of Ca, P, K^+; ↑ requirement for vitamins C, B_6, D, folate, Zn; osteopenia

Table 18-1   Nutritional effects of selected drugs—cont'd

Drug	Effect on Nutrition
Diuretics	
All	↑ Urinary excretion of Mg, Zn, K^+ (some greater than others)
Ethacrynic acid	Hypomagnesemia, hypokalemia; ↑ loss of urinary Ca
Furosemide	↓ Glucose tolerance; hyperglycemia; ↑ loss of urinary Ca
Thiazides	↓ Glucose tolerance; hyperglycemia; hypokalemia
H_2 Receptor Antagonists	
All (cimetidine, famotidine, nizatidine, ranitidine)	↓ Fe and Ca absorption caused by ↑ gastric pH
Hypocholesterolemics	
Cholestyramine	↓ Absorption of fat, vitamins A, E, D, K, B_{12}, Fe
Clofibrate	↓ Absorption of carotene, Fe, vitamin B_{12}, fat
Colestipol	↓ Absorption of fat, vitamins A, D, E, K
Laxatives	
Cathartics (e.g., senna, cascara, phenolphthalein)	↑ Fecal loss of Ca and K^+ (clinically significant only with laxative abuse)
Mineral oil	Potential for ↓ absorption of vitamins A, D, E, K, Ca^{2+}; recent evidence indicates that effects on vitamin absorption are probably not clinically significant
Levodopa	↑ Requirement for vitamin B_6
Lipid emulsions	↑ Requirement for vitamin E
Opiates	
Heroin	↓ glucose tolerance, ↓ K^+

Continued.

Table 18-1 Nutritional effects of selected drugs—cont'd

Drug	Effect on Nutrition
Oral Contraceptive Agents	↓ Serum vitamin C; possible ↓ serum vitamin B_{12}, B_6, B_2, folate, Mg, Zn; ↑ Hct, Hgb, serum Fe, Cu, vitamins A, E
Parasympatholytic Agents	
Atropine	↓ Fe absorption caused by ↑ gastric pH
Potassium Supplements	↓ Vitamin B_{12} absorption
Sedatives-Hypnotics	
Glutethimide	↓ Absorption of Ca
Uricosuric Agents*	↑ Excretion of Ca, Mg, Na, K^+, P, Cl, vitamin B_2, amino acids
Urinary Antiseptics	
Nitrofurantoin	↓ Serum folate; megaloblastic anemia

*Used in treatment of gout.

Nutritional Care

Nutritional care should be planned, as much as possible, to optimize drug therapy while minimizing nutritional impacts.

Intervention and Client Teaching

Drugs that alter appetite

If the diet history reveals that drugs appear to be stimulating or depressing appetite, the physician may be able to choose another drug with less pronounced effects on appetite. In some cases, it is possible and desirable to interrupt drug therapy periodically to promote adequate nutritional intake. For instance, methylphenidate (Ritalin), used in the treatment of children with attention deficit disorders, depresses appetite and growth. Methylphenidate is usually prescribed only during the school year, when control of

Drugs Whose Absorption is Affected by Food

Absorption Increased	Absorption Reduced
Carbamazepine (Tegretol)	Amoxicillin (Amoxil)
Griseofulvin (Fulvicin)	Ampicillin (Polycillin)
Hydralazine (Apresoline)	Aspirin
Metoprolol (Lopressor)	Astemizole (Hismanal)
Nitrofurantoin (Macrodantin)	Demeclocycline (Declomycin)
Propoxyphene (Darvon)	Doxycycline (Vibramycin)
Propranolol (Inderal)	Dipyridamole (Persantine)
Spironolactone (Aldactone)	Levodopa (Dopar)
	Methotrexate
	Oxytetracycline (Terramycin)
	Penicillin G
	Penicillin V (K)
	Phenobarbital (Luminal)
	Phenytoin (Dilantin)
	Propantheline (Pro-Banthine)
	Tetracycline (especially affected by dairy products)

From Roe DA: Drug and nutrient interactions. In Schneider HA, Anderson CE, Coursin DB, editors: Nutritional support of medical practice, Philadelphia, 1983, Harper & Row; Griffith, HW: Complete guide to prescription and nonprescription drugs, Tucson, 1985, HP Books; Physicians' Desk Reference, ed 45, Oradell, NJ, 1991, Medical Economics.

the disorder is most important. During the summer break from drug therapy, appetite improves and catch-up growth occurs.

Appetite-stimulating drugs are sometimes used when other regularly used drugs suppress appetite. Cyproheptadine (Periactin) is the most commonly used appetite stimulant. It is sometimes prescribed for patients suffering anorexia as a consequence of treatment with antineoplastic drugs.

Drugs that cause alterations in taste and smell

In some cases, dysgeusia or hypogeusia occurs because drugs cause malabsorption or increased excretion of zinc. Increased dietary zinc intake (see Appendix B) or zinc supplementation may improve sensory enjoyment of food.

Drugs that cause malabsorption or increased excretion of nutrients

Where loss of nutrients is likely to be clinically significant, plan the diet and teach the client/family to include generous amounts of those nutrients. For example, individuals receiving thiazide diuretics need several daily servings of potassium-rich foods—meats and fresh fruits and vegetables, such as oranges; bananas; melons; tomatoes; squash; carrots; and deep green, leafy vegetables.

Supplements should be used where the diet may not be adequate to replace drug-induced losses.

Drugs whose absorption is affected by food intake

Where drug absorption is affected by food intake, every dose should ideally be taken in the same relationship to food intake. This prevents fluctuations in blood levels caused by variable drug absorption.

When absorption is stimulated by food intake, the drug should be taken with a meal or snack. When absorption is decreased by food intake, it is best if the drug is taken at least 1 hour before or 2 hours after eating or receiving an intermittent tube feeding. When the client is receiving continuous tube feedings, drug levels should be monitored carefully. Drugs whose absorption is inhibited by food should never be mixed with the tube feeding.

Harmful drug and nutrient interaction

Certain drugs and foods or nutrients interact in such a way as to cause potentially serious systemic effects (Table 18-2). The interaction of monoamine oxidase inhibitors and foods containing dopamine and tyramine is among the most serious of these. The diets of individuals receiving these drugs should be planned to avoid these interactions, and they and their families should be carefully instructed in the necessity of avoiding the offending foods for as long as the drugs are used.

Table 18-2 Drugs interacting with specific foods or nutrients

Drug (Example)	Food or Nutrient	Effect
Antiacne Preparations		
Benzoyl peroxide	Cinnamon, foods containing benzoic acid or benzoate (a preservative)	Skin rash
Anticoagulant		
Coumarin (warfarin) (Coumadin)	Vitamin K-containing foods: liver, cabbage, spinach, kale, egg yolk	↓ Effect of anticoagulant
Antidepressants		
Monoamine oxidase (MAO) inhibitors Phenelzine (Nardil), Isocarboxazid (Marplan), Tranylcypromine (Parnate)	Tyramine-dopamine-containing foods: liver, dry sausage (e.g., hard salami); any pickled, aged, fermented, or smoked protein foods (e.g., pickled herring, aged cheese, yogurt); any protein food that may have been stored improperly or may have spoiled; meat extracts; commercial gravies; yeast extracts; all alcoholic beverages, including beer and wine;	Headache, hypertensive crisis, potential intracranial hemorrhage

Continued.

Table 18-2   Drugs interacting with specific foods or nutrients—cont'd

Drug (Example)	Food or Nutrient	Effect
Monoamine Oxidase (MAO) inhibitors—cont'd	sour cream; soy sauce; bananas; avocados; figs; raisins; Italian broad (fava) beans; eggplant; limit to 1 small orange/day; limit to ½ cup tomato/day	
Antineoplastic Agent Procarbazine (Matulane)		
Antihypertensive Guanadrel (Hylorel)	Caffeine-containing foods and beverages	↓ Effectiveness of the drug
Antimanic Lithium	Caffeine; sodium-restricted diet	↑ Effect of lithium; potential for lithium toxicity
Antimetabolite Methotrexate	Folate supplement Folate deficiency	↓ Effectiveness of the drug ↑ Toxicity of the drug

Anti-Parkinson's Agent		
Levodopa	Pyridoxine (vitamin B_6) supplement	↓ Effectiveness of the drug
Bronchodilator		
Isoetharine (Bronkosol)	Chocolate, caffeine	Cardiac dysrhythmia, tachycardia
Cardiac Glycosides		
Digitalis and related drugs	Potassium (K^+) depletion	↑ Toxicity of the drug
Diuretics		
Thiazides		
Chlorothiazide (Diuril), Hydrochlorothiazide (HydroDIURIL), Hydroflumethiazide (Saluron), Chlorthalidone (Hygroton)	Imported (natural) licorice	↑ K^+ excretion; cardiac dysrhythmia; sodium and water retention

From Roe DA: Drug and nutrient interactions. In Schneider HA, Anderson CE, Coursin DB, editors: *Nutritional support of medical practice*, Philadelphia, 1983, Harper & Row; Griffith HW: *Complete guide to prescription and nonprescription drugs*, Tucson, 1985, HP Books; *Drug Evaluations Annual '91*, Milwaukee, 1990, American Medical Association.

CASE STUDY

Ms. L., a 68-year-old woman, was admitted to the hospital for repair of an abdominal aortic aneurysm. As an incidental finding, it was noted that she had profound anorexia. Her weight was 80% of the standard for her height, and she stated that she had lost 5 kg (11 pounds) over the past year. During that time, she had been on maintenance digoxin therapy following an episode of congestive heart failure. Her serum digoxin level was found to be at the upper limit of the therapeutic range. This level would not cause toxicity in a younger adult, but older adults can develop toxicity at lower serum levels.

The digoxin dosage was reduced, and the client's appetite improved. Her surgery was successful, and 3 months after discharge, she had regained 3 kg and reported that her appetite was excellent.

Bibliography

Cook MC, Taren DL: Nutritional implications of medication use and misuse in elderly, *J Fla Med Assoc* 77:606, 1990.

Fagerman KE, McGuigan D, Pixley B: Potential interaction between enteral feeding solutions and oral tetracycline, *Nutr Clin Prac* 1:257, 1986.

Holtzapple PG, Schwartz SE: Drug-induced maldigestion and malabsorption. In Roe DA, Campbell TC, editors: *Drugs and nutrients: interactive effects,* New York, 1984, Marcel Dekker.

Marvel ME, Bertino JS: Comparative effects of an elemental and a complex enteral feeding formulation on the absorption of phenytoin suspension, *J Parenter Enteral Nutr* 15:316, 1991.

Mohs ME, Watson RR, Leonard-Green T: Nutritional effects of marijuana, heroin, cocaine, and nicotine, *J Am Diet Assoc* 90:1261, 1990.

Murray JJ, Healy MD: Drug-mineral interactions: a new responsibility for the hospital dietitian, *J Am Diet Assoc* 91:66, 1991.

Obesity and Weight Control 19

Overweight refers to any weight in excess of the desirable body weight. *Obesity* refers to an excess of body fat. Obesity is usually defined as 120% or more of the desirable or ideal body weight (IBW). There are three degrees of obesity: (1) mild, 120% to 140% of IBW, (2) moderate, 141% to 200% of IBW, and (3) severe or morbid, more than 200% of IBW.

Pathophysiology

Diagnosis of Obesity

There are several methods for determining whether obesity is present:

1. Comparison of weight with tables of desirable weight for height (see Appendix E)
2. Body mass index (BMI) greater than 27.8 for men or 27.3 for women; the formula for BMI is:

    Weight (kg) ÷ height^2 (m)

3. Measurement of subcutaneous fat; a triceps skinfold of 18.6 mm for males or 25.1 mm for females has been used as an indicator of obesity

Etiology

The cause of obesity is multifactorial. The following factors are involved in at least some cases of obesity:

1. *Genetics:* Children of obese parents are three to eight times as likely to be obese as children of normal-weight parents, even if they are not reared by their natural parents.
2. *Environment:* Familial influences (e.g., using food as a re-

ward, withholding dessert until the plate is clean) help develop eating habits that contribute to obesity.

3. *Psychology:* Overeating may occur as a response to loneliness, grief, or depression; it may be a response to external cues such as food advertising or the fact that it is mealtime.

4. *Physiology:* Energy expenditure declines with aging, and thus body weight often increases during middle age; in a few instances, endocrine abnormalities such as hypothyroidism are responsible for obesity.

No matter what the underlying cause(s), the primary etiologic factor of obesity is the consumption of kcal in excess of energy needs.

Health Risks Associated with Obesity

Obesity is associated with numerous health risks, which are summarized in Table 19-1. Health risks increase progressively with the severity of obesity.

Table 19-1   Health problems caused or worsened by obesity

Area or Type of Problem	Disease, Symptom, or Difficulty
Cardiovascular and respiratory	Hypertension; coronary heart disease; varicose veins; pickwickian syndrome*
Endocrine and reproductive	Non-insulin-dependent diabetes mellitus; amenorrhea, infertility; preeclampsia
Gastrointestinal	Cholecystitis and cholelithiasis; fatty liver
Psychiatric and social	Social discrimination
Musculoskeletal and skin	Osteoarthritis; skin irritation and infections, especially in fat folds; striae
Malignancies	Cancer of the colon, rectum, prostate, gallbladder, breast, uterus, and ovaries

*Hypoventilation and lethargy caused by decreased chest movement resulting from excessive weight on the chest.

Treatment and Nutritional Care in Obesity

The goals of intervention are to: (1) decrease body fat to achieve a weight within 20% of ideal, (2) develop more healthy eating habits, (3) prevent loss of lean body mass (LBM) during weight reduction, and (4) maintain weight loss.

Assessment

Assessment is summarized in Table 19-2.

Intervention

Weight reduction is achieved by consuming fewer kcal than are required to meet energy needs. Methods for achieving weight re-

Table 19-2   Assessment in obesity and weight control

Areas of Concern	Significant Findings
Factors Contributing to Obesity	*History* *Usual nutrient intake* Include: Meal and snack patterns; portion sizes; food preparation methods (frying, sauteing, adding butter or margarine as a flavoring); gravies, sauces, and beverages (including alcohol) *Conditions under which eating occurs* Keeping a food record helps the individual identify occasions that result in eating, if it includes: Who the individual eats with (alone versus with family or friends); where and when eating occurs (at the table, while watching television, while preparing meals, while studying); feelings that prompt eating (loneliness, boredom, anxiety or depression versus hunger) *Activity level* Include: Presence or absence of regularly scheduled exercise (type, frequency, duration, and intensity); activity required during work, school, housework, or hobbies

duction include diet, behavior modification, exercise, surgery, and drugs and devices. All of these will be discussed in this chapter.

Establish weight goal

In children the IBW is assumed to be the 50th percentile of weight for height on the growth charts (see Appendix F). For adults, the IBW can be established by taking the midpoint from the table of desirable weights for height (see Appendix E) or by using the formulas described in Chapter 1, p. 5).

A weight that is no more than 20% greater than ideal is associated with the least health risks. However, the obese individual should participate in setting personal weight goals. Especially in the severely obese individual, a goal of less than or equal to 120% of the IBW may seem overwhelming.

Promote weight loss, while maintaining LBM

Diet
Balanced low-kcal diets. These diets, based on common foods chosen from all food groups, though low in kcal, are adequate in all (or almost all) nutrients. They are the best choice for individuals who are less than 30% overweight and allow loss of about 0.5 to 1 kg (1 to 2 lb)/week. One pound of body fat is equivalent to approximately 3500 kcal, so weight loss is accomplished by consuming 500 to 1000 kcal less each day than are required to meet energy needs.

To calculate kcal needs:
1. Determine IBW in kilograms; if IBW is in pounds, divide by 2.2.
2. To estimate daily kcal needs for weight maintenance, multiply IBW in kilograms by: 20 to 25 kcal if sedentary, 30 kcal if engaged in moderate activity, or 35 to 50 kcal if engaged in heavy activity.
3. To determine kcal needs for weight reduction, subtract 500 to 1000 kcal/day from kcal needed for maintenance to allow 0.5 to 1 kg loss per week, respectively; intakes of less than 800 kcal/day are considered very low-calorie diets (VLCDs) and should not be used except under a physician's supervision.

The Daily Food Guide (see Appendix A) or the Exchange Lists for Meal Planning, published by the American Diabetes Association, can be used to plan balanced low-kcal diets. Diets that are low in fat and high in carbohydrate are preferred. Carbohydrate has less than half the kcal of fat (per g), and metabolism of carbohydrate causes a greater "thermic effect," or heat loss (and thus loss of kcal) than fat.

Very low-calorie diets. Very low-calorie diets (VLCDs) are those providing 400 to 800 kcal/day. Special diet formulas (e.g., Optifast) are available, with the kcal being mostly in the form of high-quality protein. This is sometimes called a *protein sparing modified fast*. The usual regimen is to follow the VLCD for 12 to 16 weeks, followed by a gradual reinstitution of regular foods over a period of 3 weeks or longer. Intake of noncaloric fluids should be at least 2 L/day to prevent dehydration. Losses of 1.5 to 2.3 kg (3.3 to 5.1 lb)/wk occur during the VLCD, with the higher losses occurring in men. These diets are designed to preserve LBM, but there is some loss of LBM during the dieting period. Therefore their use should be limited to individuals who are least 30% overweight. The severely obese not only contain more body fat but also have a greater LBM than less overweight individuals. Thus the mildly obese lose a greater proportion of their LBM during severe kcal restriction than do the severely obese.

The diets currently marketed are safer than the VLCDs marketed during the 1970s, which caused more than 70 deaths, many of them from myocardial atrophy. However, a VLCD should be begun only after a thorough medical examination including an electrocardiogram, and dieters should have electrolytes measured regularly and frequent examinations by a physician. Unsupervised dieting can lead to dehydration, electrolyte imbalance, elevation of uric acid, fatigue, dizziness, and headache; over the long term, there is a potential for ventricular dysrhythmias, as well as binge eating after the severely restricted diet is ended.

Counseling and behavioral modification is essential, since one-half to two-thirds of the weight loss is rapidly regained without it; life-style modification can reduce the amount of weight regained to about one-third of that lost.

Fad diets. Diets that promise quick weight loss are popular. Unfortunately, these diets tend to be undesirable for one or more of the following reasons: (1) they are nutritionally inadequate, (2) they require expensive foods or time-consuming food preparation, (3) they are medically unsafe, (4) they do not help the individual change poor eating habits; thus the weight lost is usually regained, (5) much of the weight lost is fluid or LBM, rather than fat. Several fad diets are described in Table 19-3.

Behavior modification

Behavior modification, in conjunction with a balanced reduction diet, helps promote lasting weight loss. It should be a part of all weight loss programs. Primary features of behavior modification programs are:

1. *Self-monitoring:* Recording exercise, food intake, and emotional and environmental circumstances at the time of food consumption to provide a basis for planning changes
2. *Stimulus control and environmental management:* Acquiring techniques to help break learned associations between environmental cues and food intake
3. *Positive reinforcement:* A reward system to encourage changes in behavior
4. *Contracts:* Signed contracts between the therapist and the individual seeking to modify behavior, outlining the consequences if various changes are made or are not made

Table 19-3   Fad weight reduction diets

Type of Diet	Examples	Comments
High-protein "ketogenic" diets	Scarsdale Diet; Dr. Atkins' Diet Revolution; Stillman Diet	These diets are very low in carbohydrate to induce ketosis; they often result in rapid weight loss caused by diuresis associated with excretion of ketones; the "water weight" lost is quickly regained; these diets are usually low in Fe, Ca, and sometimes vitamin B_2; they are high in saturated fat and cholesterol

Table 19-3   Fad weight reduction diets—cont'd

Type of Diet	Examples	Comments
Diets that rely on particular foods or hormones that are purported to help "burn fat" or alter the metabolism	Beverly Hills Diet; Grapefruit Diet; Simeon Diet	Neither grapefruit nor any other food or combinations of foods helps burn fat; the Beverly Hills Diet allows only specified fruits for the first 10 days, then a few other foods are gradually added; it is inadequate in protein, Fe, Ca, Zn, and other nutrients. The Simeon plan includes injections of human chorionic gonadotropin (hCG), which is alleged to accelerate fat loss, but the 500 kcal diet that accompanies the hCG is actually responsible for the weight loss seen with the diet
Food substitutes (diet drinks or foods substituted for regular meals)	Cambridge Diet; Carnation Slender; Sego Liquid; Pillsbury Figurines	These diets are low kcal and monotonous; they often result in weight loss; however, they do nothing to help the dieter change his or her eating habits, and the weight lost is usually rapidly regained

Modifying Behavior to Promote Weight Loss or Maintenance

1. Chew food slowly, and put utensils down between bites.
2. Never shop for food on an empty stomach.
3. Make out a grocery shopping list before starting, and do not add to it as you shop.
4. Leave a small amount of food on your plate after each meal.
5. Fill your plate in the kitchen at the start of the meal; do not put open bowls of food on the table.
6. Eat in only one or two places (e.g., the kitchen and dining room table).
7. Never eat while involved in any other activity, such as watching television.
8. Do not eat while standing.
9. Keep a diary of when and where you eat and under what circumstances (e.g., boredom, frustration, anxiety). Be aware of problem circumstances, and substitute another activity for eating.
10. Keep low-calorie snacks available at all times.
11. Reward yourself for weight loss (e.g., buy new clothes, treat yourself to concert tickets or a trip). Establish a step-wise set of goals with a reward for achieving each goal.
12. If you violate your diet on one occasion, do not use that as an excuse to go off the diet altogether. Acknowledge that setbacks happen, and return to your weight control program.
13. When confronted with an appealing food, remember that this will not be your last chance to have the food. Content yourself with a small portion.

The accompanying box provides suggestions for modifying behavior to lose and maintain weight.

Exercise

Activities involving gross movements of large muscles promote fat loss while conserving LBM. For best results, the dieter must

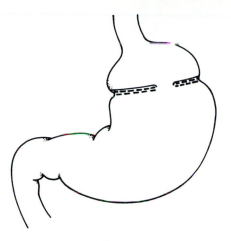

Fig. 19-1
Gastroplasty.

exercise 3 days a week, utilizing at least 300 kcal each time (or 4 days a week, using 200 kcal per session). The energy expenditures of some common exercises are shown in Table 5-1.

Surgery (gastric partitioning)

Surgery is recommended only for severely or morbidly obese individuals who have failed to lose weight via more conventional methods. Gastric partitioning creates a small (30 to 60 ml) gastric reservoir in the proximal stomach to limit the amount of food that can be consumed at one time. In *gastroplasty* (gastric stapling) (Fig. 19-1), the stomach is partitioned so that there is a small opening (10 to 12 mm) between the reservoir and the distal stomach. In *gastric bypass* (Fig. 19-2), the reservoir is connected to the jejunum, bypassing the distal stomach and the duodenum.

Results of gastric partitioning

1. Ninety percent of gastric bypass clients lose at least 50% of their excess weight.
2. Only 30% to 50% of clients will achieve a body weight less than 125% of ideal.

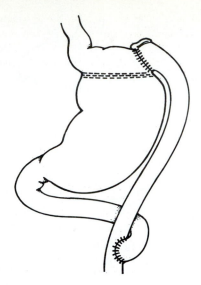

Fig. 19-2
Roux-en-Y retrocolic gastric bypass. Stomach is stapled completely horizontally; jejunum is resected from duodenum and connected to stomach entrance; distal duodenal stump is connected to jejunum to permit drainage of intestinal secretions.

3. Ninety percent of weight loss occurs during the first year after surgery, and many individuals begin to regain weight 1 to 2 years after surgery.

Specific diet and behavior modifications are required following gastric partitioning. These are discussed under Client Teaching.

Drugs and devices

Appetite suppressants such as fenfluramine (Pondimin) are sometimes prescribed as an adjunct to a reduction diet. Drug dependence can occur, and weight loss resulting from drug use is rarely maintained. Drugs, when used at all, are usually prescribed for only the first 6 to 8 weeks of dieting, to make it easier for the individual to develop new eating habits.

The gastric bubble, an inflatable plastic device inserted in the stomach to provide a feeling of fullness and satiety, is used in conjunction with diet and behavior modification. An 800 to 1000 kcal liquid or soft diet is consumed while the bubble is in place. Gastric ulcers, pyloric or intestinal obstruction, nausea and vomiting are potential complications.

Client Teaching

Achieve fat loss while maintaining LBM and retraining eating habits so that weight loss is maintained

Weight control is a lifelong process. Once weight is lost, attention must be paid to weight maintenance. Instead of thinking of weight control in terms of dieting, the client must think of it as a life-style change—the client can never return to his or her old eating habits, or the weight will be regained. This change is achieved through dieting, exercise, and behavior modification.

A. Low-kcal diet

Most adult or adolescent clients can learn to use the Exchange Lists for Meal Planning available from the American Diabetes Association, which allow flexibility and are easier than calorie counting. Clients may want to use other diet plans that are found in magazines or books or supported by various organizations. To help them evaluate these diet plans, the professional can share with clients the guidelines in the accompanying box.

Characteristics of Safe and Effective Weight Control Program

1. The diet plan includes more than 800 kcal/day.
2. The diet plan includes foods from all food groups.
3. No magical "fat burning" or appetite reducing products are recommended.
4. Claims for weight loss are no more than an average of 1 kg (~2 lb)/week.
5. Exercise is encouraged.
6. Behavior changes are incorporated.
7. The plan can be adapted to the life-style of the individual.
8. The cost of the plan is reasonable.

Preschool and young school-age children can use the "traffic light" plan. Foods less than 20 kcal/serving are green, or GO, foods and can be used freely. Green foods include seasonings and a few vegetables, such as asparagus. Yellow foods are the primary foods in the diet; they can be eaten with CAUTION. Examples are corn, oranges, baked chicken, skim milk, and English muffins. Red, or STOP, foods are high in kcal. No more than 4 servings of red foods are to be eaten per week. Some examples of red foods are scalloped potatoes, fruit in heavy syrup, fried chicken, whole milk, and doughnuts.

A few suggestions may help the dieter:

1. Dieters should weigh or measure foods initially as an aid in learning to recognize portion sizes.
2. High-fiber foods take longer to consume than low-fiber ones, and satiety (fullness or satisfaction) is achieved with fewer kcal when consuming high-fiber foods.
3. Fat is the most concentrated source of kcal. Decrease use of fats. Use lean meats or skinless poultry, and eat no more than 6 oz (about the size of two decks of cards) daily. Broil, bake, or steam rather than frying foods. Use herbs, spices, lemon juice, or other low-kcal seasonings rather than butter, margarine, olive oil, or salt pork. Choose skim milk and dairy products made with skim milk. Limit foods with "hidden" fat, such as doughnuts, pie crust, croissants, muffins and other quick breads. Choose fruit ices, fresh fruit, or low-fat cookies (gingersnaps, Newtons) rather than ice cream, cake, pie, or higher fat cookies.
4. Do not expect rapid, easy weight loss. Weight gain is usually a gradual process, and so is weight reduction. When lapses occur, do not become depressed; simply resume proper eating habits and exercise.

B. Exercise

The individual needs to establish an exercise program meeting the criteria under Interventions that can be maintained for the foreseeable future. In addition to a planned exercise program, the individual can increase energy expenditure during daily activities. Specifically, the individual can park the car farther away when shopping, walk instead of riding whenever possible, use manual instead of power appliances and tools, and use stairs rather than escalators and elevators.

C. Behavior modification

Behavior modification has been shown to be important in maintaining weight loss. Slowing the rate of eating is especially beneficial. The client should be taught to eat with friends or family and talk with them during meals, lay utensils down after each bite, chew each bite thoroughly, and eat many salads and other bulky foods. The box on p. 342 provides other behavior modification techniques that have been found to be helpful.

It has been found that certain life-style characteristics and coping mechanisms are more common among formerly obese women who maintain weight loss than among those who regain the lost weight: exercising regularly, being conscious of their eating behaviors, using available social support, confronting their problems directly, and using personally developed strategies to avoid excessive food intake. Individualized planning of interventions is thus critical to successful weight loss and maintenance.

Consume a more healthful diet

Obese individuals are often found to have poor diets, with frequent omission of breakfast and inadequate intake of minerals and vitamins. The eating habits established during weight control should change the quality of the diet in a positive way. The client should be taught that:

1. All foods can be eaten *in moderation*. However, calorie-rich extras with little nutritional value (butter, margarine, salad dressings, sugar, candy, syrups, jams, desserts, pastries, soft drinks, and fruit drinks) should be minimized. Concentrate on foods that provide large amounts of nutrients compared with the kcal they contribute.

2. Individuals consuming less than 1200 kcal/day need a vitamin-mineral supplement because of the difficulty in maintaining adequate nutrient intake within their kcal restriction.

3. Omission of meals interferes with weight loss. It often makes the individual so hungry that he or she overeats at the next meal. Furthermore, weight loss is generally facilitated by division of the allowed kcal into several smaller meals per day, rather than two or three larger ones.

Seek support

Support and reinforcement are of great importance. They can come from group or individual counseling through hospital outpatient departments, dietitians or psychologists in private practice, or lay-led community groups. These sources of support can be evaluated by the guidelines in the box on p. 345. Family members and friends are also invaluable sources of support and reinforcement.

Maintain good nutritional habits following surgery for obesity

The following measures will help the client receive optimal benefits from the surgery while avoiding complications:

1. Alteration of eating behaviors during the first 2 postoperative years is essential. During this time, the effects of surgery reinforce dieting endeavors by decreasing the amount the client can comfortably eat. After this point, the surgery has less benefit. The client should adopt techniques to slow the rate of eating (see the box, p. 342), avoid kcal-dense foods (fats, pastries, candy and sweets, and sweetened beverages), and eat regular, small meals.

2. Nausea and vomiting are the most common problems, and gastrointestinal obstruction is a possibility postoperatively. To prevent these problems, initial feedings should be liquids or blended, strained foods. Over the first 6 to 8 weeks after surgery, the diet can be progressed to soft and then regular foods. Clients should continue to chew foods well, eat slowly, and eat small meals.

3. "Dumping syndrome," with nausea, weakness, tachycardia, and diarrhea, can affect individuals with gastric bypass. This can be alleviated by avoiding concentrated sweets, eating slowly, and avoiding liquids during mealtime (after the initial postoperative period). It has been suggested that gastric bypass is preferable to gastroplasty for individuals who consume large amounts of sweets, since they lose more weight with bypass surgery. The improvement in weight loss is probably a consequence of dumping syndrome.

CASE STUDY

Mrs. S., at 157.5 cm (5'2") and 65 kg (143 lb), was anxious to lose weight to control her hypertension. A diet history showed that Mrs. S. ate three meals daily. Dessert—cake, pie, cookies, or ice cream—was a part of dinner and sometimes lunch. During the morning, Mrs. S. often snacked on pastry or doughnuts. At night, she nibbled chips or candy while watching television with her family.

Mrs. S. identified two changes she could make: (1) use of fruit, or occasionally low-fat frozen yogurt, for dessert and her morning snack, and (2) avoiding food while watching television. Although she initially insisted that she had no time for regular exercise, she finally agreed to join an aerobic walking group sponsored by her church. Three months later, Mrs. S. had lost 4.5 kg (10 lb) and was enthusiastic about continuing her diet and exercise program.

Bibliography

Doherty JU and others: Long-term evaluation of cardiac function in obese patients treated with a very-low-calorie diet: a controlled clinical study of patients without underlying cardiac disease, *Am J Clin Nutr* 53:854, 1991.

Epstein LH, Wing RR, Valoski A: Childhood obesity, *Pediatr Clin North Am* 32:363, 1985.

Fitzwater SL and others: Evaluation of long-term weight changes after a multidisciplinary weight control program, *J Am Diet Assoc* 91:421, 1991.

Grundy SM, Barnett JP: Metabolic and health complications of obesity, *Dis Mon* 36:641, 1990.

Kayman S, Bruvold W, Stern JS: Maintenance and relapse in women: behavioral aspects, *Am J Clin Nutr* 52:800, 1990.

Kendall A and others: Weight loss on a low-fat diet: consequence of the imprecision of the control of food intake in humans, *Am J Clin Nutr* 53:1124, 1991.

Kenler HA, Brolin RE, Cody RP: Changes in eating behavior after horizontal gastroplasty and Roux-en-Y gastric bypass, *Am J Clin Nutr* 52:87, 1990.

Schlundt DG and others: Obesity: a biogenetic or biobehavioral problem, *Int J Obes* 14:815, 1990.

Wadden TA, Van Itallie TB, Blackburn GL: Responsible and irresponsible use of very-low-calorie diets in the treatment of obesity, *JAMA* 263:83, 1990.

Eating Disorders 20

Anorexia nervosa and bulimia are eating disorders occurring primarily in adolescent and young adult females. Anorexia nervosa is associated with voluntary refusal to eat, extreme weight loss, body image disturbance, and an intense fear of becoming obese. The individual's activity level is commonly very high, and energy expenditure is greater than in nonanorexic individuals. Bulimia is characterized by binge-eating episodes followed by self-induced vomiting, fasting, or the use of laxatives or diuretics; these "binge-purge" episodes are often accompanied by depression or self-deprecatory thoughts. An individual may display symptoms of both disorders.

Pathophysiology

Diagnostic criteria for these two conditions are shown in the accompanying box. Table 20-1 provides additional aid in distinguishing between them.

The etiologic factors of these eating disorders are unclear. Cultural factors (e.g., the abundance of food in developed countries coupled with society's emphasis on thinness as desirable and beautiful) probably play a role. Family dysfunction may contribute to development of the disorders. Families of individuals with eating disorders have been described as overprotective, rigid, and lacking in conflict resolution skills. As a result, the children may grow up to be dependent, unassertive, excessively reliant on the approval of others, and low in self-esteem. Behavioral theorists note that anorexia nervosa is reinforced by the attention it receives. The client becomes the center of attention and manipulates her environment through her behavior.

Diagnosing Anorexia Nervosa and Bulimia

Anorexia Nervosa

1. Refusal to maintain body weight over a minimal normal weight for age and height, e.g., weight loss leading to maintenance of body weight 15% below that expected; or failure to make expected weight gain during period of growth, leading to body weight 15% below that expected
2. Intense fear of gaining weight or becoming fat, even though underweight
3. Disturbance in the way in which one's body weight, size, or shape is experienced, e.g., the person claims to "feel fat" even when emaciated
4. In females, absence of at least three consecutive menstrual cycles when otherwise expected to occur

Bulimia

1. Recurrent episodes of binge eating (rapid consumption of a large amount of food in a discrete period of time)
2. A feeling of lack of control over eating behavior during the eating binges
3. Regular engagement in either self-induced vomiting, use of laxatives or diuretics, strict dieting or fasting, or vigorous exercise in order to prevent weight gain
4. A minimum average of two binge eating episodes a week for at least 3 months
5. Persistent overconcern with body shape and weight

Modified from Diagnostic and statistical manual of mental disorders, ed 3, rev, Washington, DC, 1987, American Psychiatric Association. Used with permission.

Treatment

Treatment of anorexia nervosa and bulimia can include individual psychotherapy, group therapy, family psychotherapy, and behavioral therapy. Bulimics, in particular, appear to have a high incidence of depression. Antidepressant medications, particularly tricyclics and monoamine oxidase inhibitors (see Chapter 18), are sometimes used in therapy. Drugs such as fenfluramine and flu-

Table 20-1   Distinguishing between anorexia nervosa
and bulimia

Characteristic	Anorexia Nervosa	Bulimia
Age of onset (years)	12 to mid-30s; two peaks: 13-14 and 17-18	17-25
Attitude toward therapy	Denial that a problem exists	Often extremely secretive about bulimic behaviors, but willing to accept help once the problem is admitted
Body weight	25% or more below usual or desirable body weight	May be at or only slightly below desirable body weight
Metabolic	Amenorrhea; inability to maintain body temperature in heat or cold stress	Irregular menses, amenorrhea in fewer than 20%
Gastrointestinal	Decreased gastric emptying; constipation; elevated hepatic enzymes	Parotid enlargement; dental enamel erosion; esophagitis; Mallory-Weiss tears
Cardiovascular	Bradycardia; hypotension; dysrhythmias	Ipecac poisoning (tachycardia, cardiac dysrhythmias)
Skeletal	Decreased bone density (correlated with degree of underweight)	

oxetine, which increase brain serotonin (a neurotransmitter that inhibits eating), have also been used in an effort to prevent binge eating.

Treatment may occur on an inpatient or outpatient basis. Some indications for hospitalization are: (1) loss of 25% or more of body weight; this state is often life-threatening, and hospitalization for nutritional support and intensive psychiatric therapy is usually necessary; (2) presence or likelihood of serious electro-lyte imbalance as a result of an inability to cope with daily living without use of laxatives, diuretics, diet pills, or self-induced vomiting; (3) family tensions necessitating separation of the client and family; (4) severe depression with strong potential for suicide; and (5) inability or unwillingness to cooperate during outpatient therapy.

Nutritional Care

Goals of care are for the client to gain weight, change attitudes toward food, and develop more effective coping skills to deal with stress and conflict.

Assessment

Individuals with eating disorders may be deficient in any or all nutrients, depending on the extent of their illness. The nutritional problems addressed in Table 20-2 are the most common ones. With the exception of electrolyte disorders, nutritional deficits are more common in anorexia nervosa than in bulimia.

Intervention and Client Teaching

Treatment is based on a contract established by the client and health care team. For treatment to be successful, the following should be done:

Client and staff agree on a weight goal and a reward system for progress toward the goal

A. The goal should be no more than 1 percentile marking on the growth chart away from the percentile for height; that is, if height is at the 50th percentile, weight should be at least at the 25th.

B. Example of a reward system for an inpatient:
   1. Each day that the client gains at least 0.25 kg (the equivalent of ½ lb), she has full privileges (ambulatory status, television, use of the telephone) on the unit.
   2. If the client does not gain 0.25 kg, she can have no visitors or calls that day, and is confined to bed without access to television or reading materials.

Table 20-2 Assessment in eating disorders

Areas of Concern	Significant Findings
Fluid and electrolyte imbalance	*History* Self-induced vomiting; laxative or diuretic abuse *Physical examination* Poor skin turgor; weakness; signs of self-induced vomiting; parotid salivary gland enlargement, dental enamel erosion, esophagitis, upper GI bleeding (Mallory-Weiss tears), hoarseness or sore throat, tachycardia, cardiac dysrhythmias (ipecac poisoning, potassium [K^+] deficits); anal irritation (laxative abuse) *Laboratory analysis* Signs of prolonged or frequent vomiting: $\downarrow$ serum K^+, $\downarrow$ serum Cl^-; metabolic alkalosis (blood pH >7.45, HCO_3^- >26 mEq/L); stools turn red upon addition of NaOH (caused by presence of phenolphthalein, an ingredient in some laxatives); $\uparrow$ BUN (dehydration)
Protein Calorie Malnutrition (PCM)	*History* Severely restricted food intake (especially over a period of several months or even years); self-induced vomiting; laxative or diuretic abuse (these behaviors are often unreported, rely on physical exam; see Fluid and Electrolyte Imbalance; laxatives do not induce malabsorption severe enough to cause wt loss, their effects are usually limited to loss of fluids and electrolytes); frequent and prolonged periods of physical exercise

Table 20-2   Assessment in eating disorders—cont'd

Areas of Concern	Significant Findings
Protein Calorie Malnutrition (PCM)—cont'd	*Physical examination* Wt <90% of standard for ht (standard for adolescents = 50th percentile of growth chart) or more than 1 percentile marking < ht percentile on the growth chart (i.e., if ht is at 75th percentile, wt is <50th); BMI <19.1 (women) or 20.7 (men); triceps skinfold <5th percentile (see Appendix G); amenorrhea (can also result from psychologic stress); edema; thinning of hair, changes in hair texture *Laboratory analysis* ↓ Serum albumin, transferrin, or pre-albumin; ↓ lymphocyte count; nonreactive skin tests
Mineral Deficiencies	
Zinc (Zn)	*History* Severely restricted food intake; self-induced vomiting; laxative or diuretic abuse *Physical examination* Hypogeusia (common in anorexia nervosa), dysgeusia; alopecia *Laboratory analysis* ↓ Serum Zn
Copper (Cu)	*History* Severely restricted food intake; self-induced vomiting; laxative or diuretic abuse *Laboratory analysis* ↓ Serum Cu; ↓ Hct, Hgb, white blood cell count

Establish a dietary plan

Ideally, the client participates in establishing a dietary plan.

1. For a severely underweight individual, it may be necessary to begin at 800 kcal/day and increase the amount gradually to promote slow weight gain; dividing the food into at least four to five feedings per day, rather than only three, may help improve tolerance.

2. In the hospital, the client chooses a menu; if she does not select adequate items to equal her kcal level, the dietitian can add other items.

3. Kcal counts are done daily to ensure compliance with the treatment; one approach is to use a liquid nutritional supplement to replace any foods not consumed.

4. Bulimic individuals have a great fear of losing control of eating; to ease this fear, they need a plan providing three to four meals plus one to two snacks per day; they are asked not to eat anything not included in the meal plan; clients need to feel that the health team will help keep them from losing control.

Tube feeding or total parenteral nutrition is occasionally needed, but their use is generally limited to individuals whose weight is 35% or more below ideal or those with rapid weight loss who represent a medical emergency.

Monitor progress and behavior frequently

Inpatient monitoring (usually in anorexia nervosa):

1. Obtain daily weights at the same time each morning after the individual has voided. Weights should be done in the same light clothes (i.e., gown) each time.

2. Observe client closely during treatment to protect her and maximize therapy. Examples of client behaviors that subvert treatment include: absenting herself from group activities after meals to vomit, diluting tube feeding formulas to reduce caloric intake, surreptitiously wearing weights during weight measurement, failing to void before daily weight measurement, or hiding uneaten food.

Outpatient monitoring (especially bulimic individuals)— increased responsibility for self-monitoring:

1. Clients should weigh themselves only once weekly to interrupt unhealthy weighing behaviors accompanying their intense fear of weight gain.

2. Clients record all food eaten, along with the time, place, and amount. They should also record episodes of vomiting and diuretic or laxative use. Health professionals and the client evaluate these records for signs of progress.

Identify practices that will help client avoid binge eating

The client needs help in developing control so that binge eating is reduced or eliminated and, over the long-term, weight stabilization and a healthy life-style are achieved. To resist binging and control eating behavior:

1. Identify activities that can serve as distractions when temptations or negative emotions prompt a desire to binge, such as engaging in hobbies, taking a walk, telephoning friends, doing yard work or housework, shopping (not at a grocery store), or exercising.
2. Identify cues or stimuli that lead to overeating and alter these stimuli. For instance, if overeating is most likely to occur in the kitchen, avoid eating in the kitchen and instead eat only in the dining room.
3. Learn what an appropriate serving size is (using scales, measuring cups, or food models), and eat that amount. Many individuals with eating disorders have spent most of their lives either eating almost nothing or gorging. They may have little knowledge of normal serving sizes.
4. Eat slowly; binging is associated with rapid food intake.
5. Avoid taking repeated helpings of food. At meals, serve the food and then put leftovers away before beginning to eat. At parties, sit as far from the food as possible.
6. Plan ahead for events when excessive kcal intake can be expected. For instance, if the individual plans to go out for pizza with friends, she can reduce her intake throughout the day to compensate.
7. Limit alcohol intake, since it adds kcal and may reduce control over behavior.

Work toward increased self-esteem and coping skills

Through group or individual therapy, the individual can be helped to develop a better self-image, increased assertiveness, and better problem-solving techniques. Staff members should provide positive reinforcement for progress made toward weight goals and improving self-esteem and interactive skills.

Instruct the client in the principles of a nutritious diet

Most clients with anorexia nervosa and bulimia have misconceptions about food and nutrition. It may have been several years since they consumed a "balanced" diet. They need help in recognizing and selecting a nutritious diet. The Daily Food Guide (see Appendix A) can be used in client teaching. The diet should be moderate in protein (12% to 20%) and low in fat (less than 30%), with the balance of kcal coming from carbohydrate. The goal is to establish the habit of eating a nutritious diet, while maintaining a balance with energy expenditure so that it will not be necessary to resort to unhealthy practices such as self-induced vomiting to control weight.

CASE STUDY

Ms. J., a 19-year-old college freshman, came to the university health service at the insistence of her roommate. She admitted engaging in binging episodes three to four times per week. During the binges, she consumed mostly desserts and other high-carbohydrate foods. The binges were followed by self-induced vomiting and an overwhelming feeling of failure. The binge-purge episodes had begun shortly after she entered the university. Although she had always been an excellent student and a talented musician, she felt unable to face the scholastic and social demands of the university. Her weight was 90% of the standard for her height, and she had lost 2.3 kg (5 lb, or 4% of her usual weight) in the previous 3 months.

Ms. J. joined a bulimia self-help group conducted by the nurse practitioner and social worker from the health service. After 12 weeks, she was able to report that she had not engaged in binge-purge activities for over a month. She was consuming a balanced diet and maintaining her weight at 95% of the standard for her height. She volunteered to serve as a lay counselor for other students with bulimia and continued to do well through the time of her graduation.

Bibliography

Ainley CC and others: Zinc state in anorexia nervosa, *Br Med J* 293:992, 1986.

Bachrach LK and others: Decreased bone density in adolescent girls with anorexia nervosa, *Pediatrics* 86:440, 1990.

Casper RC and others: Total daily energy expenditure and activity level in anorexia nervosa, *Am J Clin Nutr* 53:1143, 1991.

Greene GW and others: Dietary intake and dieting practices of bulimic and non-bulimic female college students, *J Am Diet Assoc* 90:576, 1990.

Horne RL, Van-Vactor JC, Emerson S: Disturbed body image in patients with eating disorders, *Am J Psychiatry* 148:211, 1991.

Schlundt DG, Johnson WG: *Eating disorders: assessment and treatment,* Boston, 1990, Allyn & Bacon.

APPENDIXES

Appendix A
Daily Food Guide

Food Guide Pyramid
A guide to daily food choices

Fats, oils, and sweets
(use sparingly)

> **Key**
> ⊠ Fat (naturally occurring ▽ Sugars
>   and added)   (added)
>
> These symbols show fats, oils, and
> added sugars in foods.

**Milk, yogurt,
and cheese
group
2 to 3 servings**

**Meat, poultry, fish,
dry beans, eggs,
and nuts group
2 to 3 servings**

**Vegetable
group
3 to 5
servings**

**Fruit group
2 to 4
servings**

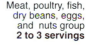

**Bread, cereal,
rice, and
pasta group
6 to 11
servings**

363

Table A-1 Food groups and servings

Food Group	Size of 1 Serving*	Suggested Number of Servings
Vegetables		3 to 5
Have dark green leafy or deep yellow vegetables often	1 cup raw leafy greens ½ cup of all others, cooked or raw	
Eat dry beans and peas often (count ½ cup of cooked dry beans or peas as a serving of vegetables *or* as 1 oz of the meat group.)		
Fruits		2 to 4
Have citrus fruits or juices, melons, or strawberries regularly	1 medium apple, orange, pear, or banana ½ cup berries, grapes, or diced fruits ¾ cup juice	
Grain products		6 to 11
Have several servings of whole-grain breads and cereals daily	1 slice bread ½ bun, bagel, or English muffin	

Food group	Serving sizes	Number of servings
	1 roll or muffin 1 oz of ready-to-eat cereal ½ cup of cooked cereals, rice, or pasta	2 to 3
Meat, poultry, fish, dry beans and peas, eggs, and nuts Total daily intake should be equivalent to about 6 oz of meat or chicken (approximately the size of two decks of cards) Trim fat from meat; take skin off poultry Use egg yolks and organ meats in moderation Use nuts, nut butters, and seeds only occasionally, because of the high fat and kcal content	2 to 3 oz meat, poultry, or fish 1 cup cooked dried beans or peas 2 eggs 3 tbsp peanut butter 3 oz of nuts 1½ oz of seeds	
Milk and milk products Choose skim or low-fat milk and fat-free or low-fat yogurt and cheese most of the time	1 cup milk or yogurt 1½ oz cheese	2 to 3 (3 to 4 during pregnancy and lactation)

*Small children may need smaller portion sizes of vegetables, fruits, grains, and meats (e.g., .3 oz of meat per day is sufficient for preschoolers). However, they should consume the equivalent of 2 to 3 cups of milk, probably in several smaller servings, in order to receive enough calcium.

Appendix B
Functions and Dietary Sources of Some Important Nutrients

Table B-1   Food sources, functions, and amounts

Function	Food Sources	Amount
Vitamins		
Vitamin A (retinol)		*retinol equivalents/ portion*
Formation and maintenance of epithelium, maintenance of light-dark visual adaptation, formation of rhodopsin (visual purple)	Liver, calf, fried, 3½ oz	6750
	Pumpkin, ⅖ cup	10,197
	Sweet potato, baked, 1 large	4380
	Spinach, cooked, ½ cup	2190
	Broccoli, frozen, chopped, ½ cup	612
	Cantaloupe, 1 cup	516
	Apricots, raw, 3	277
Vitamin B₁ (thiamin)		*mg/portion*
Coenzyme in carbohydrate metabolism	Pork chop, cooked, 3½ oz	1.18
	Bran cereal, ½ cup	0.70
	Oatmeal, instant, 1 packet	0.53
	Bread, white, enriched, 1 slice	0.11

Table B-1   Food sources, functions, and amounts—cont'd

Function	Food Sources	Amount
Vitamin B₁ (thiamin)—cont'd		mg/portion
	Bread, whole wheat, 1 slice	0.09
	Rice, white, enriched, cooked, ½ cup	0.12
	Peas, green, cooked, ⅔ cup	0.28
	Peas, black-eyed, frozen, ⅔ cup	0.40
Vitamin B₂ (riboflavin)		mg/portion
Coenzyme in carbohydrate and protein metabolism, activation of vitamin B₆ and folate	Liver, calf, cooked, 3½ oz	4.17
	Chuck, ground, cooked, 3½ oz	0.20
	Milk, 2% fat, 1 cup	0.40
	Cheese, cheddar, 1 oz	0.11
	Cheese, cottage, ½ cup	0.17
	Bran cereal, ½ cup	0.80
	Spinach, cooked, ½ cup	0.13
Niacin (nicotinic acid)		mg/portion
Coenzyme in energy release from carbohydrates, fats, and protein	Liver, calf, fried, 3½ oz	16.5
	Chicken, fried, light and dark, 3½ oz	12.4
	Chuck, ground, cooked, 3½ oz	4.0
	Peanut butter, 2 tbsp	4.4
	Soybeans, cooked, ½ cup	5.6
	Peas, green, cooked, ⅔ cup	2.3
Vitamin B₆ (pyridoxine)		mg/portion
Coenzyme in amino acid metabolism	Tuna, canned, 3 oz	0.30
	Beef round, 3½ oz	0.40
	Chicken, cooked, light and dark, 3½ oz	0.47

Continued.

Table B-1 Food sources, functions, and amounts—cont'd

Function	Food Sources	Amount
Vitamin B₆ (pyridoxine)—cont'd		*mg/portion*
	Oatmeal, instant, 1 packet	0.74
	Bran cereal, ½ cup	0.75
	Lentils, cooked, ½ cup	0.60
	Banana, 1 medium	0.66
Folic acid (folate or folacin)		*µg/portion*
Coenzyme for single carbon transfer— purines, thymine, hemoglobin	Liver, calf, fried, 3½ oz	290
	Spinach, frozen, cooked, ½ cup	153
	Broccoli, cooked, ½ cup	130
	Brussels sprouts, ⅗ cup	150
	Turnip greens, frozen, cooked, ⅗ cup	60
	Orange, 1 medium	47
Vitamin B₁₂ (cobalamin)		*µg/portion*
Coenzyme in protein synthesis; essential for RBC formation and maturation	Liver, chicken, cooked, 3½ oz	19.39
	Salmon patty, 3½ oz	3.00
	Chicken, cooked, light and dark, 3½ oz	0.33
	Milk, skim, 1 cup	0.93
	Egg, cooked, 1 large	0.60
	Cheese, cottage, ½ cup	0.65
Vitamin C (ascorbic acid)		*mg/portion*
Formation of collagen, integrity of capillaries, activation of folate	Orange, 1 medium	59-80
	Strawberries, raw, 1 cup	85
	Cantaloupe, 1 cup	68
	Broccoli, chopped, cooked, ½ cup	57

Table B-1 Food sources, functions, and amounts—cont'd

Function	Food Sources	Amount
Vitamin C (ascorbic acid)—cont'd		*mg/portion*
	Cabbage, green, raw, 1 cup	47
	Pepper, raw, 1 large	128
	Tomato, raw, 1 medium	34
Minerals		
Calcium		*mg/portion*
Formation of bone and teeth; normal muscle contraction, blood clotting, nerve transmission	Milk, whole, 1 cup	288
	Yogurt, low-fat, 1 cup	415
	Cheese, cheddar, 1 oz	204
	Ice cream, vanilla, ½ cup	88
	Cheese, cottage, ½ cup	63
	Mustard greens, cooked, ½ cup	138
	Tortillas, corn or flour, 1	44
Phosphorus		*mg/portion*
Bone and teeth formation, energy transfers, buffer system	Beef, cube steak, 3½ oz	250
	Bluefish, fried, 3½ oz	257
	Milk, whole, 1 cup	227
	Cheese, cheddar, 1 oz	145
	Oatmeal, regular, cooked, ¾ cup	133
	Bran cereal, ½ cup	160
	Cola beverages, 12 oz	40-60
Iron		*mg/portion*
Hemoglobin and myoglobin formation; cytochrome enzyme system (electron transfer)	Liver, beef, fried, 3½ oz	8.8
	Chuck, ground, cooked, 3½ oz	3.3
	Chicken, cooked, light and dark, 3½ oz	1.2

Continued.

Table B-1   Food sources, functions, and amounts—cont'd

Function	Food Sources	Amount
Iron—cont'd		*mg/portion*
	Bran cereal, ½ cup	3.5
	Oatmeal, regular, cooked, ¾ cup	1.19
	Bread, white, enriched, 1 slice	0.68
	Bread, whole wheat, 1 slice	0.86
	Lima beans, cooked, ½ cup	1.87
	Soybeans, cooked, ½ cup	2.7
	Collard greens, cooked, ½ cup	0.60
Zinc		*mg/portion*
Participates in more than 80 enzyme systems including carbonic anhydrase, alkaline phosphatase, carboxypeptidase	Oysters, raw, 3½ oz	9-75
	Beef roast, 3½ oz	5.8
	Milk, skim, 1 cup	0.98
	Egg, 1 large	0.70
	Cheese, cheddar, 1 oz	0.88
	Butter beans, ½ cup	0.73
	Spinach, frozen, ½ cup	0.32
Magnesium		*mg/portion*
Bone and teeth formation; coenzyme in carbohydrate and protein metabolism; muscle and nerve irritability	Oatmeal, regular, cooked, ¾ cup	42
	Peanut butter, 2 tbsp	44
	Cashews, 20-26	134
	Milk, skim, 1 cup	36
	Garbanzos (chickpeas), ½ cup	54
	Spinach, cooked, ½ cup	55

Appendix C
Dietary Fiber

Table C-1   Dietary fiber in selected foods

Food	Total Dietary Fiber Soluble (g)	Insoluble (g)
Grains		
All Bran, ½ cup	1.5	7.6
Cornflakes, 1¼ cup	0.1	0.4
40% Bran Flakes, ¾ cup	0.8	3.8
Oat bran	2.4	2.4
Rolled oats, uncooked, ⅓ cup	1.7	1.5
White bread, 1 slice	0.6	0.7
Whole wheat bread, 1 slice	0.8	3.1
Vegetables		
Broccoli, frozen, ½ cup	1.2	1.6
Brussels sprouts, ½ cup	1.5	2.3
Carrot, raw, 1 large	1.5	1.6
Cauliflower, frozen, ½ cup	1.0	2.0
Green beans, canned, ½ cup	0.5	1.7
Lettuce, raw, 3½ oz.	0.2	0.7
Legumes		
Kidney beans, canned, ½ cup	2.0	5.8
Lentils, cooked, ½ cup	0.8	5.8
Pinto beans, dried, cooked, ½ cup	2.2	4.7
Pork and beans, canned, ½ cup	2.7	2.9
Fruits		
Apple, 1 medium	1.0	1.7
Banana, 1 medium	0.7	1.5
Grapefruit, ½ medium	0.9	0.5
Orange, 1 medium	1.1	0.9
Pear, canned, ½ cup	0.8	3.0

Appendix D
Caffeine

Table D-1   Caffeine content of selected beverages and foods*

Food or Beverage	Caffeine (mg)
Coffee, drip, 5 fl oz	137
Coffee, percolated, 5 fl oz	117
Coffee, instant, 5 fl oz	60
Coffee, decaffeinated, 5 fl oz	3
Tea, black, 5 min brew, 5 fl oz	46
Tea, instant, 6 fl oz	33
Cola, diet or regular, 12 fl oz	30-46
Baking chocolate, 1 oz	25-35
Milk chocolate candy, 1 oz	6
Cocoa (beverage), 6 fl oz	5

*Many over-the-counter and some prescription drugs contain higher levels of caffeine than these foods and beverages. Consult the package label or a pharmacist for information about the caffeine content of drugs.

Appendix E
Weight for
Height Charts

Table E-1 Desirable weights for height

Height (ft and in)	Metropolitan 1983 Weight* (lb) (25-59 yr)		Gerontology Research Center* (Age-Specific Weight [lb] Range for Men and Women)				
	Men	Women	20-29 yr	30-39 yr	40-49 yr	50-59 yr	60-69 yr
4 10		100-131	84-111	92-119	99-127	107-135	115-142
4 11		101-134	87-115	95-123	103-131	111-139	119-147
5 0		103-137	90-119	98-127	106-135	114-143	123-152
5 1	123-145	105-140	93-123	101-131	110-140	118-148	127-157
5 2	125-148	108-144	96-127	105-136	113-144	122-153	131-163
5 3	127-151	111-148	99-131	108-140	117-149	126-158	135-168
5 4	129-155	114-152	102-135	112-145	121-154	130-163	140-173
5 5	131-159	117-156	106-140	115-149	125-159	134-168	144-179

5 6	133-163	120-160	109-144	119-154	129-164	138-174	148-184
5 7	135-167	123-164	112-148	122-159	133-169	143-179	153-190
5 8	137-171	126-167	116-153	126-163	137-174	147-184	158-196
5 9	139-175	129-170	119-157	130-168	141-179	151-190	162-201
5 10	141-179	131-173	122-162	134-173	145-184	156-195	167-207
5 11	144-183	135-176	126-167	137-178	149-190	160-201	172-213
6 0	144-187		129-171	141-183	153-195	165-207	177-219
6 1	150-192		133-176	145-188	157-200	169-213	182-225
6 2	153-197		137-181	149-194	162-206	174-219	187-232
6 3	157-202		141-186	153-199	166-212	179-225	192-238
6 4			144-191	157-205	171-218	184-231	197-244

Modified from Andres R: Morbidity and obesity: the rationale for age-specific height-weight tables. In Andres R: *Principles of geriatric medicine*, New York, 1985, McGraw-Hill.

*Values in this table are for height without shoes and weight without clothes. NOTE: These weights are "desirable" because they are associated with the lowest mortality. The age-specific Gerontology Research center weights reflect the fact that heavier weights are associated with higher mortality in younger rather than older individuals.

Appendix F
Growth Charts
for Children

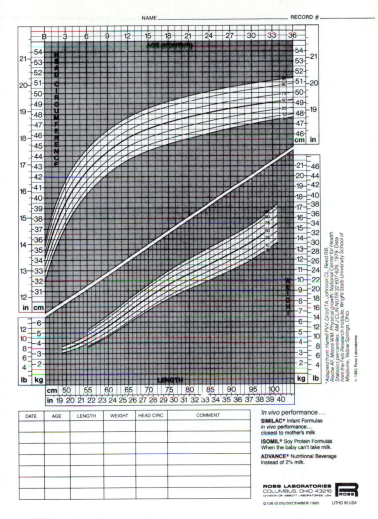

Table F-1   Girls: birth to 36 months physical growth NCHS percentiles

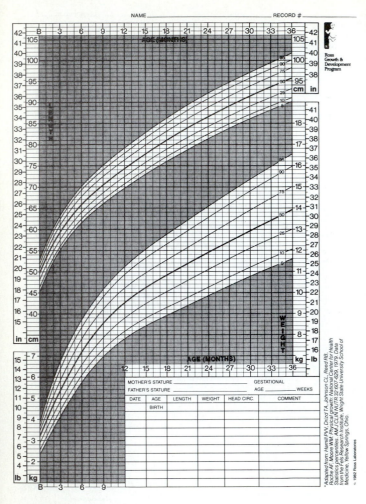

Table F-2 Girls: birth to 36 months physical growth NCHS percentiles

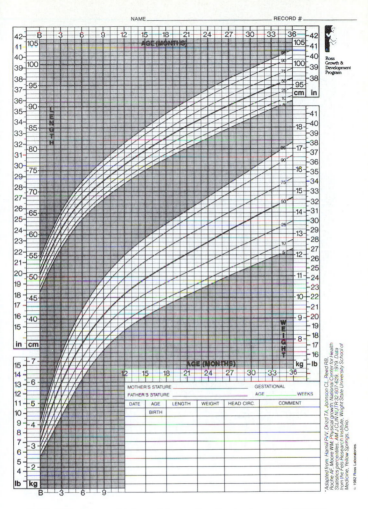

Table F-3 Boys: birth to 36 months physical growth NCHS percentiles

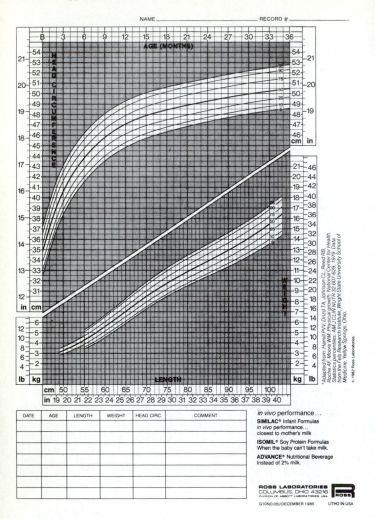

DATE	AGE	LENGTH	WEIGHT	HEAD CIRC.	COMMENT

in vivo performance...
SIMILAC® Infant Formulas
in vivo performance...
closest to mother's milk.

ISOMIL® Soy Protein Formulas
When the baby can't take milk.

ADVANCE® Nutritional Beverage
Instead of 2% milk.

ROSS LABORATORIES
COLUMBUS, OHIO 43216
DIVISION OF ABBOTT LABORATORIES, USA

G105(0.05)/DECEMBER 1985   LITHO IN USA

Table F-4 Boys: birth to 36 months physical growth NCHS
percentiles

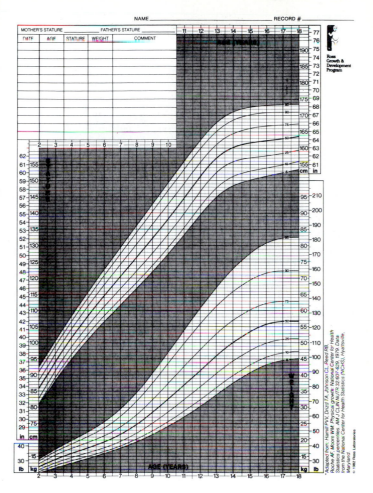

Table F-5 Girls: 2 to 18 years physical growth NCHS percentiles

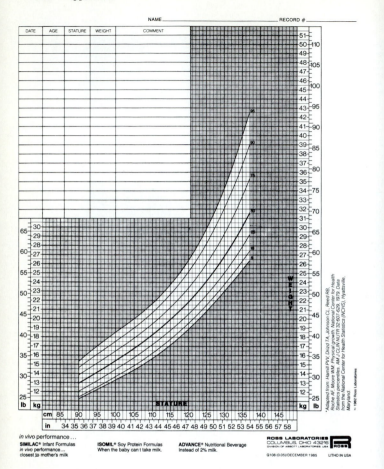

Table F-6 Girls: prepubescent physical growth NCHS percentiles

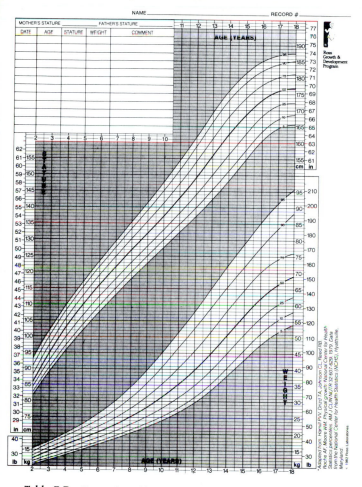

Table F-7   Boys: 2 to 18 years physical growth NCHS percentiles

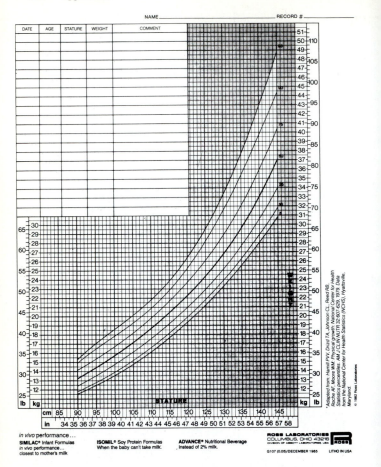

Table F-8 Boys: prepubescent physical growth NCHS percentiles

Appendix G
TSF and AMC
Percentiles

Table G-1 Triceps skinfold (TSF) and arm muscle circumference (AMC) percentiles for females

	TSF (mm)		AMC (cm)	
Age (Yr)	5th Percentile	95th Percentile	5th Percentile	95th Percentile
1	6	15.5	10.5	14.3
2	7	15	11.1	14.7
3	7	15	11.3	15.2
4	7.5	16	11.5	15.7
5	6	17.5	12.5	16.5
6	6.5	17.5	13	17.1
7	7	17.5	12.9	17.6
8	7	22	13.8	19.4
9	7.5	22	14.7	19.8
10	7.5	23	14.8	19.7
11	8	28.5	15	22.3
12	8	26	16.2	22
13	7	28.5	16.9	24
14	9	33	17.4	24.7
15	9	28.5	17.5	24.4
16	10	32.1	17	24.9
17	10	35	17.5	25.7
18-24	10	34	17.9	24.9
25-34	11	36.5	18.3	26.4
35-44	12	38.5	18.6	27.2
45-54	13	39.5	18.7	27.4
55-64	11.5	38	18.7	28
65-74	12	35.5	18.5	27.9

Modified from National Center for Health Statistics, Department of Health and Human Services, Health and Nutrition Examination Survey 1, 1971-1974; Frisancho AR: New norms of upper limb fat and muscle areas for assessment of nutritional status, *Am J Clin Nutr* 34:2540, 1981.

Table G-2 Triceps skinfold (TSF) and arm muscle circumference (AMC) percentiles for males

	TSF (mm)		AMC (cm)	
Age (Yr)	5th Percentile	95th Percentile	5th Percentile	95th Percentile
1	7	16.5	11	14.7
2	6	14.7	11.1	15
3	6.5	14.5	11.7	15.3
4	6	14	12.3	15.9
5	6	15	12.8	16.9
6	5.5	14	13.1	17.7
7	5	17	13.7	19
8	5	18	14	19.5
9	5.5	19	15.1	20.2
10	5.5	19.5	15.6	22.1
11	6	24.5	15.9	23
12	6	27	16.7	24.1
13	5	25.5	17.2	24.5
14	4	24	18.9	26.4
15	4	24	19.9	27.2
16	4	22	21.3	29.6
17	4.5	19	22.4	31.2
18-24	4	23	22.6	32.4
25-34	5	24	24.3	32.6
35-44	5	23	24.7	32.7
45-54	5.5	26	23.9	32.6
55-64	5	21	23.6	32
65-74	5	22	22.3	30.6

Appendix H
Laboratory Values

Table H-1 Laboratory reference values

Parameter	Units	Reference Range	
		Adult	Pediatric*
Blood Analyses			
Albumin	g/dl	3.5-5.0	<1 yr: 3.0-5.0; 1-15 yr: 3.2-5.0
Alkaline phosphatase	U/ml	30-85	<6 yr: 95-231; 6-12 yr: 122-323; 12-19 yr: 27-367
Ascorbic acid			
Serum	mg/dl	0.4-1.5	
Leukocyte	mg/dl	>15	
Bilirubin			
Total	mg/dl	≤1.0	NB: 1-12
Direct	mg/dl	≤0.4	NB: ≤1.0
Calcium			
Total	mg/dl	8.5-10.5	1-2 yr: 10-12; 2-16 yr: 9-11.5
Ionized	mg/dl	3.9-4.6	4.4-5.4
Carotene	μg/dl	50-200	<1 yr: 7-340; >3 yr: 100-150
Ceruloplasmin	mg/dl	27-37	20-40
Chloride	mEq/L	90-110	94-106

Cholesterol	mg/dl	120-220	70-200
Complete blood count			
Hematocrit	%	M: 42-52; F: 37-48; Pregnancy: >33	NB: 46-62; >1 mo: 31-43
Hemoglobin	g/dl	M: 13-18; F: 12-16; Pregnancy: >11	NB: 14-24; >1 mo: 11-16
Erythrocyte (RBC) count	$10^7/mm^3$	4.2-5.9	NB: 4.8-7.1; >1 mo: 3.8-5.5
Leukocyte (WBC) count	$10^3/mm^3$	4.3-1.08	NB: 4-35; <2: 6-18
Lymphocyte count	$10^3/mm^3$	>1.2	
Mean corpuscular volume (MCV)	μm^3	80-94	NB: 96-108
Mean corpuscular hemoglobin (MCH)	pg	27-32	NB: 32-34
Mean corpuscular hemoglobin concentration (MCHC)	%	32-36	NB: 32-33

Continued.

Meites S, editor: *Pediatric clinical chemistry*, ed. 2, Washington, 1981, American Association for Clinical Chemistry; Sauberlich HE and others: *Laboratory tests for the assessment of nutritional status*, Cleveland, 1976, CRC Press; Scully RE and others, editors: Normal reference laboratory values, *N Engl J Med* 302:37, 1980.

*Where no value is given for pediatrics, it is assumed to be similar to the adult value.
NB, newborn; *M*, male; *F*, female; *RBC*, red blood cell; *WBC*, white blood cell.

Table H-1 Laboratory reference values — cont'd

Parameter	Units	Reference Range Adult	Reference Range Pediatric*
Copper	μg/dl	100-200	6 mo-5 yr: 50-120
Creatinine	mg/dl	0.6-1.5	0.5-1.2
Ferritin	ng/ml	M: 10-273	7-144
		F: 5-99	
Folic acid			
Serum	ng/ml	≥6	
RBC	ng/ml	≥160	
Glucose			
Fasting	mg/dl	70-110	NB: 40-110; <16 yr: 60-105
2-hr postprandial	mg/dl	<140	
Glycosylated hemoglobin (Hb A$_{1c}$)			
Nondiabetic	%	2.2-4.8	1.8-4
Good diabetic control	%	2.5-6	
Fair control	%	6.1-8	
Poor control	%	>8	

Iron	μg/dl	50-150	30-120
Magnesium	mEq/L	1.5-2	1.4-1.9
Manganese	μg/dl	0.8-2.1	
Prealbumin	mg/dl	>15	
Osmolality (serum)	$mOsm/kgH_2O$	285-295	
Phenylalanine	mg/dl	0-2	NB: <4
Phosphorus	mg/dl	3-4.5	3.5-6.8
Potassium	mEq/L	3.5-5	3.6-5.2
Prothrombin time	seconds	<2 second deviation from control	
Sodium	mEq/L	135-145	
Total iron binding capacity (TIBC)	μg/dl	250-410	
Transferrin	mg/dl	170-250	
Triglycerides	mg/dl	40-150	
Urea nitrogen (BUN)	mg/dl	8-25	5-25
Vitamin A (retinol)	μg/dl	20-80	
Vitamin B_1 (thiamin pyrophosphate stimulation)	None	<1.23	

Continued.

Table H-1 Laboratory reference values—cont'd

Parameter	Units	Reference Range	
		Adult	Pediatric*
Vitamin B$_2$ (erythrocyte glutathione reductase)	None	<1.2	
Vitamin B$_6$ (erythrocyte glutamic-oxaloacetic transaminase)	None	<1.89	
Vitamin B$_{12}$	pg/ml	130-785	
Vitamin D			
25-Hydroxyvitamin D	ng/ml	≥7	NB: 19-23
1,25-Dihydroxyvitamin D	pg/ml	27-31	<16 yr: 40-46
Vitamin E (tocopherol)	mg/dl	0.5-1.2	
D-Xylose (absorption, 2 hr after ingestion of 25 g of xylose)	mg/dl	40	

Zinc	μg/ml	60-160	
Urine Analyses			
Creatinine	mg/kg body weight	M: 23 F: 17	20
Niacin	mg/g creatinine	≥1.6	
Specific gravity		1.005-1.030	NB: <1.020
Sugars (reducing substances)	%	0	
Urea nitrogen	g/day	6-17	
D-Xylose (absorption)	g/5 hr	5-8	
Stool Analyses			
Fat			
Excretion	g/day	≤5	
Absorption	% of intake	≥95	NB: 80-85; 1-2 yr: >93
Nitrogen	g/day	<2	
Sugars (reducing substance)	%	<0.25	

Appendix I
RDAs and Average
Energy Allowance

Table I-1   Food and Nutrition Board, National Academy allowances,[a] revised 1989 (designed for the maintenance States)

Category	Age (yr)	Weight[b] (kg)	Weight[b] (lb)	Height[b] (cm)	Height[b] (in)
Infants	0.0-0.5	6	13	60	24
	0.5-1.0	9	20	71	28
Children	1-3	13	29	90	35
	4-6	20	44	112	44
	7-10	28	62	132	52
Males	11-14	45	99	157	62
	15-18	66	145	176	69
	19-24	72	160	177	70
	25-50	79	174	176	70
	51+	77	170	173	68
Females	11-14	46	101	157	62
	15-18	55	120	163	64
	19-24	58	128	164	65
	25-50	63	138	163	64
	51+	65	143	160	63
Pregnant/ Lactating	1st 6 mo				
	2nd 6 mo				

Modified from National Academy of Sciences: *Recommended dietary allowances,* ed 10, Washington DC, 1989, National Academy Press. Reprinted with permission.

[a]The allowances, expressed as average daily intakes over time, are intended to provide for individual variations among most normal persons as they live in the United States under usual environmental stresses. Diets should be based on a variety of common foods in order to provide other nutrients for which human requirements have been less well defined.

of Sciences: National Research Council recommended dietary
of good nutrition of practically all healthy people in the United

Protein (g)	Fat-soluble Vitamins			
	A (μg RE)[c]	D (μg)[d]	E (mg α-TE)[e]	K (μg)
13	375	7.5	3	5
14	375	10	4	10
16	400	10	6	15
24	500	10	7	20
28	700	10	7	30
45	1000	10	10	45
59	1000	10	10	65
58	1000	10	10	70
63	1000	5	10	80
63	1000	5	10	80
46	800	10	8	45
44	800	10	8	55
46	800	10	8	60
50	800	5	8	65
50	800	5	8	65
60	800	10	10	65
65	1300	10	12	65
62	1200	10	11	65

[b]Weights and heights of reference adults are actual medians for the U.S. population
of the designated age, as reported by NHANES II. The median weights and heights
of those under 19 years of age were taken from Hamill et al. (1979). The use of
these figures does not imply that the height-to-weight ratios are ideal.

[c]Retinol equivalents. 1 retinol equivalent = 1 μg retinol or 6 μg β-carotene.

[d]As cholecalciferol. 10 μg cholecalciferol = 400 IU of vitamin D.

[e]α-Tocopherol equivalents. 1 mg d-α tocopherol = 1 α-TE.

[f]1 NE (niacin equivalent) is equal to 1 mg of niacin or 60 mg of dietary tryptophan.

Continued.

Table I-1   Food and Nutrition Board, National Academy of Sciences — cont'd

		Water-soluble Vitamins						
Category	Age (yr)	C (mg)	Thiamin (mg)	Riboflavin (mg)	Niacin (mg NE)[f]	B_6 (mg)	Folate (μg)	B_{12} (μg)
Infants	0.0-0.5	30	0.3	0.4	5	0.3	25	0.3
	0.5-1.0	35	0.4	0.5	6	0.6	35	0.5
Children	1-3	40	0.7	0.8	9	1.0	50	0.7
	4-6	45	0.9	1.1	12	1.1	75	1.0
	7-10	45	1.0	1.2	13	1.4	100	1.4
Males	11-14	50	1.3	1.5	17	1.7	150	2.0
	15-18	60	1.5	1.8	20	2.0	200	2.0
	19-24	60	1.5	1.7	19	2.0	200	2.0
	25-50	60	1.5	1.7	19	2.0	200	2.0
	51+	60	1.2	1.4	15	2.0	200	2.0
Females	11-14	50	1.1	1.3	15	1.4	150	2.0
	15-18	60	1.1	1.3	15	1.5	180	2.0
	19-24	60	1.1	1.3	15	1.6	180	2.0
	25-50	60	1.1	1.3	15	1.6	180	2.0
	51+	60	1.0	1.2	13	1.6	180	2.0
		70	1.5	1.6	17	2.2	400	2.2
Pregnant/		95	1.6	1.8	20	2.1	280	2.6
Lactating	1st 6 mo	90	1.6	1.7	20	2.1	260	2.6
	2nd 6 mo							

Minerals						
Ca (mg)	P (mg)	Mg (mg)	Fe (mg)	Zn (mg)	I (μg)	Se (μg)
400	300	40	6	5	40	10
600	500	60	10	5	50	15
800	800	80	10	10	70	20
800	800	120	10	10	90	20
800	800	170	10	10	120	30
1200	1200	270	12	15	150	40
1200	1200	400	12	15	150	50
1200	1200	350	10	15	150	70
800	800	350	10	15	150	70
800	800	350	10	15	150	70
1200	1200	280	15	12	150	45
1200	1200	300	15	12	150	50
1200	1200	280	15	12	150	55
800	800	280	15	12	150	55
800	800	280	10	12	150	55
1200	1200	320	30	15	175	65
1200	1200	355	15	19	200	75
1200	1200	340	15	16	200	75

Table I-2 Median heights and weights and recommended energy intake

Category	Age (yr)	Weight		Height		REE* (kcal/day)	Average Energy Allowance (kcal)†		
		(kg)	(lb)	(cm)	(in)		Multiples of REE	Per kg	Per day
Infants	0.0-0.5	6	13	60	24	320		108	650
	0.5-1.0	9	20	71	28	500		98	850
Children	1-3	13	29	90	35	740		102	1300
	4-6	20	44	112	44	950		90	1800
	7-10	28	62	132	52	1130		70	2000
Males	11-14	45	99	157	62	1440	1.70	55	2500
	15-18	66	145	176	69	1760	1.67	45	3000
	19-24	72	160	177	70	1780	1.67	40	2900
	25-50	79	174	176	70	1800	1.60	37	2900
	51+	77	170	173	68	1530	1.50	30	2300

Females	11-14	46	101	157	62	1310	1.67	47	2200
	15-18	55	120	163	64	1370	1.60	40	2200
	19-24	58	128	164	65	1350	1.60	38	2200
	25-50	63	138	163	64	1380	1.55	36	2200
	51+	65	143	160	63	1280	1.50	30	1900
Pregnant	1st trimester								+0
	2nd trimester								+300
	3rd trimester								+300
Lactating	1st 6 mo								+500
	2nd 6 mo								+500

Modified from National Academy of Sciences: *Recommended dietary allowances*, ed 10, Washington DC, 1989, National Academy Press. Reprinted with permission.

*Resting energy expenditure.

†Light to moderate activity.

Index

I